Therapeutic Radionuclides in Nuclear Medicine

Therapeutic Radionuclides in Nuclear Medicine

Guest Editors

Marc Pretze
Jörg Kotzerke

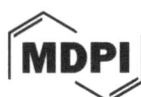

Basel • Beijing • Wuhan • Barcelona • Belgrade • Novi Sad • Cluj • Manchester

Guest Editors

Marc Pretze
Department of Nuclear Medicine
University Hospital
Carl Gustav Carus
Dresden
Germany

Jörg Kotzerke
Department of Nuclear Medicine
University Hospital
Carl Gustav Carus
Dresden
Germany

Editorial Office
MDPI AG
Grosspeteranlage 5
4052 Basel, Switzerland

This is a reprint of the Special Issue, published open access by the journal *Pharmaceuticals* (ISSN 1424-8247), freely accessible at: www.mdpi.com/journal/pharmaceuticals/special_issues/M8TAS21VQU.

For citation purposes, cite each article independently as indicated on the article page online and using the guide below:

Lastname, A.A.; Lastname, B.B. Article Title. *Journal Name* **Year**, *Volume Number*, Page Range.

ISBN 978-3-7258-2938-5 (Hbk)
ISBN 978-3-7258-2937-8 (PDF)
https://doi.org/10.3390/books978-3-7258-2937-8

© 2025 by the authors. Articles in this book are Open Access and distributed under the Creative Commons Attribution (CC BY) license. The book as a whole is distributed by MDPI under the terms and conditions of the Creative Commons Attribution-NonCommercial-NoDerivs (CC BY-NC-ND) license (https://creativecommons.org/licenses/by-nc-nd/4.0/).

Contents

Preface vii

Matthias Miederer, Martina Benešová-Schäfer, Constantin Mamat, David Kästner, Marc Pretze and Enrico Michler et al.
Alpha-Emitting Radionuclides: Current Status and Future Perspectives
Reprinted from: *Pharmaceuticals* **2024**, *17*, 76, https://doi.org/10.3390/ph17010076 1

Wael Jalloul, Vlad Ghizdovat, Cati Raluca Stolniceanu, Teodor Ionescu, Irena Cristina Grierosu and Ioana Pavaleanu et al.
Targeted Alpha Therapy: All We Need to Know about ^{225}Ac's Physical Characteristics and Production as a Potential Theranostic Radionuclide
Reprinted from: *Pharmaceuticals* **2023**, *16*, 1679, https://doi.org/10.3390/ph16121679 21

Bryce J. B. Nelson, John Wilson, Jan D. Andersson and Frank Wuest
Theranostic Imaging Surrogates for Targeted Alpha Therapy: Progress in Production, Purification, and Applications
Reprinted from: *Pharmaceuticals* **2023**, *16*, 1622, https://doi.org/10.3390/ph16111622 41

Marc Pretze, Enrico Michler, Roswitha Runge, Kerstin Wetzig, Katja Tietze and Florian Brandt et al.
Influence of the Molar Activity of $^{203/212}$Pb-PSC-PEG$_2$-TOC on Somatostatin Receptor Type 2-Binding and Cell Uptake
Reprinted from: *Pharmaceuticals* **2023**, *16*, 1605, https://doi.org/10.3390/ph16111605 61

Paul M. D. Gape, Michael K. Schultz, Graeme J. Stasiuk and Samantha Y. A. Terry
Towards Effective Targeted Alpha Therapy for Neuroendocrine Tumours: A Review
Reprinted from: *Pharmaceuticals* **2024**, *17*, 334, https://doi.org/10.3390/ph17030334 72

Roswitha Runge, Falco Reissig, Nora Herzog, Liane Oehme, Claudia Brogsitter and Joerg Kotzerke
Combining Cisplatin with Different Radiation Qualities—Interpretation of Cytotoxic Effects In Vitro by Isobolographic Analysis
Reprinted from: *Pharmaceuticals* **2023**, *16*, 1720, https://doi.org/10.3390/ph16121720 98

Kerstin Michalski, Wiebke Schlötelburg, Philipp E. Hartrampf, Aleksander Kosmala, Andreas K. Buck and Stefanie Hahner et al.
Radiopharmaceuticals for Treatment of Adrenocortical Carcinoma
Reprinted from: *Pharmaceuticals* **2023**, *17*, 25, https://doi.org/10.3390/ph17010025 110

Alexander Bellendorf, Nicolai Mader, Stefan P. Mueller, Samer Ezziddin, Andreas Bockisch and Hong Grafe et al.
Safety and Efficacy of Selective Internal Radionuclide Therapy with ^{90}Y Glass Microspheres in Patients with Progressive Hepatocellular Carcinoma after the Failure of Repeated Transarterial Chemoembolization
Reprinted from: *Pharmaceuticals* **2024**, *17*, 101, https://doi.org/10.3390/ph17010101 119

Marco D'Arienzo, Emilio Mezzenga, Amedeo Capotosti, Oreste Bagni, Luca Filippi and Marco Capogni et al.
The Importance of Uncertainty Analysis and Traceable Measurements in Routine Quantitative ^{90}Y-PET Molecular Radiotherapy: A Multicenter Experience
Reprinted from: *Pharmaceuticals* **2023**, *16*, 1142, https://doi.org/10.3390/ph16081142 131

Kevin J. H. Allen, Ohyun Kwon, Matthew R. Hutcheson, Joseph J. Grudzinski, Stuart M. Cain and Frederic A. Cruz et al.
Image-Based Dosimetry in Dogs and Cross-Reactivity with Human Tissues of IGF2R-Targeting Human Antibody
Reprinted from: *Pharmaceuticals* **2023**, *16*, 979, https://doi.org/10.3390/ph16070979 . . . . **146**

Güllü Davarci, Carmen Wängler, Klaus Eberhardt, Christopher Geppert, Ralf Schirrmacher and Robert Freudenberg et al.
Radiosynthesis of Stable ^{198}Au-Nanoparticles by Neutron Activation of $\alpha_v\beta_3$-Specific AuNPs for Therapy of Tumor Angiogenesis
Reprinted from: *Pharmaceuticals* **2023**, *16*, 1670, https://doi.org/10.3390/ph16121670 . . . . **158**

Preface

The field of radionuclide therapies and targeted drug delivery continues to rapidly evolve, offering renewed hope for patients with various cancers and other diseases. The recent studies featured in this Special Issue reflect the dynamic and rapidly advancing field of radionuclide therapy. From SIRT and PRRT to innovative combinations with chemotherapy and the development of new theranostic agents, these advancements hold promise in significantly improving cancer treatment outcomes. Continued research and clinical trials will be essential to fully realize the potential of these therapies, paving the way for more effective and personalized cancer care.

The study by Runge et al. explored the cytotoxic effects of combining cisplatin with various radiation qualities, including alpha-emitter ^{223}Ra and beta-emitter ^{188}Re [1]. Their isobolographic analyses highlighted the potential of ^{223}Ra to enhance cisplatin's efficacy, suggesting a promising approach for more effective cancer treatments. This combination could offer a new therapeutic strategy, particularly for cancers resistant to conventional therapies. D'Arienzo et al. addressed the importance of uncertainty analysis and traceable measurements in ^{90}Y-PET molecular radiotherapy [2]. Their multicenter study provided a framework for ensuring quantitative accuracy in PET scans, which is vital for precise dose estimation and effective treatment planning. Nelson et al. highlighted the development of diagnostic imaging surrogates for TAT [3]. These surrogates are crucial for improving diagnostic accuracy and facilitating research in radionuclide therapy. The integration of imaging surrogates enhances the ability to monitor and optimize treatment, ensuring better patient outcomes. These studies represented just a fraction of the ongoing research in radionuclide therapies and targeted drug delivery. As our understanding of disease mechanisms deepens and technology advances, we can expect to see more personalized and effective treatment options emerge.

In our study, we found the target upregulation by the epigenetic stimulation [4] of tumor-specific receptors (e.g. SSTR2 [5] and PSMA [6]) to be very exciting because the nuclear medicine approach could shift from palliative to curative after increasing the target by a factor of 40, with a significant reduction in the side effects on the critical organs [7]. It is also worth noting that one case report illustrated that radiation is always effective, while chemotherapy creates resistance that requires a change in agent [8].

There is already an emerging number of radiopharmaceuticals with approval for patient therapy (e.g. Xofigo, Luthathera, and Pluvicto, to name some), and more are currently in clinical phase II or even phase III. However, those radiopharmaceuticals were already widely used for individual patient therapies in many hospitals in accordance with the German Pharmaceutical Act §13.2b. It is known that the tumor accumulation and biodistribution in organs at risk of those well-studied radiopharmaceuticals is not at its optimum levels. Therefore, further developments in radiochemistry might enhance tumor accumulation while maintaining or even lowering the accumulation in organs at risk. A promising approch is the functionalization of already-known radio ligands to SuFEx moieties, enabling them to covalently bind to the tumor-specific receptor proteins or other binding sites to dramatically improve tumor binding [9].

A second improvement would be the functionalization of ligands with albumin binder to reach a higher blood circulation of the radio ligand and, therefore, a higher tumor accumulation. It has to be considered that, while preserving the kidneys, the albumin binder leads to a higher blood toxicity.

One emerging field in radionuclide therapy are alpha emitters, which can overcome radio-resistance against beta-minus therapy and extend the life and well-being of palliative patients [10,11]. One case report about ^{225}Ac-PSMA-617 shows that a 5-year complete remission is possible when the patients have a good tumor response to the radiopharmaceutical [12]. It must be said that such long-term treatments with high alpha dose might lead to chronic side effects like xerostomia or kidney insufficency. The ejection of three alpha particles in a short series from ^{225}Ac dramatically reduces the activity used for peptide receptor-targeted therapy by a factor of 1000 [13] and the ejection of, in sum, one alpha particle from ^{212}Pb reduces the activity by a factor of 20–30 [14] while maintaining or even improving the therapeutic outcome. The cytotoxic nature of the alpha particles is mainly due to the destruction of Golgi, endoplasmic reticulum, mitochondria, or other structures within the cell plasma rather than direct DNA double-strand breaks, as often cited in the literature [15], since the ^{212}Pb- and ^{225}Ac-labeled peptides certainly do not reach the cell nuclei but are able to pass the cell membrane to some extent.

New chelators like lead-specific chelator (PSC) for ^{212}Pb and macropa (MCP) for ^{225}Ac are known to bind the respective alpha nuclides even at room temperature, with up to factor 50 lower precursor amounts, compared to standard chelators like DOTA and DOTAGA. Therefore, a certain amount of safe unlabeled precursor could even lead to a rechelation of daughter nuclides like ^{212}Bi (to PSC) or ^{213}Bi (to MCP) within the final patient solution.

Theoretically, the combination of the above-mentioned albumin binder and improved chelators would increase the tumor accumulation of known radiopharmaceuticals because of longer blood circulation and higher molar activities. This might lead to the same therapeutical outcome like for standard therapies but at much lower doses. Technically, a therapy with ^{225}Ac might be performed with just 1 MBq instead of 10 MBq. Ultimately, the toxicity to blood and organs at risk should significantly decline using therapeutic applications of 1 MBq ^{225}Ac.

The diversity of the approaches being explored—from optimizing existing therapies to developing entirely new delivery systems—underscores the dynamic nature of pharmaceutical research. It is crucial that we continue to support and invest in these areas of study, as they hold the potential to significantly improve patient outcomes and quality of life. As we move forward, it will be essential to conduct rigorous clinical trials to validate these promising approaches and translate them into clinical practice. Collaboration between researchers, clinicians, and industry partners will be key to ac-celerating progress and bringing these innovative therapies to patients in need. As the Guest Editors, we hope that the findings included in this Special Issue will inspire further investigations in this challenging field.

References

1. Runge, R.; Reissig, F.; Herzog, N.; Oehme, L.; Brogsitter, C.; Kotzerke, J. Combining Cisplatin with Different Radiation Qualities-Interpretation of Cytotoxic Effects In Vitro by Isobolographic Analysis. *Pharmaceuticals (Basel)* 2023, 16, doi:10.3390/ph16121720

2. D'Arienzo, M.; Mezzenga, E.; Capotosti, A.; Bagni, O.; Filippi, L.; Capogni, M.; Indovina, L.; Sarnelli, A. The Importance of Uncertainty Analysis and Traceable Measurements in Routine Quantitative ^{90}Y-PET Molecular Radiotherapy: A Multicenter Experience. *Pharmaceuticals (Basel)* 2023, 16, doi:10.3390/ph16081142

3. Nelson, B.J.B.; Wilson, J.; Andersson, J.D.; Wuest, F. Theranostic Imaging Surrogates for Targeted Alpha Therapy: Progress in Production, Purification, and Applications. *Pharmaceuticals (Basel)* 2023, 16, doi:10.3390/ph16111622.

4. Taelman, V.F.R., P.; Marincek, N.; Ben-Shlomo, A.; Grotzky, A.; Olariu, C.I.; Perren, A.; Stettler, C.; Krause, T.; Meier, L.P.; et al. . Upregulation of Key Molecules for Targeted Imaging and Therapy. *J. Nucl. Med.* 2016, 57, 1805–1810

5. Veenstra, M.J.; van Koetsveld, P.M.; Dogan, F.; Farrell, W.E.; Feelders, R.A.; Lamberts, S.W.J.; de Herder, W.W.; Vitale, G.; Hofland, L.J. Epidrug-induced upregulation of functional somatostatin type 2 receptors in human pancreatic neuroendocrine tumor cells. . *Oncotarget* 2018, 9, 14791–14802

6. Runge, R.; Naumann, A.; Miederer, M.; Kotzerke, J.; Brogsitter, C. Up-Regulation of PSMA Expression In Vitro as Potential Application in Prostate Cancer Therapy. *Pharmaceuticals (Basel)* 2023, 16, 538, doi:10.3390/ph16040538

7. Kotzerke, J.; Buesser, D.; Naumann, A.; Runge, R.; Huebinger, L.; Kliewer, A.; Freudenberg, R.; Brogsitter, C. Epigenetic-like stimulation of receptor expression in SSTR2 transfected HEK293 cells as a new therapeutic strategy. *Cancers* 2022, 14, 2513, doi:10.3390/cancers14102513

8. Brogsitter, C.; Hartmann, H.; Wunderlich, G.; Schottelius, M.; Wester, H.J.; Kotzerke, J. Twins in spirit part IV - [^{177}Lu] high affinity DOTATATE. A promising new tracer for peptide receptor radiotherapy? *Nuklearmedizin* 2017, 56, 1–8, doi:10.3413/Nukmed-0860-16-11

9. Cui, X.Y.; Li, Z.; Kong, Z.; Liu, Y.; Meng, H.; Wen, Z.; Wang, C.; Chen, J.; Xu, M.; Li, Y., et al. Covalent targeted radioligands potentiate radionuclide therapy. *Nature* 2024, 630, 206–213, doi:10.1038/s41586-024-07461-6

10. Feuerecker, B.; Tauber, R.; Knorr, K.; Heck, M.; Beheshti, A.; Seidl, C.; Bruchertseifer, F.; Pickhard, A.; Gafita, A.; Kratochwil, C., et al. Activity and Adverse Events of Actinium-225-PSMA-617 in Advanced Metastatic Castration-resistant Prostate Cancer After Failure of Lutetium-177-PSMA. *Eur. Urol.* 2021, 79, 343–350, doi:10.1016/j.eururo.2020.11.013

11. Sathekge, M.M.; Lawal, I.O.; Bal, C.; Bruchertseifer, F.; Ballal, S.; Cardaci, G.; Davis, C.; Eiber, M.; Hekimsoy, T.; Knoesen, O., et al. Actinium-225-PSMA radioligand therapy of metastatic castration-resistant prostate cancer (WARMTH Act): a multicentre, retrospective study. *Lancet Oncol.* 2024, 25, 175–183, doi:10.1016/S1470-2045(23)00638-1

12. Rathke, H.; Bruchertseifer, F.; Kratochwil, C.; Keller, H.; Giesel, F.L.; Apostolidis, C.; Haberkorn, U.; Morgenstern, A. First patient exceeding 5-year complete remission after ^{225}Ac-PSMA-TAT. *Eur. J. Nucl. Med. Mol. Imaging* 2021, 48, 311–312, doi:10.1007/s00259-020-04875-y.

13. Kratochwil, C.; Bruchertseifer, F.; Giesel, F.L.; Weis, M.; Verburg, F.A.; Mottaghy, F.; Kopka, K.; Apostolidis, C.; Haberkorn, U.; Morgenstern, A. ^{225}Ac-PSMA-617 for PSMA-targeted α-radiation therapy of metastatic castration-resistant prostate cancer. *J. Nucl. Med.* 2016, 57, 1941–1944, doi:10.2967/jnumed.116.178673

14. Delpassand, E.S.; Tworowska, I.; Esfandiari, R.; Torgue, J.; Hurt, J.; Shafie, A.; Núñez, R. Targeted α-emitter therapy with ^{212}Pb-DOTAMTATE for the treatment of metastatic SSTR-expressing neuroendocrine tumors: first-in-humans dose-escalation clinical trial. *J. Nucl. Med.* 2022, 63, 1326–1333, doi:10.2967/jnumed.121.263230

15. Graf, F.; Fahrer, J.; Maus, S.; Morgenstern, A.; Bruchertseifer, F.; Venkatachalam, S.; Fottner, C.; Weber, M.M.; Huelsenbeck, J.; Schreckenberger, M., et al. DNA double strand breaks as predictor of efficacy of the alpha-particle emitter Ac-225 and the electron emitter Lu-177 for somatostatin receptor targeted radiotherapy. *PLoS One* 2014, 9, e88239, doi:10.1371/journal.pone.0088239.

Marc Pretze and Jörg Kotzerke
Guest Editors

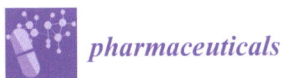

Review

Alpha-Emitting Radionuclides: Current Status and Future Perspectives

Matthias Miederer [1,2,3,4,*], Martina Benešová-Schäfer [5], Constantin Mamat [6,7], David Kästner [8], Marc Pretze [8], Enrico Michler [8], Claudia Brogsitter [8], Jörg Kotzerke [2,8], Klaus Kopka [6,7,9,10], David A. Scheinberg [11] and Michael R. McDevitt [12,13]

1. Department of Translational Imaging in Oncology, National Center for Tumor Diseases (NCT/UCC), 01307 Dresden, Germany
2. Medizinische Fakultät and University Hospital Carl Gustav Carus, Technische Universität Dresden, 01307 Dresden, Germany
3. German Cancer Research Center (DKFZ), 69120 Heidelberg, Germany
4. Helmholtz-Zentrum Dresden-Rossendorf (HZDR), 01328 Dresden, Germany
5. Research Group Molecular Biology of Systemic Radiotherapy, German Cancer Research Center (DKFZ), 69120 Heidelberg, Germany; m.benesova@dkfz-heidelberg.de
6. Helmholtz-Zentrum Dresden-Rossendorf, Institute of Radiopharmaceutical Cancer Research, Bautzner Landstr. 400, 01328 Dresden, Germany
7. School of Science, Faculty of Chemistry and Food Chemistry, Technische Universität Dresden, 01062 Dresden, Germany
8. Department of Nuclear Medicine, University Hospital Carl Gustav Carus, Technische Universität Dresden, Fetscherstraße 74, 01307 Dresden, Germany; david.kaestner@ukdd.de (D.K.); claudia.brogsitter@ukdd.de (C.B.)
9. National Center for Tumor Diseases (NCT) Dresden, University Hospital Carl Gustav Carus, Fetscherstraße 74, 01307 Dresden, Germany
10. German Cancer Consortium (DKTK), Partner Site Dresden, Fetscherstraße 74, 01307 Dresden, Germany
11. Molecular Pharmacology Program, Sloan Kettering Institute, New York, NY 10065, USA; scheinbd@mskcc.org
12. Molecular Imaging and Therapy Service, Department of Radiology, Memorial Sloan Kettering Cancer Center, New York, NY 10065, USA
13. Department of Radiology, Weill Cornell Medical College, New York, NY 10065, USA
* Correspondence: matthias.miederer@nct-dresden.de

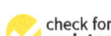

Citation: Miederer, M.; Benešová-Schäfer, M.; Mamat, C.; Kästner, D.; Pretze, M.; Michler, E.; Brogsitter, C.; Kotzerke, J.; Kopka, K.; Scheinberg, D.A.; et al. Alpha-Emitting Radionuclides: Current Status and Future Perspectives. *Pharmaceuticals* **2024**, *17*, 76. https://doi.org/10.3390/ph17010076

Academic Editor: Hirofumi Hanaoka

Received: 28 November 2023
Revised: 27 December 2023
Accepted: 28 December 2023
Published: 8 January 2024

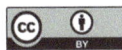

Copyright: © 2024 by the authors. Licensee MDPI, Basel, Switzerland. This article is an open access article distributed under the terms and conditions of the Creative Commons Attribution (CC BY) license (https://creativecommons.org/licenses/by/4.0/).

Abstract: The use of radionuclides for targeted endoradiotherapy is a rapidly growing field in oncology. In particular, the focus on the biological effects of different radiation qualities is an important factor in understanding and implementing new therapies. Together with the combined approach of imaging and therapy, therapeutic nuclear medicine has recently made great progress. A particular area of research is the use of alpha-emitting radionuclides, which have unique physical properties associated with outstanding advantages, e.g., for single tumor cell targeting. Here, recent results and open questions regarding the production of alpha-emitting isotopes as well as their chemical combination with carrier molecules and clinical experience from compassionate use reports and clinical trials are discussed.

Keywords: alpha emitter; targeted alpha therapy; actinium-225; high let; theranostic

1. Introduction

The ensemble between diagnostic and therapeutic radionuclides has opened a rapidly growing area for individualized targeted radionuclide theranostics. Recent developments and increasing knowledge in the field of radiation biology, radiochemistry, radiopharmaceutical sciences, nuclear medicine, and oncology are currently making steps forward to several more, highly relevant therapy options. One distinct research field is that of the therapeutic use of alpha particle-emitting radionuclides (alpha emitters). With their unique physical properties, it has been hypothesized that principles known, e.g., from external proton irradiation can be transferred to a systemic targeted internal radiotherapy, also called targeted endoradiotherapy, down to treating single cells. The physical properties of alpha emitters determining their biological potential are their short range in tissue with 50–80 μm and their high linear energy transfer (LET) along this track (Figure 1). With typical particle energies of 5–9 MeV, the resulting LET is approximately 80–100 keV/μm, which is orders of magnitude higher compared to beta or gamma radiation.

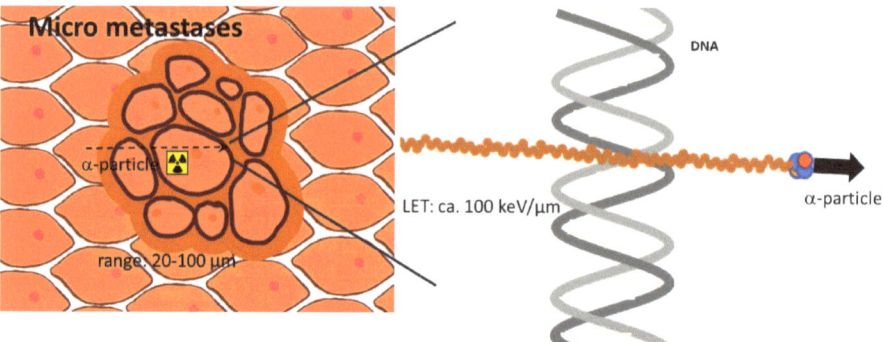

Figure 1. Scheme visualizing the prominent advantages of alpha-emitting radionuclides treating singles cells or a small tumor cell cluster. Due to the high linear energy transfer, alpha-induced DNA damage is higher than for other radiation like gamma or beta radiation.

The main target of radiation is the cell nucleus and when comparing alpha to beta particles, 2 to 10-fold higher relative biological effectiveness can be measured [1,2]. High LET radiation results in both extremely high radiotoxicity per alpha particle and thus in a cytotoxic effect that is at least partly independent of the formation of reactive oxygen species. This has been known to be advantageous, particularly for the treatment of hypoxic tumors. The alpha particle-induced DNA damage often leads to complex double-strand breaks (DSBs). These DSBs are the assumed mechanism that drives an exponential curve of dose–response to alpha radiation. This is in contrast to beta or gamma irradiation, which induces cell death with a dose–response relationship described by a linear quadratic model. The high LET also leads to the strongly reduced dependency of a damaging effect on oxygenation. Thus, for hypoxic and radio-resistant cells, alpha radiation has further advantages as a targeted therapeutic agent over other forms of radiation.

For clinical development and application, the theranostic pairing of diagnostic and therapeutic isotopes has posed certain limitations when applied to the use of therapeutic alpha emitters. Diagnostic radionuclides can be utilized to characterize key pharmacokinetic parameters such as tumor uptake, clearance, and any accumulation in off-target organs and tissues. Furthermore, these diagnostic radionuclides can yield additional biological information about the tumor target and dosimetry predictions of therapeutic radionuclides. However, dosimetry predictions for internal targeted alpha therapy (TAT) have limitations. This is due to possible additional factors that are partly unique for alpha radiation. One is that the heterogeneity of activity distribution on a microscopic level has a much higher impact on efficacy, since the range of alpha particles is limited to a few cell diameters. Another obstacle preventing the accurate prediction of effects from imaging is the common use of alpha-emitting isotopes derived from in vivo isotope generators. That is, after the decay of the original targeted isotope, additional alpha emitting as well as beta emitting daughter nuclides are released which contribute to cytotoxic effects. Typically, these daughter radionuclides have independent and often difficult to model pharmacokinetic profiles due to local protein or cell binding and heterogeneous clearance [3].

Here, we review current strategies on ways that alpha particle-emitting radionuclides (Figure 2) can be provided on recent developments of the chemistry to radiolabel them to molecules functioning as binding vectors including the new hypothesis of matched radionuclide pairs that might foster clinical development and on the currently available clinical experience.

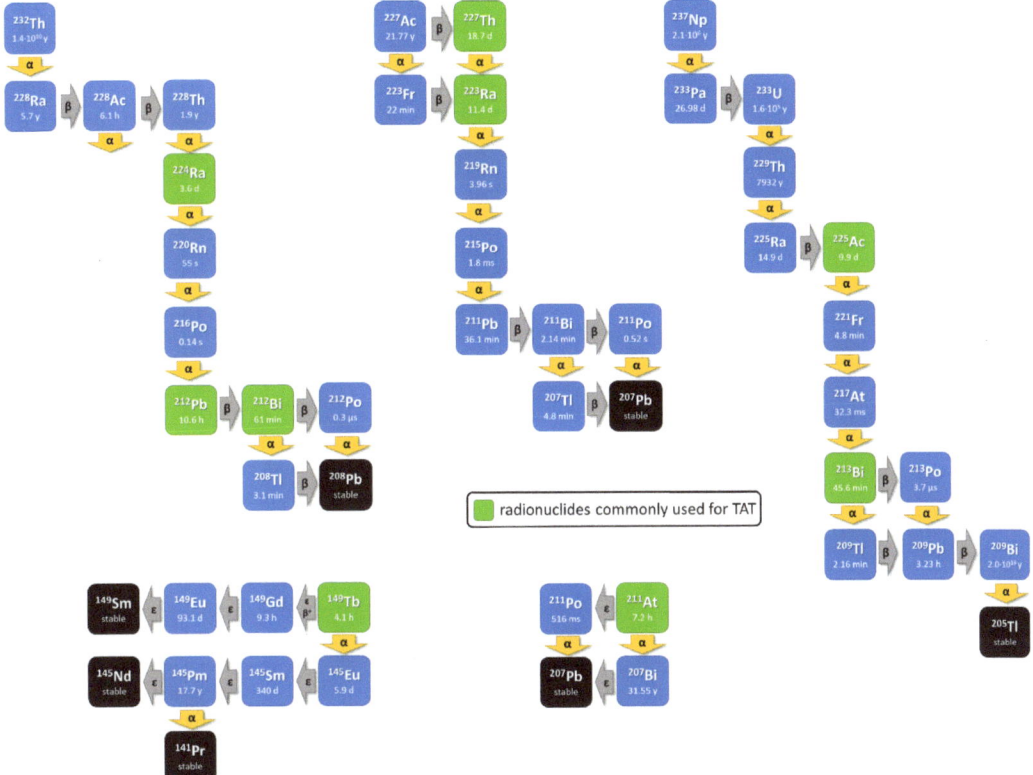

Figure 2. The principle of internal alpha radiation is enhanced with approaches that use radionuclides decaying via a short decay chain including further alpha-emitting isotopes. The decay schemes of the commonly used in vivo alpha radionuclides (green box).

2. Current Production and Availability of Alpha-Particle-Emitting Radionuclides

Actinium-225 (^{225}Ac) could be seen as the most critical radionuclide because of its high demand and limited availability. The primary source of ^{225}Ac comes from uranium-233 (^{233}U, $\tau_{\frac{1}{2}} = 1.59\ldots10^5$ y) waste which was generated in the frame of nuclear weapons development 80 years ago. ^{233}U decays to thorium-229 (^{229}Th; $\tau_{\frac{1}{2}} = 7.88\ldots10^3$ y), which serves as a parent radionuclide for radionuclide generators and provides a robust source of ^{225}Ac each month [4].

Unfortunately, the amount of available ^{233}U/^{229}Th is sufficient to generate ^{225}Ac in MBq/mCi quantities, enabling less than a thousand of targeted alpha therapies per year [5]. This issue comes hand in hand with not only uncertain ^{225}Ac availability, but also higher costs and limited research options which hamper the widespread translation and application of targeted alpha therapies. Thus, solving this shortage by alternative production routes became one of the main priorities in the community involving both scientists and physicians. The current focus lies on the cyclotron and reactor production with accompanying purification strategies while employing existing infrastructure and approaches as well as securing other infrastructural and technical alternatives. One concrete example might be demonstrated by the joint effort of Brookhaven, Los Alamos, and Oak Ridge National Laboratories to deliver accelerator-produced ^{225}Ac [6].

There are various nuclear reactions either producing ^{225}Ac directly or providing the parent radionuclide thorium-232, thorium-229 or radium-225, alternatively. These include but are not limited to: ^{226}Ra(γ,,n)^{225}Ra → ^{225}Ac (accelerator, electrons); ^{226}Ra(p,2n)^{225}Ac, ^{226}Ra(α,n)^{229}Th, ^{232}Th(p,x)^{229}Th, ^{226}Ra(p,pn)^{225}Ra, (accelerator, low-energy particles); ^{232}Th(p,x)^{225}Ac, ^{232}Th(p,x)^{225}Ra → ^{225}Ac (accelerator, high-energy particles); and ^{226}Ra(3n,γ)^{229}Ra → ^{229}Ac → ^{229}Th (reactor, thermal neutrons) [7–9].

The main complication of ^{225}Ac production via the accelerator applying higher energies results in the co-production of actinium-224 ($\tau_{\frac{1}{2}}$ = 2.78 h), actinium-226 ($\tau_{\frac{1}{2}}$ = 29.37 h), and actinium-227 ($\tau_{\frac{1}{2}}$ = 21.77 y)—which cannot be separated from the desired actinium-225. Since the half-lives of actinium-224 and -226 are very short, both are eliminated by natural decay. On the other hand, the long half-life of actinium-227 significantly complicates its related waste disposal, dosimetry, and radiation safety [10]. The actinium-225/actinium-227 ratio improves with increasing proton energy, but degrades with a longer irradiation time and careful balance between these two parameters has to be set. In addition, the irradiation of a highly radiotoxic and not so easily accessible radium-226 ($\tau_{\frac{1}{2}}$ = 1.600 y) in a cyclotron needs a more sophisticated target with gas-trapping filters and/or leak-tight equipment due to the presence of radioactive noble gas radon-222 ($\tau_{\frac{1}{2}}$ = 3.82 d) [11]. It is also important to note that the accelerator-produced ^{225}Ac differs slightly in comparison to the one obtained from the radionuclide generator, which, e.g., requires separate drug master files.

Another possibility is also to focus on the development, evaluation, and application of another alpha in vivo nanogenerator, thorium-227 (^{227}Th, $\tau_{\frac{1}{2}}$ = 18.9 d) [12]. There is, however, one significant difference between ^{227}Th and ^{225}Ac, which is that they have concretely different equilibria. ^{225}Ac forms a so-called secular equilibrium ($\tau_{\frac{1}{2}}$, parent >>> $\tau_{\frac{1}{2}}$, decay nuclide) with its decay radionuclide francium-221 having the half-life of 5 min. ^{227}Th forms a so-called transient equilibrium ($\tau_{\frac{1}{2}}$, parent > $\tau_{\frac{1}{2}}$, decay nuclide) with its decay radionuclide radium-223 having the half-life 11.4 d. By the direct comparison of the 5 min half-life of francium-221 with the 11.4 d half-life of 11.4 d results in the fact that ^{227}Th does not deliver so many alpha particles as quickly as ^{225}Ac and, by that, it has a much higher radiobiological effectiveness, which is clearly desired for targeted alpha therapies [13].

3. Radiochemistry and Concept of Theranostic Matched Radionuclide Pairs

A fundamental requirement of using alpha emitters for treatment is their selective delivery in vivo to a cancer cell target. This is ideally pursued with molecules used as binding vectors that display high target accumulation and low interactions with off-target sites. Also, it is essential that the sufficient stability of the labeling is ensured along with minimal influence on the initial pharmacokinetic properties of the carrier. By matched radionuclide pairs, theranostics allow the combination of diagnostic imaging using, for example, positron-emitting radionuclides with the therapeutic approach using particle-emitting radionuclides. Matched radionuclide pairs are generally a crucial component of radionuclide theranostics since the pharmacokinetics of the binding vector and the availability of the tumor targets are the main factors that determine the efficacy of radioligand-mediated endoradiotherapy. Theranostic pairs consist of the same binding vector molecule and matching radionuclides that share in best case identical or at least similar chemical properties, making them ready to label one and the same precursor compound. Therefore, the exact prediction of the therapeutic radionuclide distribution can be derived from the more suited imaging.

The key criteria for the choice of alpha-particle-emitting radionuclides are the half-life, the stable binding to a chelating system, the particle energy, the possible decay chain properties, and the kinetics of the daughters, as well as the costs and availability. These features result in a small number of radionuclides that are suitable, including thorium-227, actinium-225, radium-223/-224, bismuth-212/-213, astatine-211, and terbium-149 [14,15].

Additionally, lead-212 can be mentioned in this list, while delivering one beta particle prior to the alpha decay. Some attempts were made to use the concomitant gamma radiation of the alpha radionuclides as the diagnostic modality, but this has been met with limited success in human applications, mostly due to the activities used for alpha radionuclide therapy that are orders of magnitude lower than they are for imaging. To fulfill the theranostic concept, the respective matching radionuclides for imaging were previously developed using the same conjugate or precursor compound.

3.1. Matched Radionuclide Pair Lanthanum-133/Actinium-225

All isotopes of actinium are radioactive. Among them, ^{225}Ac has favorable nuclear properties such as a half-life of 9.9 days and a decay chain delivering 4 alpha and 2 beta particles [16]. Lanthanum has similar coordination properties and can be used as a nonradioactive match for the design of new radioconjugates and as a diagnostic reference isotope. Recently, two ß$^+$ emitters were introduced with lanthanum-132 (^{132}La) and lanthanum-133 (^{133}La) as theranostic matches [17].

Actinium mainly exists as a cation in the oxidation state +3. Different chelating compounds were developed in the past, especially for radiopharmaceutical applications. As a hard cation according to the hard–soft acid–base (HSAB) concept, the Ac^{3+} cation prefers oxygen donor atoms for complexation in coordination numbers of >10, but oxygen and nitrogen mixed ligands were mostly applied. The most sufficient complex stability is found with open-chain ligands of high denticity like DTPA which is increased when changing to macrocyclic ligands like DOTA [16] (Figure 3).

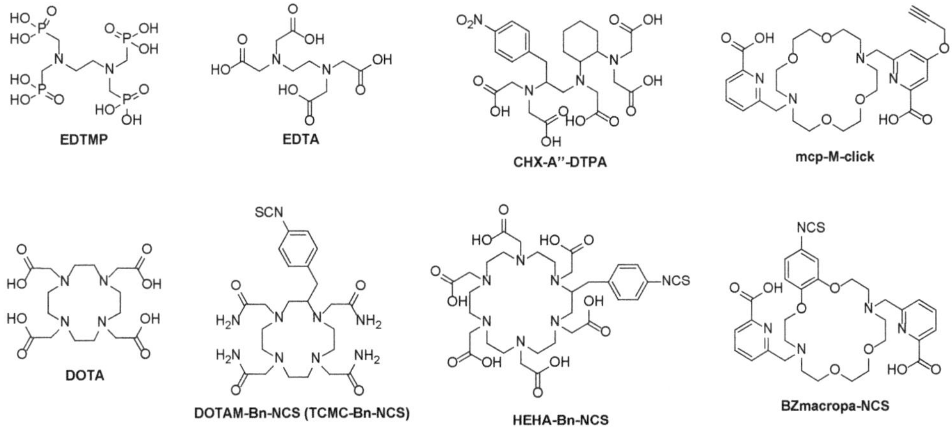

Figure 3. Examples of open-chain (EDTMP, EDTA, CHX-A″–DTPA) and macrocyclic chelators (DOTA, DOTAM–Bn-NCS, HEHA–Bn–NCS, BZmacropa–NCS) for ^{225}Ac and its diagnostic radiometal matches.

The first attempts to determine the in vivo behavior of ^{225}Ac complexes were made using citrate, DTPA, and EDTMP as ligands [18]. A rapid radiolabeling kinetic is found with these acyclic ligands, allowing a fast complexation of the radiometal at ambient temperatures within minutes. However, these formed complexes are kinetically labile, leading to a release of the radiometal in vivo. As a result, significant amounts of ^{225}Ac as well as of its (grand)daughters were found in the liver and the femur [19,20]. A higher stability can be reached when using ligands with a higher donor number. For example, the more stable 2^{25}Ac complex is formed using CHX-A″–DTPA with eight donor functions in contrast to EDTA with six donor positions. Additionally, the steric effect and the certain pre-organization of the backbone of the CHX-A″–DTPA ligand have a positive effect on the complex stability [19].

The aforementioned pre-organization of the chelating system is always found in macrocyclic compounds and is known as a macrocyclic effect, mostly leading to the higher stability of the complexes [21]. In this regard, macrocycles such as HEHA, PEPA, TETA, TETPA, and DOTPA were employed for ^{225}Ac complexation. These all differ in cavity size and donor numbers, but the stability of the formed ^{225}Ac complexes may still be lacking. For instance, the ^{225}Ac–HEHA complex is more stable in vivo compared to DOTA due to the higher donor number of 12 and the larger cavity for the metal ion. In contrast, the functionalized HEHA–NCS, which was used for antibody labeling with ^{225}Ac, has a low in vivo stability and decomposed to 50% after 24 h when tested in fetal bovine serum [22].

Due to the convenient availability, most experience is cumulated with the macrocyclic chelator DOTA (1,4,7,10-tetraazacyclododecane-N,N',N'',N'''-tetraacetic acid) used in a series of radiopharmaceuticals suitable for clinical use [23]. DOTA is a 12-membered macrocycle containing four tertiary amine nitrogen donors and four pendent arms with carboxylate functional groups that altogether provide an octadentate coordination. Due to the ability to stably bind the hard cations of charge +3, DOTA is expected to work well as a chelating agent for Ac^{3+} [24].

The DOTA chelator [25] has been widely used for the alpha-emitting radionuclides actinium-225, bismuth-213, and terbium-149, frequently for thorium-227, and some trials were made for radium-223 [12,26–28]. Elevated temperatures of up to 90–100 °C and a labeling time of 15–30 min were typically required for labeling, making this chelator unfavorable for sensitive biomacromolecules like proteins or antibodies. For this purpose, a robust clinical labeling method was developed, consisting of a two-step labeling strategy (pre-labeling) [29].

A variety of trivalent radiometal cations for diagnostic applications like ^{111}In, $^{43/44}$Sc, or ^{68}Ga were also stably complexed with DOTA, forming matched pairs with ^{225}Ac and even with the therapeutic beta emitter ^{177}Lu, but also mostly under the same unfavorable labeling conditions [25]. Several EMA- and FDA-approved radioconjugates, such as [^{68}Ga]Ga-DOTA-TATE, [^{177}Lu]Lu-DOTA-TATE, or [^{177}Lu]Lu-PSMA-617, are known to contain DOTA as a chelating motif.

The sufficient in vivo stability was pointed out in a preliminary biodistribution study of [^{225}Ac]Ac–DOTA in normal BALB/c mice only showing a slight accumulation in the liver (3.29% ID/g) and bone (2.87% ID/g) after 5 days [20]. The high efficiency of the ^{225}Ac chelation was further demonstrated using DOTA–NCS in a two-step labeling procedure to create ^{225}Ac–DOTA-modified IgG antibodies to avoid denaturation during radiolabeling [29]. In the first step, ^{225}Ac–DOTA–NCS was prepared from 2B–DOTA–NCS at 55–50 °C within 30 min. In the second step, ^{225}Ac–DOTA–NCS was conjugated to the antibody at 37 °C for 52 min via a free lysine function. Notably, the ^{225}Ac–DOTA complex showed a slow dissociation with a loss of 10% over one half-life. Several antibodies such as HuM195 (antiCD33), B4 (anti-CD19), trastuzumab (anti-HER2/neu), and J591 (anti-PSMA), which target leukemia, lymphoma, breast/ovarian cancer, and prostate cancer, respectively, were ^{225}Ac-labeled using this procedure and tested in vivo [30]. One recent innovation is the development of a live-cell-based theranostic carrier, in which a chimeric antigen receptor (CAR) T cell can chelate the PET diagnostic and ^{225}Ac therapeutic isotopes for delivery to the tumor cell and live tracking in vivo [31–33]. These promising initial results triggered a wave of investigations that resulted in numerous clinical trials [34].

3.2. Chelator Design to Improve the In Vivo Stability of ^{225}Ac Complexes

In 2017, a new chelating macrocycle called macropa (N,N'-bis[(6-carboxy-2-pyridyl) methyl]-4,13-diaza-18-crown-6) was introduced, allowing radiolabeling within a 5 min labeling time at room temperature with >99% RCC and leading to remarkably stable in vivo ^{225}Ac–macropa complexes [35] (Table 1). Subsequently, an NCS-modified and two clickable derivatives were prepared, allowing the conjugation to target vector molecules [36,37].

Table 1. Chelating systems for ^{225}Ac to pair with diagnostic radionuclides.

Chelator	Labeling Conditions	In Vivo Stability	Diagnostic RN
EDTA/DTPA	40 °C, 30 min	Failed	^{68}Ga, $^{43/44}$Sc
HEHA, PEPA, TETA, TETPA, and DOTPA	95 °C, 60 min (HEHA) 40 °C, 30 min (PEPA)	Failed	^{68}Ga, $^{43/44}$Sc, ^{111}In
DOTA	90 °C, 30 min	Sufficient	^{68}Ga, $^{43/44}$Sc, ^{111}In, ($^{132/133}$La)
DO3APic	25 °C, 30 min	Sufficient to low	$^{132/133}$La
Macropa	rt, 5–15 min	High	$^{132/133}$La

In vitro and in vivo studies showed the remarkable stability of the ^{225}Ac-mcp-radioconjugates over a period of 10 days and a high tumor accumulation combined with a fast renal excretion in LNCaP-tumor bearing mice. In 2022, a ^{225}Ac-radioconjugate based on the anti-EGFR antibody ch806 was presented, showing high stability when challenged with La^{3+} and EDTA in human serum. High tumor accumulation was found in U87MG.de2–7 xenografts. A therapy study showed 100% survival of the tumor-bearing treatment group over 80 days post-injection [38]. Recently, [^{225}Ac]Ac–MACROPATATE, the macropa-variant of DOTATATE based on the Tyr^3-octreotate peptide, was developed to treat neuroendocrine tumors [39]. The remarkable radiotracer stability of 10 days in human serum was confirmed and a high accumulation in SSTR-positive tumors was pointed out in mice bearing SSTR-positive H69 tumor xenografts. However, a higher off-target accumulation of [^{225}Ac]Ac–MACROPATATE was found.

[^{225}Ac]Ac–crown–αMSH was developed containing a chelator with a tetraazacrown-6 backbone with four pendant acetate side arms, which is connected to a peptide to target the melanocortin 1 receptor (MC1R) in specifically expressed primary and metastatic melanoma [40]. The radiolabeling worked under mild conditions (pH 5–7, rt, 10 min, c = 10^{-7} M, >98% RCY). However, the in vivo stability of the resulting tracer was lacking, which was indicated from the time-dependent HPLC experiments over 16 h. A different biodistribution profile was obtained when using freshly prepared the ^{225}Ac-crown-αMSH in contrast to the overnight prepared sample, showing the insufficient in vitro stability of this chelator.

Furthermore, BZmacropa–NCS was developed containing a benzyl moiety in the macrocyclic ring to investigate this modification on the complexation stability. A respective antibody conjugate GC33-BZmacropa was preclinically investigated showing a slightly reduced in vivo stability and higher uptake in the liver and femur [41].

One drawback of the macropa-based chelators is the absence of diagnostic radionuclides, because the standard radionuclides used for DOTA failed here. Thus, the radioisotopes of lanthanum, namely ^{132}La ($\tau_{\frac{1}{2}}$ = 4.6 h, E$_{\beta+,mean}$ = 1.29 MeV) and ^{133}La ($\tau_{\frac{1}{2}}$ = 3.9 h, E$_{\beta+,mean}$ = 0.46 MeV) were utilized as β$^+$ emitters for PET [17]. Lanthanum has a similar coordination chemistry to actinium and therefore acts as a surrogate (ionic radii: 1.12 Å for Ac^{3+} and 1.032 Å for La^{3+} in six-fold coordination). Highly apparent molar activities up to 330 GBq/μmol and a high in vivo stability were observed for ^{133}La–macropa complexes using a macropa concentration down to 10^{-7} M [42–44]. PET phantom images were performed, pointing out that the spatial resolution and contrast of ^{133}La is superior to those of ^{44}Sc, ^{68}Ga, and ^{132}La, but comparable to ^{89}Zr (E$_{\beta+,mean}$ = 0.396 MeV) [45].

^{13X}La-radioconjugates, namely [^{133}La]La–PSMA–I&T, [^{133}La]La–macropa–DUPA, [^{133}La]La–DO2APic–DUPA, [^{132}La]La–NM600 and [^{133}La]La–mcp–M–PSMA were prepared on the basis of DOTA, DO3APic, and macropa as chelators [42,43,45,46].

4. Radioisotopes of Lead for Theranostics

Radioisotopes of lead, ^{212}Pb (β emitter, $\tau_{\frac{1}{2}}$ = 10.6 h), and ^{203}Pb (γ emitter, $\tau_{\frac{1}{2}}$ = 51.9 h) as the true matched pair have gained attention for TAT, because ^{212}Pb functions as an in vivo generator for the release of ^{212}Bi ($\tau_{\frac{1}{2}}$ = 1.01 h), which is the actual α emitter [47,48]. ^{212}Pb can be obtained as the decay nuclide from ^{224}Ra. Different chromatographic generator systems were developed to isolate ^{212}Pb based either on ^{228}Th as the mother nuclide or directly on ^{224}Ra [49]. ^{203}Pb is available via cyclotron irradiation of enriched ^{203}Tl [49,50]. As a borderline cation according to the hard–soft acid–base concept, Pb^{2+} is found in complexes with oxygen, nitrogen, and sulfur donor atoms and coordination numbers between 2 and 10 [51]. In aqueous environments, Pb is primarily found as a bivalent cation in the oxidation state +2. The most frequently used chelators for radioconjugate preparation are DOTA [52] and TCMC or DOTAM (1,4,7,10-tetraaza-1,4,7,10-tetra(2-carbamoylmethyl)cyclododecane) and the derivatives thereof, whereas DOTAM seems to have a higher in vivo stability compared to DOTA [14]. A total CN of 8 was found in the Pb complexes of the standard chelators DOTA, DOTAM, or DTPA with high log K values of >18. In addition to the true match ^{203}Pb, other standard diagnostic radionuclides like $^{43/44}$Sc, ^{68}Ga, or ^{111}In can possibly be used for diagnostic purposes depending on the chelating system.

Recently, $^{203/212}$Pb came into focus by several first in-human theranostic applications. In 2014, [^{212}Pb]Pb–TCMC–trastuzumab was used for patients with human epidermal growth factor receptor type 2 (HER-2)-expressing malignancies [53]. The antibody was modified with DOTAM as a chelator with preference over DOTA. The in vitro and animal model testing of [^{212}Pb]Pb–TCMC–trastuzumab to investigate the therapeutic behavior prior to the human trials was performed to give an explicit preference of DOTAM as the chelator over DOTA [54].

To treat metastatic SSTR-expressing neuroendocrine tumors, the radioconjugate [^{212}Pb]Pb–DOTAMTATE was used in a first-in-human dose-escalation clinical trial with 10 patients [55]. However, the diagnostic imaging was performed with [^{68}Ga]Ga–DOTATATE, whereas [^{203}Pb]Pb–DOTAMTATE was used for human dose calculations. The activity dose was administered in four circles leading to an effective reduction in tumor lesions. Additionally, the Tyr^3–octreotide (TOC) variant VMT-α-NET was used for human applications as a conjugate for $^{203/212}$Pb that shows high chelation properties [56]. SPECT/CT images (low dose, 224 MBq) using [^{203}Pb]Pb–VMT-α-NET were acquired to assess the feasibility of the [^{212}Pb]Pb–VMT-α-NET therapy. A higher NET uptake combined with a rapid renal excretion within the first hour was observed.

Ligands with the PSMA-617-binding motif containing the chelators p-SCN–Bn–DOTAM or DO3AM were used for preclinical studies with ^{203}Pb [57]. Interestingly, the slightly different coordination behaviors of the chelating ligands to Pb^{2+} resulted in a different tumor uptake and internalization in vitro. [^{203}Pb]Pb–PSMA–CA012 was found to be the best candidate showing a high tumor uptake and internalization combined with a fast renal excretion.

Astatine-211: The Alpha-Emitting Therapeutic Big Brother of Radioiodine

Since the first discovery of ^{211}At in 1940, several reports on human therapy treatments with ^{211}At are known [58]. A 100% alpha emission with only one alpha particle emitted per decay was found for ^{211}At which prevented the unpredictable dose localization caused by the formation for radioactive daughters. ^{211}At is cyclotron-produced by the irradiation of ^{209}Bi with α-particles accelerated at ~28 MeV. Its chemistry resembles iodine; however, its covalent bonds are more instable. Furthermore, it also has a tendency to behave like a metalloid. Nonetheless, naturally occurring ^{127}I is used as a nonradioactive reference and the radioisotopes of iodine like ^{123}I or ^{124}I function as diagnostic matches. Oxidation states from +7 to −1 are possible, but −1 oxidation state is probably the most clearly established form of astatine with strong similarity to iodide [59]. It can easily be converted into the +1 oxidation state using mild oxidizing agents, such as Chloramine-T, Iodogen, or N-halosuccinimide to generate electrophilic I$^+$ or At$^+$ to perform electrophilic reactions. In this regard, labeling strategies are related to the formation of covalent bonds with carbon in most the cases. However, the carbon–astatine bond is much weaker compared to the carbon–iodine bond, but with a higher stability of astatine–aryl compounds over astatine–alkyl compounds, as expressed in Table 2.

Table 2. Comparison of bond energies of iodinated and astatine–alkyl and –aryl compounds.

	Alkyl Derivatives	Aryl Derivatives
C–I bond energy	220 kJ/mol	270 kJ/mol
C–At bond energy	160 kJ/mol	200 kJ/mol

Several clinical trials were made in the past, with Na [^{211}At]At itself (thyroid cancer) or small organic molecules like [^{211}At]At-MABG (*meta*-[^{211}At]astatobenzylguanidine) to treat malignant pheochromocytoma, but also with ^{211}At-labeled biomacromolecules like proteins and antibodies [58]. In contrast to direct radiolabeling procedures with I$^+$ using the tyrosine residues of the respective biomacromolecule, direct labeling with At$^+$ is not possible. Differently labeled building blocks like *N*-succinimidyl 3-[^{211}At]astatobenzoate ([^{211}At]SAB) [60,61] were used in a two-step labeling approach. To further improve the labeling efficiency, one-step approaches were developed in which the radionuclide is directly reacted with a pre-conjugated biomacromolecule. *N*-succinimidyl 3-(trimethylstannyl)benzoate was first conjugated to the antibody (trastuzumab) and then labeled with ^{211}At$^+$ leading to a high RCY and A$_S$ in a reduced procedure time. An improved approach using a cysteine coupling approach with an analogous maleimide-based precursor provides a more homogeneous bioconjugation to thiol instead of lysine residue [62]. Further improvements to raise the radioconjugate stability were made using guanidine-based building blocks like [^{211}At]At-SAGMB [63] (Figure 4).

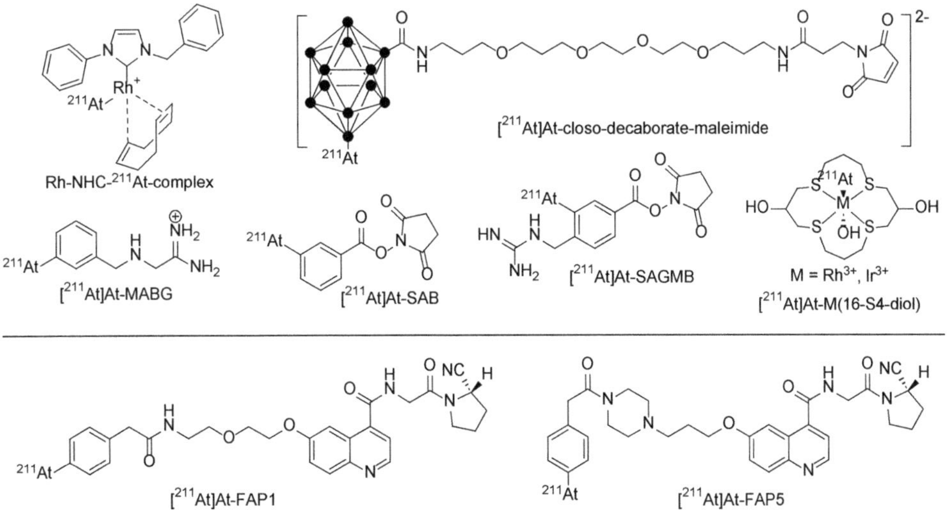

Figure 4. Different chemical strategies using prosthetic labeling groups to stably bind ^{211}At for a later conjugation to the target molecule and two promising small-molecule ^{211}At-radiotherapeutics [^{211}At]At-FAPI1 and [^{211}At]At-FAPI5.

Recently, four new ^{211}At-containing small-molecule radiotherapeutics based on the FAPI binding motif with different linkers (PEG, piperazine) were developed [64]. Cell uptake was performed using FAP-transfected HEK293/FAPα and A549/FAPα cell lines, and biodistribution on PANC-1-cell-bearing mice. Control experiments were performed with ^{131}I-labeled derivatives. [^{211}At]At-FAPI1 and [^{211}At]At-FAPI5 were the most promising with the highest tumor uptake and the best therapeutic effect.

In order to limit uptake in thyroid or stomach tissues, alternative attempts were made towards the use of alternatives to astatine bound to carbon using three-dimensional carboranes [65], which form thermodynamically stable boron–astatine bonds. The bond enthalpy is estimated to be approximately 50% higher than the aryl–At bond [66]. This radiolabeling approach has been transferred in several successful preclinical therapy studies using monoclonal antibodies as carriers [58]. The frequently reported activity retention in the liver and kidney is a limit of these boron–At clusters, especially when using molecules that are smaller than monoclonal antibodies.

Alternatively, At–metal complexes became more prominent for astatine labeling due to the soft base character of the At–anion. The first investigations considered the formation of mercury complexes. Later, complexes with Rh^{3+} or Ir^{3+} as a central cation included in macrocyclic ligands were developed [67]. However, in vivo studies have not successfully proven these approaches adequate yet for further (pre)clinical applications [68]. Softer metal cations like Rh^+ could improve the in vivo stability when N-heterocyclic carbenes are used as ligands [64,69].

5. Use of Carrier Molecules for Selective Delivery of Alpha Particle-Emitting Nuclides

The properties of alpha emitters are suitably matched to uses involving the targeting of various moieties ranging from small molecules over peptides to antibodies that are capable of selectively targeting receptors or antigens on cancer cells. A unique biological target that has been successfully addressed by targeted endoradiotherapy is the sodium–iodine symporter in thyroid cancer, which has been used for decades for radio-iodine therapy and can also be coopted for radioastatine-211 therapy since astatine chemically resembles iodine. When it comes to targeting in a broader sense, other synthetic binding vectors are introduced to facilitate target-specific transport in vivo (Figure 5). In nuclear medicine, several approaches for diagnostics and therapy are currently in clinical practice, namely the targets SSTR2, PSMA, CXCR4, $\alpha v \beta 3$, $\alpha v \beta 6$, and FAPα, among others [70,71]. Extensive experience of using pharmacokinetics with such small molecules has been documented in the literature and useful biological targets across several tumor entities are available. Based on the wide experience of measuring the uptake of these carriers by PET, robust data exist with regard to target availability that can be applied to targeted alpha therapies.

Other attractive carriers—taken from biological templates—are monoclonal antibodies. Theranostic approaches have also been suggested towards commonly known targets like Her2/neu [72]. The utilization of monoclonal antibodies as carriers for alpha-emitting radionuclides were widely used in the past and are promising for ongoing clinical trials [4,73]. Although monoclonal antibodies are associated with very good binding properties and a broad range of availability, their size limits renal elimination and therefore long circulation times are observed, which are associated with relevant toxicity. In contrast, small molecules can rapidly diffuse to targets leading to rapid accumulation together with fast excretion. This is then typically associated with a larger window between toxicity and efficacy for small molecules in contrast to monoclonal antibodies.

For example, the beta-emitting radionuclide lutetium-177 (^{177}Lu) was used for labeling the PSMA-binding antibody J591, which displayed efficacy at a dose activity of two applications of 1.67 GBq/m^2 myelosuppression as dose-limiting toxicity [74]. In contrast, ^{177}Lu, which was used for labeling PSMA-617, was reported as safe in a phase 3 clinical trial when 4–6 cycles of 7.4 GBq were applied [75]. Small antibody-derived molecules such as nanobodies or antibody fragments might combine fast pharmacokinetics with retained high in vivo tumor binding. However, such approaches are still rarely applied in clinical trials. Also, the concept of separating tumor-binding pharmacokinetics from radionuclide-carrying pharmacokinetic pre-targeting approaches in order to reduce toxicity has rarely reached clinical trials to date.

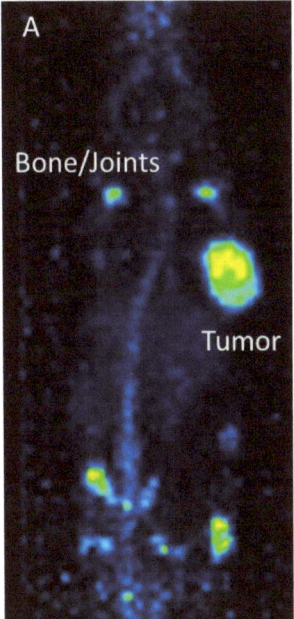 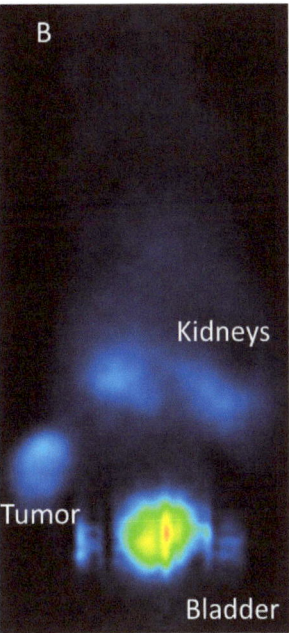

Figure 5. Preclinical examples for targeting with monoclonal antibodies or peptides. (**A**): [^{89}Zr]Zr–Trastuzumab targeting Her2/neu in a mouse model carrying subcutaneous BT474 tumors. PET imaging was conducted 7 days after radiotracer application. (**B**): [^{68}Ga]Ga–DOTA–TOC targeting the somatostatin receptor in a mouse model with subcutaneous AR42J tumor. PET imaging was performed one hour after tracer application.

6. Clinical Overview and Perspectives

Clinically, one commonly used alpha particle-emitting radionuclide is radium-223, with a randomized clinical trial in metastasized castration-resistant prostate cancer (mCRPC) showing a significant benefit in terms of overall survival compared to placebo, leading to the approval of radium-223 (^{223}Ra, Xofigo®) in this indication. The approved activity is 55 kBq/kg, administered for six cycles every 4 weeks [76]. However, due to the indirect targeting mechanism aimed at bone remodeling and the insufficient ability to couple radium-223 with binding vector molecules, radium-223 has not been successfully used in other indications [77]. Nevertheless, the side effect profile of this treatment is low and its combination with targeted beta-emitting therapy is possible [78]. With the introduction of an alpha-emitting radionuclide into clinical routine, radiation safety has been addressed in particular. Possible doses that might arise from contamination with radium-223 were calculated. Also, theoretical estimations and measurements for clinical routines were performed. Although precautionary measures are dependent on the local regulatory authority, the application of radium-223 does not pose any significant radiation safety issue [79,80]. At the level of clinical trials or compassionate use programs, there is also firm experience for the use of many other alpha-emitters for several other indications.

In hematologic diseases, where tumor cells are readily accessible for carrier molecules and single cells are the main cause of tumor manifestations, the isotope bismuth-213 ($\tau_{\frac{1}{2}} = 46$ min) and the 9.9-day half-life radionuclide ^{225}Ac were used to couple to the CD33-binding antibody lintuzumab (HuM195), and leukemia-inhibitory activity was reported [81–83]. In this case, the radioligand-constructs consisting of an alpha emitter and a monoclonal antibody were administered intravenously. The cellular target for lintuzumab is the myeloid-specific transmembrane receptor CD33, which has high availability on leukemia cells while lacking expression in hematologic stem cells. A maximum tolerated dose of 37 MBq/kg was reported for a sequential protocol with cytarabine followed by [^{213}Bi]Bi–lintuzumab. The optimized targeting of lintuzumab was achieved by the administration of 250 µg unlabeled antibody before the administration of [^{225}Ac]Ac-lintuzumab at activity levels between 18.4 and 148 kBq/kg. Based on a grade 3 hyperbilirubinemia and one episode of syncope complicated by subarachnoid hemorrhage toxicity, and both patients experiencing infections in the 148 kBq/kg dose group, the maximum tolerated dose was estimated at 111 kBq/kg as a single infusion of [^{225}Ac]Ac–lintuzumab. With doses exceeding 37 kBq/kg, peripheral blasts were eliminated in most patients. However, in this small, severely therapy-refractory cohort, the measurement of strong efficacy, such as complete remissions, was not achieved [83]

Since ^{223}Ra cannot be reliably chelated and then coupled to binding vector molecules, its parent nuclide thorium-227, with a half-life of 18.7 days, was used in a first human clinical trial for targeted alpha therapy with monoclonal antibodies against CD22 in lymphomas. In this study, the octadentate chelator 3,2-hydroxypyridinone (3,2-HOPO) was used. A small number of patients (n = 21) were treated with a maximum cumulative activity of 13.8 MBq, and complete remission (CR) was observed in one patient treated with 3.1 MBq and partial remission (PR) was observed in four patients treated with 1.5–4.6 MBq [84]. ^{225}Ac was conjugated to the monoclonal antibody J591 targeting PSMA in prostate cancer is under investigation in a phase I clinical trial (ClinicalTrials.gov Identifier: NCT03276572).

However, in general, peptides as carrier molecules for alpha–emitting radionuclides are currently more commonly applied for solid tumors. The intravenous injection of longer half-lived radionuclides might reduce the background radiation of the carrier molecules show rapid renal elimination [85,86]. Consequently, the combination of the rapidly distributing somatostatin analogue with the short-lived radionuclide ^{213}Bi was focused on intra-arterial application taking advantage of a high first-pass effect [87]. Patients that were refractory to beta-emitting radionuclides were treated with the cumulative activities of up to 20 GBq [^{213}Bi]Bi–DOTA–TOC over several treatment cycles. During the follow-up, one patient (1/7) developed MDS and acceptable renal function impairment was observed. For the parent nuclide ^{225}Ac, cumulative doses of up to 60–80 MBq [^{225}Ac]Ac–DOTA–TOC resulted in acute hematologic toxicity with a platelet and leucocyte count nadir at 4–6 weeks with subsequent recovery. No hematological malignancies were observed, but renal toxicity was observed and two long-term survivors developed terminal kidney failure [88]. Based on the experience with ^{225}Ac, clinical trials targeting the somatostatin receptor by [^{225}Ac]Ac–DOTA–TOC are under way (ClinicalTrials.gov Identifier: NCT05477576) [89].

Furthermore, not only is [^{225}Ac]Ac–DOTA–TOC under investigation, but there is also increasing experience with [^{225}Ac]Ac–DOTA–TATE [90,91]. In a pilot study in metastatic paragangliomas, the [^{225}Ac]Ac–DOTA–TATE ((100 kBq/kg) body weight per cycle at 8-weekly intervals up to a cumulative activity of ~74 MBq), in combination with the radiosensitizer capezetabine, achieved disease control in 8 of 9 patients treated [91].

In the future, it is expected that combined immuno- and endoradiotherapies will gain significance in personalized medicine, especially for established tumor mutations like BRCA, RET, and BRAF. A favorable outcome was recently reported in a patient with a G3 BRCA-mutated neuroendocrine tumor through a successful combination of olaparib and [^{225}Ac]Ac–DOTA–TATE (see Figure 6). To further elucidate the effectiveness, safety, and efficacy of the aforementioned treatments, clinical trials are necessary.

In a clinical trial treating NET patients without prior peptide receptor radiotherapy with four cycles of 2.50 MBq/kg [^{212}Pb]Pb–DOTAM–TATE, objective radiological responses were observed in most patients. However, diagnostic imaging was performed with [^{68}Ga]Ga–DOTA–TATE, whereas [^{203}Pb]Pb–DOTAM–TATE was used for human dose calculations [55]. Additionally, the Tyr^3-octreotide (TOC) variant VMT-α-NET was used for human applications as a conjugate for $^{203/212}$Pb with high chelation properties [56]. SPECT/CT images (low dose, 224 MBq) with [^{203}Pb]Pb–VMT-α-NET were acquired to assess the feasibility of [^{212}Pb]Pb–VMT-α-NET therapy. A recent study demonstrated the post-treatment imaging of [^{212}Pb]Pb–VMT-α-NET in a patient with metastatic NET [92]. The advantages of [^{212}Pb]Pb–VMT-α-NET therapy are rapid renal clearance with potentially less nephrotoxicity than the standard radiopharmaceuticals and the possibility of dosimetry prediction using the elementally matched isotope ^{203}Pb as an imaging surrogate (Figure 7).

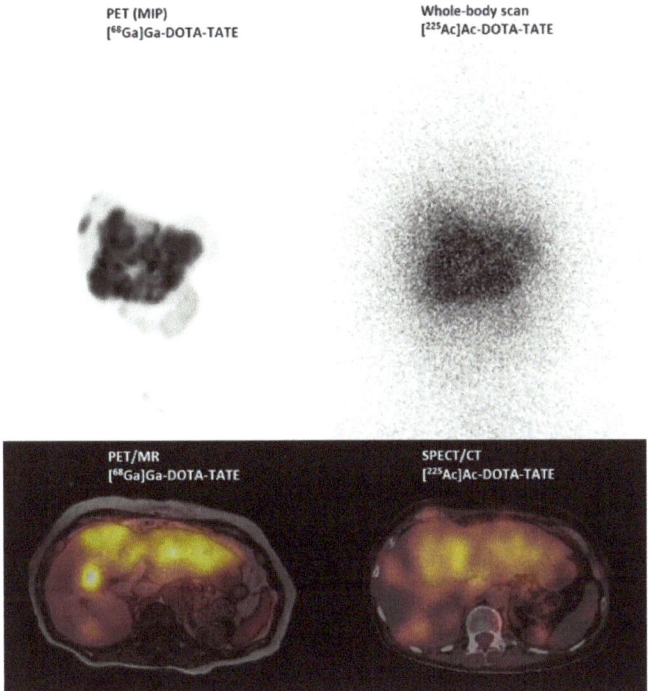

Figure 6. [^{68}Ga]Ga–DOTA–TATE PET/MR (maximum intensity projection (MIP) and PET/MR fusion image) and post-therapy scintigraphic imaging (whole body and SPECT/CT fusion image) 24 h after injection of 6.5 MBq [^{225}Ac]Ac–DOTA–DATE in a patient with a G3 neuroendocrine tumor.

With other solid tumors, target availability is typically a major challenge. Therefore, many attempts to introduce alpha particle-emitting radionuclides into clinical application followed locoregional applications where pharmacokinetics in the whole body are less relevant. A variety of applications have been proposed, for example, to treat the peritoneal cavity, the urinary bladder, or the intracerebral operation cavities after the resection of malignant cerebral tumors. Here, a broader choice of nuclides is possible because target-to-background is already high due to the route of application. ^{211}At coupled to MX35-F(ab')2 was applied to the peritoneal cavity for treating ovarian cancer with activities up to 355 MBq and no signs of radiation-induced toxicity were reported [93]. Also, ^{212}Pb ($\tau_{\frac{1}{2}}$ = 10.6 days) coupled to the Her2/neu binding monoclonal antibody trastuzumab was considered safe for patients with peritoneal carcinomatosis up to 27 MBq/m^2 [94]. ^{213}Bi was proved to be safe in loco-regional treatment for in situ bladder carcinoma up to 821 MBq [95]. Other clinical approaches targeted residual tumor cells of high-grade brain tumors after operation. Here, the radionuclides ^{213}Bi or ^{225}Ac were labeled to substance-P and applied after surgical resection and considered as safe and well tolerated [96–98].

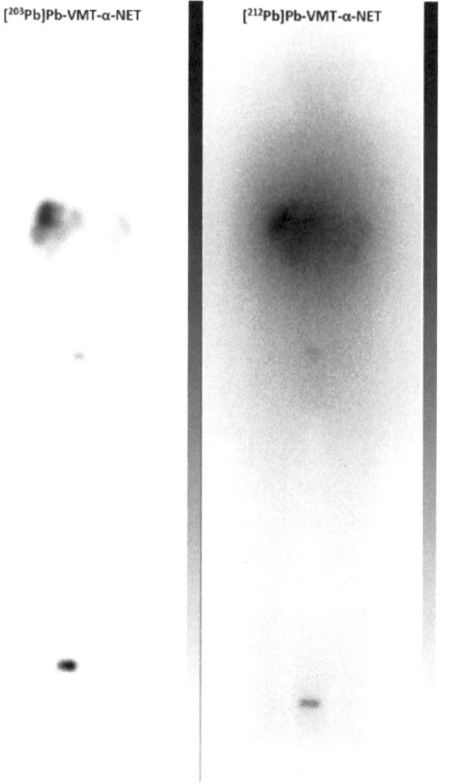

Figure 7. Clinical example of the scintigraphic imaging of the theranostic pair ^{203}Pb and ^{212}Pb: Pretreatment whole body scan of [^{203}Pb]Pb–VMT-α-NET (348 MBq, 2 h p.i.) and post-treatment imaging of [^{212}Pb]Pb–VMT-α-NET (86 MBq, 2 h p.i.) in a patient with a G3 hepatic metastatic neuroendocrine tumor.

For systemic therapy, typically administered by i.v. route, the properties and availability of the molecular target are undoubtedly dominating factors for successful internal targeted endoradiotherapy. With the prostate-specific membrane antigen (PSMA), a highly expressed carboxypeptidase and a well available target on the cell surface is available and targeted alpha therapy is expected to contribute to further improvements in treating prostate carcinoma. Here, clinical data mainly from ^{225}Ac were reported, but the radionuclide ^{227}Th has also been suggested. ^{227}Th transported by a monoclonal antibody targeting PSMA showed preclinical efficacy in several subcutaneous mouse models and is a candidate for clinical translation [99]. In thirteen patients treated with [^{225}Ac]Ac-PSMA-617, the median overall survival was 8.5 months with a majority of patients showing prostate-specific antigen (PSA) responses [100]. By standardized quality of life questionnaires, a moderate improvement in the global health status was documented. One patient even reported exceeding a 5-year complete remission after [^{225}Ac]Ac–PSMA-617 treatment [101]. In addition to PSMA-617, other PSMA-binding small molecules were also used as binding vectors in clinical application [102]. For example, [^{225}Ac]Ac–PSMA–I&T applied in 1–5 cycles (6–8.5 MBq) was compassionately used in 18 patients, among which seven were experiencing a PSA response with the lowest PSA levels, which were < 50% to baseline. Despite being a well-suited target and although imaging has become increasingly applied in the therapeutic management of PSMA-targeted therapies, the imaging of ^{225}Ac after therapy is—in contrast to the imaging of ^{177}Lu—not well suited for diagnostic purposes.

Low therapeutic activities and gamma ray emissions coming from the daughter nuclides preclude the quantification of targeting and post-therapeutic imaging might be mainly suited for quality control (Figure 8). Although the PSA response rates might be high in these patient cohorts, a number of patients did not show a response to PSMA-targeted alpha therapy. A molecular analysis of the non-responding tumor tissue with sufficient PSMA expression from seven patients after therapy with ^{225}Ac-labeled PSMA-617 shows a high rate of alterations in the DNA damage-repair or cell cycle checkpoint [103]. This underlies the importance of the relationship between the tumor biology and targeted alpha therapy.

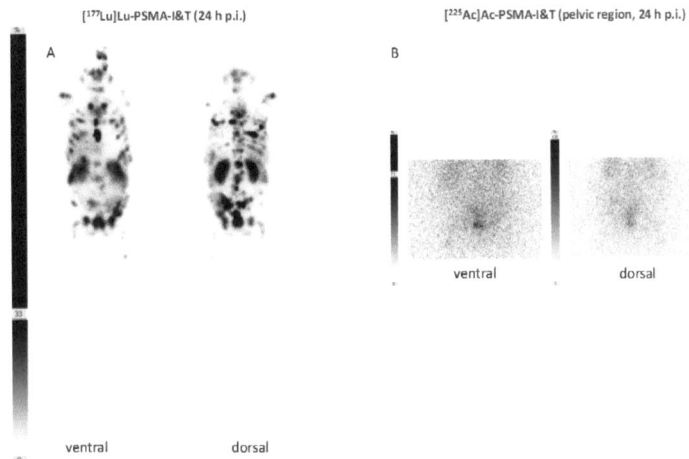

Figure 8. Anterior and posterior scintigraphic imaging of a patient treated with 5 GBq [^{177}Lu]Lu–PSMA–I&T (**A**) and subsequently—due to rising PSA levels combined with reduced bone marrow reserve—with 8 MBq [^{225}Ac]Ac–PSMA–I&T 6 months afterwards (**B**).

Taken together, advances in the development of therapeutic radiopharmaceuticals likely will trigger the vast expansion of clinical trials in the future. Clinical data from controlled, non-controlled trials, or clinical observations will be valuable to determine the extent of therapeutic effects in comparison, for example, to clinical experience and other reported clinical trials. Although prospective randomized trials are needed, such trials will be further complemented by, e.g., establishing broad safety profiles and dose–response relationships from compassionate use applications. In particular, with the aim of developing newly approved therapies, future randomized clinical trials might further elucidate the exact role of alpha emitters in patient care.

7. Outlook

One major field of application of α-radionuclide radiopharmaceuticals will be the clinical validation of several unique aspects that are described in the theoretical models and preclinical work. The exact impact of off-target and daughter redistribution on a clinical effect might depend on the pharmacokinetic details of the carrier, its individual variation, and the extent of internalization upon cell binding, and must be addressed in future work. In addition, the cytotoxic effects on tumors displaying a different biology and a different extent on biological variation are fields to be addressed for different tumor entities. Clinical trial design with regard to individual aspects like dosimetry including micro-dosimetric aspects will also remain challenging. Another major field will be the incorporation of imaging and a more sophisticated analysis like the parameters of heterogeneity and radiomics. In this regard, new tools such as artificial intelligence might contribute to both trial design and individualization by imaging guidance. Future developments will also need to address the role of alpha-emitting endoradiotherapy in several aspects where synergistic effects are expected. Several examples can be hypothesized like adjuvant systemic or locoregional treatment to maximize the advantage arising from the short high-LET pathways of alpha particles for single-tumor-cell diseases. Other highly promising scenarios include the combination of systemic alpha therapy with other approaches like chemotherapy or immune modulation therapy or the combination of internal with external radiation.

Author Contributions: Conceptualization, M.M. and M.R.M.; writing—original draft preparation, M.M., M.B.-S., C.M., D.K., M.P., E.M., C.B., J.K., K.K., D.A.S. and M.R.M.; writing—review and editing, M.M., M.B.-S., C.M., D.K., M.P., E.M., C.B., J.K., K.K., D.A.S. and M.R.M. All authors have read and agreed to the published version of the manuscript.

Funding: This research received no external funding.

Institutional Review Board Statement: Not applicable.

Informed Consent Statement: Not applicable.

Data Availability Statement: Data sharing not applicable.

Conflicts of Interest: MSKCC has filed for IP protection on behalf of Scheinberg for various inventions discussed herein. Relevant licenses exist between MSKCC and Abbott and Actinium. D.A.S. is a consultant to, on BOD of, or has equity in Pfizer, Actinium, Eureka, and Lantheus. Sloan Kettering has filed for IP protection for inventions described herein in which M.R.M. is an inventor. M.R.M. was a consultant for Actinium Pharmaceuticals, Regeneron, Progenics, and General Electric. M.M. has received personal fees from Novartis, Roche, and TELIX outside the submitted work. The other authors do not report any relevant financial or non-financial interests that are relevant to the content of this article.

References

1. Chan, H.S.; de Blois, E.; Morgenstern, A.; Bruchertseifer, F.; de Jong, M.; Breeman, W.; Konijnenberg, M. In Vitro comparison of ^{213}Bi- and ^{177}Lu-radiation for peptide receptor radionuclide therapy. *PLoS ONE* **2017**, *12*, e0181473. [CrossRef]
2. Graf, F.; Fahrer, J.; Maus, S.; Morgenstern, A.; Bruchertseifer, F.; Venkatachalam, S.; Fottner, C.; Weber, M.M.; Huelsenbeck, J.; Schreckenberger, M.; et al. DNA double strand breaks as predictor of efficacy of the alpha-particle emitter Ac-225 and the electron emitter Lu-177 for somatostatin receptor targeted radiotherapy. *PLoS ONE* **2014**, *9*, e88239. [CrossRef]
3. Miederer, M.; McDevitt, M.R.; Sgouros, G.; Kramer, K.; Cheung, N.K.; Scheinberg, D.A. Pharmacokinetics, dosimetry, and toxicity of the targetable atomic generator, 225Ac-HuM195, in nonhuman primates. *J. Nucl. Med.* **2004**, *45*, 129–137.
4. Miederer, M.; Scheinberg, D.A.; McDevitt, M.R. Realizing the potential of the Actinium-225 radionuclide generator in targeted alpha particle therapy applications. *Adv. Drug Deliv. Rev.* **2008**, *60*, 1371–1382. [CrossRef]
5. Robertson, A.K.H.; Ramogida, C.F.; Schaffer, P.; Radchenko, V. Development of ^{225}Ac Radiopharmaceuticals: TRIUMF Perspectives and Experiences. *Curr. Radiopharm.* **2018**, *11*, 156–172. [CrossRef]
6. Apostolidis, C.; Molinet, R.; Rasmussen, G.; Morgenstern, A. Production of Ac-225 from Th-229 for targeted alpha therapy. *Anal. Chem.* **2005**, *77*, 6288–6291. [CrossRef]
7. Engle, J.W. The Production of Ac-225. *Curr. Radiopharm.* **2018**, *11*, 173–179. [CrossRef]
8. Melville, G.; Meriarty, H.; Metcalfe, P.; Knittel, T.; Allen, B.J. Production of Ac-225 for cancer therapy by photon-induced transmutation of Ra-226. *Appl. Radiat. Isot.* **2007**, *65*, 1014–1022. [CrossRef]
9. Higashi, T.; Nagatsu, K.; Tsuji, A.B.; Zhang, M.R. Research and Development for Cyclotron Production of Ac from Ra-The Challenges in a Country Lacking Natural Resources for Medical Applications. *Processes* **2022**, *10*, 1215. [CrossRef]
10. Sgouros, G.; He, B.; Ray, N.; Ludwig, D.L.; Frey, E.C. Dosimetric impact of Ac-227 in accelerator-produced Ac-225 for alpha-emitter radiopharmaceutical therapy of patients with hematological malignancies: A pharmacokinetic modeling analysis. *EJNMMI Phys.* **2021**, *8*, 60. [CrossRef]
11. Nagatsu, K.; Suzuki, H.; Fukada, M.; Ito, T.; Ichinose, J.; Honda, Y.; Minegishi, K.; Higashi, T.; Zhang, M.R. Cyclotron production of ^{225}Ac from an electroplated ^{226}Ra target. *Eur. J. Nucl. Med. Mol. Imaging* **2021**, *49*, 279–289. [CrossRef]
12. Karlsson, J.; Schatz, C.A.; Wengner, A.M.; Hammer, S.; Scholz, A.; Cuthbertson, A.; Wagner, V.; Hennekes, H.; Jardine, V.; Hagemann, U.B. Targeted thorium-227 conjugates as treatment options in oncology. *Front. Med.* **2022**, *9*, 1071086. [CrossRef]
13. Roscher, M.; Bakos, G.; Benesova, M. Atomic Nanogenerators in Targeted Alpha Therapies: Curie's Legacy in Modern Cancer Management. *Pharmaceuticals* **2020**, *13*, 76. [CrossRef]
14. Grieve, M.L.; Paterson, B.M. The Evolving Coordination Chemistry of Radiometals for Targeted Alpha Therapy. *Aust. J. Chem.* **2022**, *75*, 65–88. [CrossRef]
15. Eychenne, R.; Cherel, M.; Haddad, F.; Guerard, F.; Gestin, J.F. Overview of the Most Promising Radionuclides for Targeted Alpha Therapy: The "Hopeful Eight". *Pharmaceutics* **2021**, *13*, 906. [CrossRef]

16. Thiele, N.A.; Wilson, J.J. Actinium-225 for Targeted alpha Therapy: Coordination Chemistry and Current Chelation Approaches. *Cancer Biother. Radiopharm.* **2018**, *33*, 336–348. [CrossRef]
17. Nelson, B.J.B.; Andersson, J.D.; Wuest, F. Radiolanthanum: Promising theranostic radionuclides for PET, alpha, and Auger-Meitner therapy. *Nucl. Med. Biol.* **2022**, *110–111*, 59–66. [CrossRef]
18. Price, E.W.; Orvig, C. Matching chelators to radiometals for radiopharmaceuticals. *Chem. Soc. Rev.* **2014**, *43*, 260–290. [CrossRef]
19. Davis, I.A.; Glowienka, K.A.; Boll, R.A.; Deal, K.A.; Brechbiel, M.W.; Stabin, M.; Bochsler, P.N.; Mirzadeh, S.; Kennel, S.J. Comparison of 225actinium chelates: Tissue distribution and radiotoxicity. *Nucl. Med. Biol.* **1999**, *26*, 581–589. [CrossRef]
20. Deal, K.A.; Davis, I.A.; Mirzadeh, S.; Kennel, S.J.; Brechbiel, M.W. Improved in vivo stability of actinium-225 macrocyclic complexes. *J. Med. Chem.* **1999**, *42*, 2988–2992. [CrossRef]
21. Duatti, A. The DOTA macrocyclic cavity in metallic radiopharmaceuticals: Mythology or reality? *EJNMMI Radiopharm. Chem.* **2023**, *8*, 17. [CrossRef]
22. Chappell, L.L.; Deal, K.A.; Dadachova, E.; Brechbiel, M.W. Synthesis, conjugation, and radiolabeling of a novel bifunctional chelating agent for ^{225}Ac radioimmunotherapy applications. *Bioconjug. Chem.* **2000**, *11*, 510–519. [CrossRef]
23. Baranyai, Z.; Tircso, G.; Rosch, F. The Use of the Macrocyclic Chelator DOTA in Radiochemical Separations. *Eur. J. Inorg. Chem.* **2020**, *2020*, 36–56. [CrossRef]
24. Khabibullin, A.R.; Karolak, A.; Budzevich, M.M.; McLaughlin, M.L.; Morse, D.L.; Woods, L.M. Structure and properties of DOTA-chelated radiopharmaceuticals within the ^{225}Ac decay pathway. *Medchemcomm* **2018**, *9*, 1155–1163. [CrossRef]
25. Beyer, G.J.; Offord, R.; Kunzi, G.; Aleksandrova, Y.; Ravn, U.; Jahn, S.; Barker, J.; Tengblad, O.; Lindroos, M.; The ISOLDE Collaboration. The influence of EDTMP-concentration on the biodistribution of radio-lanthanides and 225-Ac in tumor-bearing mice. *Nucl. Med. Biol.* **1997**, *24*, 367–372. [CrossRef]
26. Ahenkorah, S.; Cassells, I.; Deroose, C.M.; Cardinaels, T.; Burgoyne, A.R.; Bormans, G.; Ooms, M.; Cleeren, F. Bismuth-213 for Targeted Radionuclide Therapy: From Atom to Bedside. *Pharmaceutics* **2021**, *13*, 599. [CrossRef]
27. Muller, C.; Vermeulen, C.; Koster, U.; Johnston, K.; Turler, A.; Schibli, R.; van der Meulen, N.P. Alpha-PET with terbium-149: Evidence and perspectives for radiotheragnostics. *EJNMMI Radiopharm. Chem.* **2017**, *1*, 5. [CrossRef]
28. Ivanov, A.S.; Simms, M.E.; Bryantsev, V.S.; Benny, P.D.; Griswold, J.R.; Delmau, L.H.; Thiele, N.A. Elucidating the coordination chemistry of the radium ion for targeted alpha therapy. *Chem. Commun.* **2022**, *58*, 9938–9941. [CrossRef]
29. McDevitt, M.R.; Ma, D.; Simon, J.; Frank, R.K.; Scheinberg, D.A. Design and synthesis of ^{225}Ac radioimmunopharmaceuticals. *Appl. Radiat. Isot.* **2002**, *57*, 841–847. [CrossRef]
30. McDevitt, M.R.; Ma, D.; Lai, L.T.; Simon, J.; Borchardt, P.; Frank, R.K.; Wu, K.; Pellegrini, V.; Curcio, M.J.; Miederer, M.; et al. Tumor therapy with targeted atomic nanogenerators. *Science* **2001**, *294*, 1537–1540. [CrossRef]
31. Maguire, W.F.; McDevitt, M.R.; Smith-Jones, P.M.; Scheinberg, D.A. Efficient 1-step radiolabeling of monoclonal antibodies to high specific activity with ^{225}Ac for alpha-particle radioimmunotherapy of cancer. *J. Nucl. Med.* **2014**, *55*, 1492–1498. [CrossRef]
32. Kurtz, K.; Eibler, L.; Dacek, M.M.; Carter, L.M.; Veach, D.R.; Lovibond, S.; Reynaud, E.; Qureshy, S.; McDevitt, M.R.; Bourne, C.; et al. Engineering CAR-T cells for radiohapten capture in imaging and radioimmunotherapy applications. *Theranostics* **2023**, *13*, 5469–5482. [CrossRef]
33. Arndt, C.; Bergmann, R.; Striese, F.; Merkel, K.; Mathe, D.; Loureiro, L.R.; Mitwasi, N.; Kegler, A.; Fasslrinner, F.; Gonzalez Soto, K.E.; et al. Development and Functional Characterization of a Versatile Radio-/Immunotheranostic Tool for Prostate Cancer Management. *Cancers* **2022**, *14*, 1996. [CrossRef]
34. Kratochwil, C.; Bruchertseifer, F.; Giesel, F.L.; Weis, M.; Verburg, F.A.; Mottaghy, F.; Kopka, K.; Apostolidis, C.; Haberkorn, U.; Morgenstern, A. ^{225}Ac-PSMA-617 for PSMA-Targeted alpha-Radiation Therapy of Metastatic Castration-Resistant Prostate Cancer. *J. Nucl. Med.* **2016**, *57*, 1941–1944. [CrossRef]
35. Thiele, N.A.; Brown, V.; Kelly, J.M.; Amor-Coarasa, A.; Jermilova, U.; MacMillan, S.N.; Nikolopoulou, A.; Ponnala, S.; Ramogida, C.F.; Robertson, A.K.H.; et al. An Eighteen-Membered Macrocyclic Ligand for Actinium-225 Targeted Alpha Therapy. *Angew. Chem. Int. Ed. Engl.* **2017**, *56*, 14712–14717. [CrossRef]
36. Reissig, F.; Bauer, D.; Zarschler, K.; Novy, Z.; Bendova, K.; Ludik, M.C.; Kopka, K.; Pietzsch, H.J.; Petrik, M.; Mamat, C. Towards Targeted Alpha Therapy with Actinium-225: Chelators for Mild Condition Radiolabeling and Targeting PSMA-A Proof of Concept Study. *Cancers* **2021**, *13*, 1974. [CrossRef] [PubMed]
37. Reissig, F.; Zarschler, K.; Novy, Z.; Petrik, M.; Bendova, K.; Kurfurstova, D.; Bouchal, J.; Ludik, M.C.; Brandt, F.; Kopka, K.; et al. Modulating the pharmacokinetic profile of Actinium-225-labeled macropa-derived radioconjugates by dual targeting of PSMA and albumin. *Theranostics* **2022**, *12*, 7203–7215. [CrossRef]
38. Wichmann, C.; Morgan, K.; Guo, N.; Gan, H.; Burvenich, I.; Donnelly, P.; Scott, A. Conjugation and radiolabelling of [Ac]Ac-macropa-tzPEGSq-ch806, a tumour-specific anti-EGFR antibody, and preclinical evaluation in a murine glioma model. *Intern. Med. J.* **2022**, *52*, 6–7.
39. King, A.P.; Gutsche, N.T.; Raju, N.; Fayn, S.; Baidoo, K.E.; Bell, M.M.; Olkowski, C.S.; Swenson, R.E.; Lin, F.I.; Sadowski, S.M.; et al. ^{225}Ac-MACROPATATE: A Novel alpha-Particle Peptide Receptor Radionuclide Therapy for Neuroendocrine Tumors. *J. Nucl. Med.* **2023**, *64*, 549–554. [CrossRef]
40. Yang, H.; Zhang, C.; Yuan, Z.; Rodriguez-Rodriguez, C.; Robertson, A.; Radchenko, V.; Perron, R.; Gendron, D.; Causey, P.; Gao, F.; et al. Synthesis and Evaluation of a Macrocyclic Actinium-225 Chelator, Quality Control and In Vivo Evaluation of ^{225}Ac-crown-alphaMSH Peptide. *Chemistry* **2020**, *26*, 11435–11440. [CrossRef]

41. Kadassery, K.J.; King, A.P.; Fayn, S.; Baidoo, K.E.; MacMillan, S.N.; Escorcia, F.E.; Wilson, J.J. H$_2$BZmacropa-NCS: A Bifunctional Chelator for Actinium-225 Targeted Alpha Therapy. *Bioconjug. Chem.* **2022**, *33*, 1222–1231. [CrossRef] [PubMed]
42. Aluicio-Sarduy, E.; Thiele, N.A.; Martin, K.E.; Vaughn, B.A.; Devaraj, J.; Olson, A.P.; Barnhart, T.E.; Wilson, J.J.; Boros, E.; Engle, J.W. Establishing Radiolanthanum Chemistry for Targeted Nuclear Medicine Applications. *Chemistry* **2020**, *26*, 1238–1242. [CrossRef] [PubMed]
43. Bruhlmann, S.A.; Kreller, M.; Pietzsch, H.J.; Kopka, K.; Mamat, C.; Walther, M.; Reissig, F. Efficient Production of the PET Radionuclide ^{133}La for Theranostic Purposes in Targeted Alpha Therapy Using the ^{134}Ba(p,2n)^{133}La Reaction. *Pharmaceuticals* **2022**, *15*, 1167. [CrossRef] [PubMed]
44. Blei, M.K.; Waurick, L.; Reissig, F.; Kopka, K.; Stumpf, T.; Drobot, B.; Kretzschmar, J.; Mamat, C. Equilibrium Thermodynamics of Macropa Complexes with Selected Metal Isotopes of Radiopharmaceutical Interest. *Inorg. Chem.* **2023**, *62*, 20699–20709. [CrossRef] [PubMed]
45. Nelson, B.J.B.; Wilson, J.; Andersson, J.D.; Wuest, F. High yield cyclotron production of a novel $^{133/135}$La theranostic pair for nuclear medicine. *Sci. Rep.* **2020**, *10*, 22203. [CrossRef] [PubMed]
46. Aluicio-Sarduy, E.; Barnhart, T.E.; Weichert, J.; Hernandez, R.; Engle, J.W. Cyclotron-Produced ^{132}La as a PET Imaging Surrogate for Therapeutic ^{225}Ac. *J. Nucl. Med.* **2021**, *62*, 1012–1015. [CrossRef] [PubMed]
47. Li, M.; Sagastume, E.A.; Lee, D.; McAlister, D.; DeGraffenreid, A.J.; Olewine, K.R.; Graves, S.; Copping, R.; Mirzadeh, S.; Zimmerman, B.E.; et al. $^{203/212}$Pb Theranostic Radiopharmaceuticals for Image-guided Radionuclide Therapy for Cancer. *Curr. Med. Chem.* **2020**, *27*, 7003–7031. [CrossRef]
48. Edem, P.E.; Fonslet, J.; Kjaer, A.; Herth, M.; Severin, G. In Vivo Radionuclide Generators for Diagnostics and Therapy. *Bioinorg. Chem. Appl.* **2016**, *2016*, 6148357. [CrossRef]
49. Kokov, K.V.; Egorova, B.V.; German, M.N.; Klabukov, I.D.; Krasheninnikov, M.E.; Larkin-Kondrov, A.A.; Makoveeva, K.A.; Ovchinnikov, M.V.; Sidorova, M.V.; Chuvilin, D.Y. ^{212}Pb: Production Approaches and Targeted Therapy Applications. *Pharmaceutics* **2022**, *14*, 189. [CrossRef]
50. McNeil, B.L.; Robertson, A.K.H.; Fu, W.; Yang, H.; Hoehr, C.; Ramogida, C.F.; Schaffer, P. Production, purification, and radiolabeling of the ^{203}Pb/^{212}Pb theranostic pair. *EJNMMI Radiopharm. Chem.* **2021**, *6*, 6. [CrossRef]
51. Li, M.; Baumhover, N.J.; Liu, D.; Cagle, B.S.; Boschetti, F.; Paulin, G.; Lee, D.; Dai, Z.; Obot, E.R.; Marks, B.M.; et al. Preclinical Evaluation of a Lead Specific Chelator (PSC) Conjugated to Radiopeptides for ^{203}Pb and ^{212}Pb-Based Theranostics. *Pharmaceutics* **2023**, *15*, 414. [CrossRef] [PubMed]
52. Tosato, M.; Lazzari, L.; Marco, V.D. Revisiting Lead(II)-1,4,7,10-tetraazacyclododecane-1,4,7,10-tetraacetic Acid Coordination Chemistry in Aqueous Solutions: Evidence of an Underestimated Thermodynamic Stability. *ACS Omega* **2022**, *7*, 15596–15602. [CrossRef]
53. Meredith, R.; Torgue, J.; Shen, S.; Fisher, D.R.; Banaga, E.; Bunch, P.; Morgan, D.; Fan, J.; Straughn, J.M., Jr. Dose escalation and dosimetry of first-in-human alpha radioimmunotherapy with 212Pb-TCMC-trastuzumab. *J. Nucl. Med.* **2014**, *55*, 1636–1642. [CrossRef]
54. Meredith, R.F.; Torgue, J.; Azure, M.T.; Shen, S.; Saddekni, S.; Banaga, E.; Carlise, R.; Bunch, P.; Yoder, D.; Alvarez, R. Pharmacokinetics and imaging of 212Pb-TCMC-trastuzumab after intraperitoneal administration in ovarian cancer patients. *Cancer Biother. Radiopharm.* **2014**, *29*, 12–17. [CrossRef] [PubMed]
55. Delpassand, E.S.; Tworowska, I.; Esfandiari, R.; Torgue, J.; Hurt, J.; Shafie, A.; Nunez, R. Targeted alpha-Emitter Therapy with ^{212}Pb-DOTAMTATE for the Treatment of Metastatic SSTR-Expressing Neuroendocrine Tumors: First-in-Humans Dose-Escalation Clinical Trial. *J. Nucl. Med.* **2022**, *63*, 1326–1333. [CrossRef]
56. Muller, D.; Herrmann, H.; Schultz, M.K.; Solbach, C.; Ettrich, T.; Prasad, V. ^{203}Pb-VMT-alpha-NET Scintigraphy of a Patient With Neuroendocrine Tumor. *Clin. Nucl. Med.* **2023**, *48*, 54–55. [CrossRef] [PubMed]
57. Dos Santos, J.C.; Schafer, M.; Bauder-Wust, U.; Lehnert, W.; Leotta, K.; Morgenstern, A.; Kopka, K.; Haberkorn, U.; Mier, W.; Kratochwil, C. Development and dosimetry of ^{203}Pb/^{212}Pb-labelled PSMA ligands: Bringing "the lead" into PSMA-targeted alpha therapy? *Eur. J. Nucl. Med. Mol. Imaging* **2019**, *46*, 1081–1091. [CrossRef] [PubMed]
58. Albertsson, P.; Back, T.; Bergmark, K.; Hallqvist, A.; Johansson, M.; Aneheim, E.; Lindegren, S.; Timperanza, C.; Smerud, K.; Palm, S. Astatine-211 based radionuclide therapy: Current clinical trial landscape. *Front. Med.* **2022**, *9*, 1076210. [CrossRef]
59. Sergentu, D.C.; Teze, D.; Sabatie-Gogova, A.; Alliot, C.; Guo, N.; Bassal, F.; Silva, I.D.; Deniaud, D.; Maurice, R.; Champion, J.; et al. Advances on the Determination of the Astatine Pourbaix Diagram: Predomination of AtO(OH)$_2^-$ over At$^-$ in Basic Conditions. *Chemistry* **2016**, *22*, 2964–2971. [CrossRef]
60. Zalutsky, M.R.; Reardon, D.A.; Akabani, G.; Coleman, R.E.; Friedman, A.H.; Friedman, H.S.; McLendon, R.E.; Wong, T.Z.; Bigner, D.D. Clinical experience with alpha-particle emitting 211At: Treatment of recurrent brain tumor patients with 211At-labeled chimeric antitenascin monoclonal antibody 81C6. *J. Nucl. Med.* **2008**, *49*, 30–38. [CrossRef]
61. Andersson, H.; Cederkrantz, E.; Back, T.; Divgi, C.; Elgqvist, J.; Himmelman, J.; Horvath, G.; Jacobsson, L.; Jensen, H.; Lindegren, S.; et al. Intraperitoneal alpha-particle radioimmunotherapy of ovarian cancer patients: Pharmacokinetics and dosimetry of ^{211}At-MX35 F(ab')2—A phase I study. *J. Nucl. Med.* **2009**, *50*, 1153–1160. [CrossRef] [PubMed]
62. Aneheim, E.; Gustafsson, A.; Albertsson, P.; Back, T.; Jensen, H.; Palm, S.; Svedhem, S.; Lindegren, S. Synthesis and Evaluation of Astatinated N-[2-(Maleimido)ethyl]-3-(trimethylstannyl)benzamide Immunoconjugates. *Bioconjug. Chem.* **2016**, *27*, 688–697. [CrossRef] [PubMed]

63. Vaidyanathan, G.; Affleck, D.J.; Bigner, D.D.; Zalutsky, M.R. N-succinimidyl 3-[211At]astato-4-guanidinomethylbenzoate: An acylation agent for labeling internalizing antibodies with alpha-particle emitting 211At. *Nucl. Med. Biol.* **2003**, *30*, 351–359. [CrossRef]
64. Aso, A.; Nabetani, H.; Matsuura, Y.; Kadonaga, Y.; Shirakami, Y.; Watabe, T.; Yoshiya, T.; Mochizuki, M.; Ooe, K.; Kawakami, A.; et al. Evaluation of Astatine-211-Labeled Fibroblast Activation Protein Inhibitor (FAPI): Comparison of Different Linkers with Polyethylene Glycol and Piperazine. *Int. J. Mol. Sci.* **2023**, *24*, 8701. [CrossRef]
65. Wilbur, D.S.; Chyan, M.K.; Hamlin, D.K.; Vessella, R.L.; Wedge, T.J.; Hawthorne, M.F. Reagents for astatination of biomolecules. 2. Conjugation of anionic boron cage pendant groups to a protein provides a method for direct labeling that is stable to in vivo deastatination. *Bioconjug. Chem.* **2007**, *18*, 1226–1240. [CrossRef] [PubMed]
66. Ayed, T.; Pilme, J.; Teze, D.; Bassal, F.; Barbet, J.; Cherel, M.; Champion, J.; Maurice, R.; Montavon, G.; Galland, N. ^{211}At-labeled agents for alpha-immunotherapy: On the in vivo stability of astatine-agent bonds. *Eur. J. Med. Chem.* **2016**, *116*, 156–164. [CrossRef] [PubMed]
67. Pruszynski, M.; Bilewicz, A.; Zalutsky, M.R. Preparation of Rh[16aneS4-diol](211)At and Ir[16aneS4-diol](211)At complexes as potential precursors for astatine radiopharmaceuticals. Part I: Synthesis. *Bioconjug. Chem.* **2008**, *19*, 958–965. [CrossRef]
68. Pruszynski, M.; Lyczko, M.; Bilewicz, A.; Zalutsky, M.R. Stability and in vivo behavior of Rh[16aneS4-diol]211 at complex: A potential precursor for astatine radiopharmaceuticals. *Nucl. Med. Biol.* **2015**, *42*, 439–445. [CrossRef]
69. Rajerison, H.; Faye, D.; Roumesy, A.; Louaisil, N.; Boeda, F.; Faivre-Chauvet, A.; Gestin, J.F.; Legoupy, S. Ionic liquid supported organotin reagents to prepare molecular imaging and therapy agents. *Org. Biomol. Chem.* **2016**, *14*, 2121–2126. [CrossRef]
70. Buck, A.K.; Serfling, S.E.; Kraus, S.; Samnick, S.; Dreher, N.; Higuchi, T.; Rasche, L.; Einsele, H.; Werner, R.A. Theranostics in Hematooncology. *J. Nucl. Med.* **2023**, *64*, 1009–1016. [CrossRef]
71. Cankaya, A.; Balzer, M.; Amthauer, H.; Brenner, W.; Spreckelmeyer, S. Optimization of ^{177}Lu-labelling of DOTA-TOC, PSMA-I&T and FAPI-46 for clinical application. *EJNMMI Radiopharm. Chem.* **2023**, *8*, 10. [CrossRef] [PubMed]
72. Koehler, C.; Sauter, P.F.; Klasen, B.; Waldmann, C.; Pektor, S.; Bausbacher, N.; Lemke, E.A.; Miederer, M. Genetic Code Expansion for Site-Specific Labeling of Antibodies with Radioisotopes. *ACS Chem. Biol.* **2023**, *18*, 443–448. [CrossRef] [PubMed]
73. Miederer, M.; McDevitt, M.R.; Borchardt, P.; Bergman, I.; Kramer, K.; Cheung, N.K.; Scheinberg, D.A. Treatment of neuroblastoma meningeal carcinomatosis with intrathecal application of alpha-emitting atomic nanogenerators targeting disialo-ganglioside GD2. *Clin. Cancer Res.* **2004**, *10*, 6985–6992. [CrossRef] [PubMed]
74. Tagawa, S.T.; Vallabhajosula, S.; Christos, P.J.; Jhanwar, Y.S.; Batra, J.S.; Lam, L.; Osborne, J.; Beltran, H.; Molina, A.M.; Goldsmith, S.J.; et al. Phase 1/2 study of fractionated dose lutetium-177-labeled anti-prostate-specific membrane antigen monoclonal antibody J591 (^{177}Lu-J591) for metastatic castration-resistant prostate cancer. *Cancer* **2019**, *125*, 2561–2569. [CrossRef] [PubMed]
75. Sartor, O.; de Bono, J.; Chi, K.N.; Fizazi, K.; Herrmann, K.; Rahbar, K.; Tagawa, S.T.; Nordquist, L.T.; Vaishampayan, N.; El-Haddad, G.; et al. Lutetium-177-PSMA-617 for Metastatic Castration-Resistant Prostate Cancer. *N. Engl. J. Med.* **2021**, *385*, 1091–1103. [CrossRef] [PubMed]
76. Parker, C.; Nilsson, S.; Heinrich, D.; Helle, S.I.; O'Sullivan, J.M.; Fossa, S.D.; Chodacki, A.; Wiechno, P.; Logue, J.; Seke, M.; et al. Alpha emitter radium-223 and survival in metastatic prostate cancer. *N. Engl. J. Med.* **2013**, *369*, 213–223. [CrossRef] [PubMed]
77. Deandreis, D.; Maillard, A.; Zerdoud, S.; Bournaud, C.; Vija, L.; Sajous, C.; Terroir, M.; Leenhardt, L.; Schlumberger, M.; Borget, I.; et al. RADTHYR: An open-label, single-arm, prospective multicenter phase II trial of Radium-223 for the treatment of bone metastases from radioactive iodine refractory differentiated thyroid cancer. *Eur. J. Nucl. Med. Mol. Imaging* **2021**, *48*, 3238–3249. [CrossRef]
78. Kostos, L.; Buteau, J.P.; Yeung, T.; Iulio, J.D.; Xie, J.; Cardin, A.; Chin, K.Y.; Emmerson, B.; Owen, K.L.; Parker, B.S.; et al. AlphaBet: Combination of Radium-223 and [^{177}Lu]Lu-PSMA-I&T in men with metastatic castration-resistant prostate cancer (clinical trial protocol). *Front. Med.* **2022**, *9*, 1059122. [CrossRef]
79. Dauer, L.T.; Williamson, M.J.; Humm, J.; O'Donoghue, J.; Ghani, R.; Awadallah, R.; Carrasquillo, J.; Pandit-Taskar, N.; Aksnes, A.K.; Biggin, C.; et al. Radiation safety considerations for the use of ^{223}RaCl$_2$ DE in men with castration-resistant prostate cancer. *Health Phys.* **2014**, *106*, 494–504. [CrossRef]
80. Stabin, M.G.; Siegel, J.A. Radiation Dose and Hazard Assessment of Potential Contamination Events During Use of 223Ra Dichloride in Radionuclide Therapy. *Health Phys.* **2015**, *109*, 212–217. [CrossRef]
81. Jurcic, J.G.; Larson, S.M.; Sgouros, G.; McDevitt, M.R.; Finn, R.D.; Divgi, C.R.; Ballangrud, A.M.; Hamacher, K.A.; Ma, D.; Humm, J.L.; et al. Targeted alpha particle immunotherapy for myeloid leukemia. *Blood* **2002**, *100*, 1233–1239. [CrossRef] [PubMed]
82. Rosenblat, T.L.; McDevitt, M.R.; Mulford, D.A.; Pandit-Taskar, N.; Divgi, C.R.; Panageas, K.S.; Heaney, M.L.; Chanel, S.; Morgenstern, A.; Sgouros, G.; et al. Sequential cytarabine and alpha-particle immunotherapy with bismuth-213-lintuzumab (HuM195) for acute myeloid leukemia. *Clin. Cancer Res.* **2010**, *16*, 5303–5311. [CrossRef]
83. Rosenblat, T.L.; McDevitt, M.R.; Carrasquillo, J.A.; Pandit-Taskar, N.; Frattini, M.G.; Maslak, P.G.; Park, J.H.; Douer, D.; Cicic, D.; Larson, S.M.; et al. Treatment of Patients with Acute Myeloid Leukemia with the Targeted Alpha-Particle Nanogenerator Actinium-225-Lintuzumab. *Clin. Cancer Res.* **2022**, *28*, 2030–2037. [CrossRef]
84. Linden, O.; Bates, A.T.; Cunningham, D.; Hindorf, C.; Larsson, E.; Cleton, A.; Pinkert, J.; Huang, F.; Bladt, F.; Hennekes, H.; et al. ^{227}Th-Labeled Anti-CD22 Antibody (BAY 1862864) in Relapsed/Refractory CD22-Positive Non-Hodgkin Lymphoma: A First-in-Human, Phase I Study. *Cancer Biother. Radiopharm.* **2021**, *36*, 672–681. [CrossRef] [PubMed]

85. Miederer, M.; Henriksen, G.; Alke, A.; Mossbrugger, I.; Quintanilla-Martinez, L.; Senekowitsch-Schmidtke, R.; Essler, M. Preclinical evaluation of the alpha-particle generator nuclide ^{225}Ac for somatostatin receptor radiotherapy of neuroendocrine tumors. *Clin. Cancer Res.* **2008**, *14*, 3555–3561. [CrossRef] [PubMed]
86. Drecoll, E.; Gaertner, F.C.; Miederer, M.; Blechert, B.; Vallon, M.; Muller, J.M.; Alke, A.; Seidl, C.; Bruchertseifer, F.; Morgenstern, A.; et al. Treatment of peritoneal carcinomatosis by targeted delivery of the radio-labeled tumor homing peptide bi-DTPA-[F3]2 into the nucleus of tumor cells. *PLoS ONE* **2009**, *4*, e5715. [CrossRef]
87. Kratochwil, C.; Giesel, F.L.; Bruchertseifer, F.; Mier, W.; Apostolidis, C.; Boll, R.; Murphy, K.; Haberkorn, U.; Morgenstern, A. ^{213}Bi-DOTATOC receptor-targeted alpha-radionuclide therapy induces remission in neuroendocrine tumours refractory to beta radiation: A first-in-human experience. *Eur. J. Nucl. Med. Mol. Imaging* **2014**, *41*, 2106–2119. [CrossRef]
88. Kratochwil, C.; Apostolidis, L.; Rathke, H.; Apostolidis, C.; Bicu, F.; Bruchertseifer, F.; Choyke, P.L.; Haberkorn, U.; Giesel, F.L.; Morgenstern, A. Dosing ^{225}Ac-DOTATOC in patients with somatostatin-receptor-positive solid tumors: 5-year follow-up of hematological and renal toxicity. *Eur. J. Nucl. Med. Mol. Imaging* **2021**, *49*, 54–63. [CrossRef]
89. Rubira, L.; Deshayes, E.; Santoro, L.; Kotzki, P.O.; Fersing, C. ^{225}Ac-Labeled Somatostatin Analogs in the Management of Neuroendocrine Tumors: From Radiochemistry to Clinic. *Pharmaceutics* **2023**, *15*, 1051. [CrossRef]
90. Demirci, E.; Alan Selcuk, N.; Beydagi, G.; Ocak, M.; Toklu, T.; Akcay, K.; Kabasakal, L. Initial Findings on the Use of [^{225}Ac]Ac-DOTATATE Therapy as a Theranostic Application in Patients with Neuroendocrine Tumors. *Mol. Imaging Radionucl. Ther.* **2023**, *32*, 226–232. [CrossRef]
91. Yadav, M.P.; Ballal, S.; Sahoo, R.K.; Bal, C. Efficacy and safety of ^{225}Ac-DOTATATE targeted alpha therapy in metastatic paragangliomas: A pilot study. *Eur. J. Nucl. Med. Mol. Imaging* **2022**, *49*, 1595–1606. [CrossRef] [PubMed]
92. Michler, E.; Kastner, D.; Brogsitter, C.; Pretze, M.; Hartmann, H.; Freudenberg, R.; Schultz, M.K.; Kotzerke, J. First-in-human SPECT/CT imaging of [^{212}Pb]Pb-VMT-alpha-NET in a patient with metastatic neuroendocrine tumor. *Eur. J. Nucl. Med. Mol. Imaging* **2023**. [CrossRef] [PubMed]
93. Hallqvist, A.; Bergmark, K.; Back, T.; Andersson, H.; Dahm-Kahler, P.; Johansson, M.; Lindegren, S.; Jensen, H.; Jacobsson, L.; Hultborn, R.; et al. Intraperitoneal alpha-Emitting Radioimmunotherapy with ^{211}At in Relapsed Ovarian Cancer: Long-Term Follow-up with Individual Absorbed Dose Estimations. *J. Nucl. Med.* **2019**, *60*, 1073–1079. [CrossRef] [PubMed]
94. Meredith, R.F.; Torgue, J.J.; Rozgaja, T.A.; Banaga, E.P.; Bunch, P.W.; Alvarez, R.D.; Straughn, J.M., Jr.; Dobelbower, M.C.; Lowy, A.M. Safety and Outcome Measures of First-in-Human Intraperitoneal alpha Radioimmunotherapy with ^{212}Pb-TCMC-Trastuzumab. *Am. J. Clin. Oncol.* **2018**, *41*, 716–721. [CrossRef]
95. Autenrieth, M.E.; Seidl, C.; Bruchertseifer, F.; Horn, T.; Kurtz, F.; Feuerecker, B.; D'Alessandria, C.; Pfob, C.; Nekolla, S.; Apostolidis, C.; et al. Treatment of carcinoma in situ of the urinary bladder with an alpha-emitter immunoconjugate targeting the epidermal growth factor receptor: A pilot study. *Eur. J. Nucl. Med. Mol. Imaging* **2018**, *45*, 1364–1371. [CrossRef]
96. Krolicki, L.; Bruchertseifer, F.; Kunikowska, J.; Koziara, H.; Krolicki, B.; Jakucinski, M.; Pawlak, D.; Apostolidis, C.; Mirzadeh, S.; Rola, R.; et al. Prolonged survival in secondary glioblastoma following local injection of targeted alpha therapy with ^{213}Bi-substance P analogue. *Eur. J. Nucl. Med. Mol. Imaging* **2018**, *45*, 1636–1644. [CrossRef]
97. Krolicki, L.; Bruchertseifer, F.; Kunikowska, J.; Koziara, H.; Pawlak, D.; Kulinski, R.; Rola, R.; Merlo, A.; Morgenstern, A. Dose escalation study of targeted alpha therapy with [^{225}Ac]Ac-DOTA-substance P in recurrence glioblastoma—Safety and efficacy. *Eur. J. Nucl. Med. Mol. Imaging* **2021**, *48*, 3595–3605. [CrossRef]
98. Miederer, M. Alpha emitting nuclides in nuclear medicine theranostics. *Nuklearmedizin* **2022**, *61*, 273–279. [CrossRef]
99. Hammer, S.; Hagemann, U.B.; Zitzmann-Kolbe, S.; Larsen, A.; Ellingsen, C.; Geraudie, S.; Grant, D.; Indrevoll, B.; Smeets, R.; von Ahsen, O.; et al. Preclinical Efficacy of a PSMA-Targeted Thorium-227 Conjugate (PSMA-TTC), a Targeted Alpha Therapy for Prostate Cancer. *Clin. Cancer Res.* **2020**, *26*, 1985–1996. [CrossRef]
100. van der Doelen, M.J.; Mehra, N.; van Oort, I.M.; Looijen-Salamon, M.G.; Janssen, M.J.R.; Custers, J.A.E.; Slootbeek, P.H.J.; Kroeze, L.I.; Bruchertseifer, F.; Morgenstern, A.; et al. Clinical outcomes and molecular profiling of advanced metastatic castration-resistant prostate cancer patients treated with ^{225}Ac-PSMA-617 targeted alpha-radiation therapy. *Urol. Oncol.* **2021**, *39*, 729.e7–729.e16. [CrossRef]
101. Rathke, H.; Bruchertseifer, F.; Kratochwil, C.; Keller, H.; Giesel, F.L.; Apostolidis, C.; Haberkorn, U.; Morgenstern, A. First patient exceeding 5-year complete remission after ^{225}Ac-PSMA-TAT. *Eur. J. Nucl. Med. Mol. Imaging* **2021**, *48*, 311–312. [CrossRef] [PubMed]
102. Zacherl, M.J.; Gildehaus, F.J.; Mittlmeier, L.; Boning, G.; Gosewisch, A.; Wenter, V.; Unterrainer, M.; Schmidt-Hegemann, N.; Belka, C.; Kretschmer, A.; et al. First Clinical Results for PSMA-Targeted alpha-Therapy Using ^{225}Ac-PSMA-I&T in Advanced-mCRPC Patients. *J. Nucl. Med.* **2021**, *62*, 669–674. [CrossRef] [PubMed]
103. Kratochwil, C.; Giesel, F.L.; Heussel, C.P.; Kazdal, D.; Endris, V.; Nientiedt, C.; Bruchertseifer, F.; Kippenberger, M.; Rathke, H.; Leichsenring, J.; et al. Patients Resistant Against PSMA-Targeting alpha-Radiation Therapy Often Harbor Mutations in DNA Damage-Repair-Associated Genes. *J. Nucl. Med.* **2020**, *61*, 683–688. [CrossRef] [PubMed]

Disclaimer/Publisher's Note: The statements, opinions and data contained in all publications are solely those of the individual author(s) and contributor(s) and not of MDPI and/or the editor(s). MDPI and/or the editor(s) disclaim responsibility for any injury to people or property resulting from any ideas, methods, instructions or products referred to in the content.

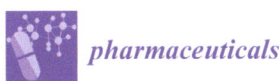 pharmaceuticals

Review

Targeted Alpha Therapy: All We Need to Know about ^{225}Ac's Physical Characteristics and Production as a Potential Theranostic Radionuclide

Wael Jalloul [1,2,*], Vlad Ghizdovat [1,2], Cati Raluca Stolniceanu [1,2], Teodor Ionescu [3], Irena Cristina Grierosu [1], Ioana Pavaleanu [4], Mihaela Moscalu [5] and Cipriana Stefanescu [1,2]

1. Department of Biophysics and Medical Physics-Nuclear Medicine, "Grigore T. Popa" University of Medicine and Pharmacy, 700115 Iasi, Romania
2. North East Regional Innovative Cluster for Structural and Molecular Imaging (Imago-Mol), 700115 Iasi, Romania
3. Department of Morpho-Functional Sciences (Pathophysiology), "Grigore T. Popa" University of Medicine and Pharmacy, 700115 Iasi, Romania
4. Department of Mother and Child, "Grigore T. Popa" University of Medicine and Pharmacy, 700115 Iasi, Romania
5. Department of Preventive Medicine and Interdisciplinarity, "Grigore T. Popa" University of Medicine and Pharmacy, 700115 Iasi, Romania
* Correspondence: jalloul.wael@umfiasi.ro

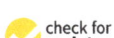

Citation: Jalloul, W.; Ghizdovat, V.; Stolniceanu, C.R.; Ionescu, T.; Grierosu, I.C.; Pavaleanu, I.; Moscalu, M.; Stefanescu, C. Targeted Alpha Therapy: All We Need to Know about ^{225}Ac's Physical Characteristics and Production as a Potential Theranostic Radionuclide. *Pharmaceuticals* **2023**, *16*, 1679. https://doi.org/10.3390/ph16121679

Academic Editors: Hirofumi Hanaoka, Marc Pretze and Jörg Kotzerke

Received: 31 October 2023
Revised: 24 November 2023
Accepted: 30 November 2023
Published: 2 December 2023

Correction Statement: This article has been republished with a minor change. The change does not affect the scientific content of the article and further details are available within the backmatter of the website version of this article.

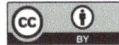

Copyright: © 2023 by the authors. Licensee MDPI, Basel, Switzerland. This article is an open access article distributed under the terms and conditions of the Creative Commons Attribution (CC BY) license (https://creativecommons.org/licenses/by/4.0/).

Abstract: The high energy of α emitters, and the strong linear energy transfer that goes along with it, lead to very efficient cell killing through DNA damage. Moreover, the degree of oxygenation and the cell cycle state have no impact on these effects. Therefore, α radioisotopes can offer a treatment choice to individuals who are not responding to β− or gamma-radiation therapy or chemotherapy drugs. Only a few α-particle emitters are suitable for targeted alpha therapy (TAT) and clinical applications. The majority of available clinical research involves ^{225}Ac and its daughter nuclide ^{213}Bi. Additionally, the ^{225}Ac disintegration cascade generates γ decays that can be used in single-photon emission computed tomography (SPECT) imaging, expanding the potential theranostic applications in nuclear medicine. Despite the growing interest in applying ^{225}Ac, the restricted global accessibility of this radioisotope makes it difficult to conduct extensive clinical trials for many radiopharmaceutical candidates. To boost the availability of ^{225}Ac, along with its clinical and potential theranostic applications, this review attempts to highlight the fundamental physical properties of this α-particle-emitting isotope, as well as its existing and possible production methods.

Keywords: targeted alpha therapy; ^{225}Ac; physical properties; production routes; theranostic application

1. Introduction

At the end of the 1800s, Pierre and Marie Curie, along with Alexander Graham Bell in the early 1900s, conducted research linked to cancer-targeted α therapy (TAT), which represented one of the earliest non-surgical cancer treatments [1]. Furthermore, α-particle emitters have significant curative effects, particularly in patients with limited therapeutic options and metastatic spread [2–4]. They can target very small clusters of metastatic cancer cells.

There are many benefits of using these radioisotopes in cancer therapy over common methods. α particles can selectively destroy tumour cells while preserving adjacent normal tissues due to their narrow extent in human tissue, corresponding to less than 0.1 mm [5]. Meanwhile, highly efficient cell destruction through DNA double-strand and DNA cluster damage is caused by the high energy of α emitters, in addition to the strong linear energy transfer (LET) (80 keV/μm) that goes along with it. These effects are mainly unaffected by the state of the cell cycle and oxygenation [6–8]. Thus, α radioisotopes can provide a therapeutic option for patients who are resistant to therapy with β− or gamma radiation or chemotherapeutic medications [9–11]. According to research estimations, tens of thousands of β− particles are needed to reach a single-cell killing rate of 99.99%, whereas only a few α decays are needed to accomplish a similar killing potential [4,12].

The high-LET radiation's biological efficacy is explained by its tendency to cause complex multiple clusters and double-strand or single-strand breaks in a target cells' DNA, rendering cellular repair mechanisms ineffective [4,13]. Additionally, reactive oxygen species (ROS), which are produced when emitted particles interact with water, can react with biomolecules such as proteins, phospholipids, RNA, and DNA, leading to permanent cell deterioration [14]. Moreover, during this type of therapy, the primary tumour and any additional cancerous lesions in the body that the radiation did not directly target may decrease as a result of "the abscopal effect" [14]. It is thought that the immune system is a key player in this process, even though the precise biological mechanisms underlying the phenomenon are as yet unknown [4,15,16] (Figure 1).

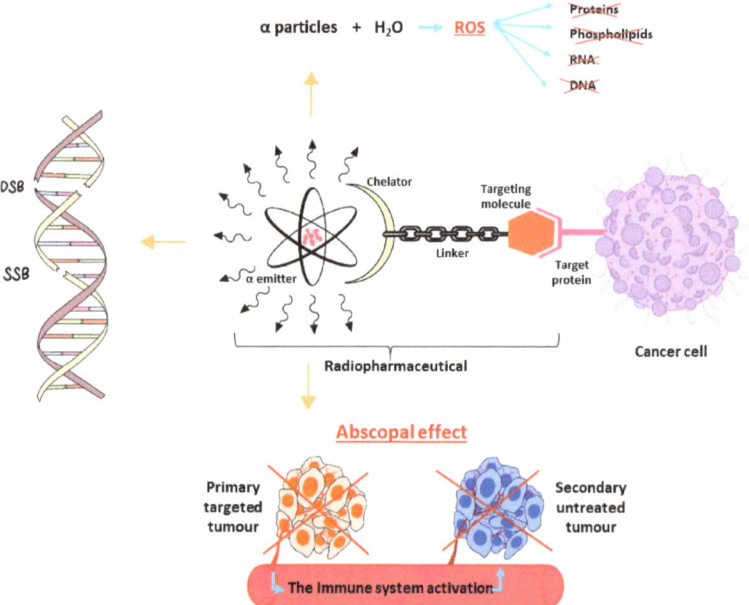

Figure 1. Schematic representation of the biological effects following the use of α-particle emitter radiopharmaceutical for cancer therapy. SSD = Single-Strand Break, DSB = Double-Strand Break, ROS = Reactive Oxygen Species.

Considering the clinical application of TAT, only a limited number of α-particle emitters are appropriate [17]. The use of ^{225}Ac and its short-lived daughter nuclide ^{213}Bi represents the vast majority of available experience in clinical research [5]. Furthermore, applying γ decays, which are produced during the radioactive ^{225}Ac cascade [5] in SPECT imaging, raises the possibility of theranostic nuclear medicine applications.

Although interest in using ^{225}Ac as an α-emitting radiolabel has been steadily increasing [18], substantial clinical investigations of many radiopharmaceutical candidates cannot be supported due to ^{225}Ac's limited worldwide accessibility [19]. Notwithstanding the significant financial investments made by numerous laboratories to establish production pathways, the widespread use of ^{225}Ac-labeled radiopharmaceuticals in human patients is still not achievable [19]. This ongoing shortage in ^{225}Ac supply can be explained by the practical production techniques that need difficult logistical tasks, such as using controlled nuclear materials or highly irradiating radioactive accelerator targets [19].

In order to increase the availability of ^{225}Ac and thus boosting the clinical use of α-particle-emitter therapeutics and potential theranostic applications, this review aims to outline the fundamental physical characteristics of ^{225}Ac in addition to its existing and potential production routes.

2. ^{225}Ac: Physical Characteristics

Actinium is a radioactive component with atomic number 89 [20]. Only two of its 32 isotopes, ^{228}Ac and ^{227}Ac, are naturally produced as a result of the disintegration of ^{232}Th and ^{235}U, respectively [20,21]. With its long half-life of 21.7 years and predominant β− emissions decay, ^{227}Ac represents the most common actinium isotope. However, ^{228}Ac, which is also a β− emitter, is highly uncommon [20,21].

^{225}Ac is the initial element in the actinide family, and its radioactive parents are parts of the now-extinct "neptunium series" [19,21]. This α-emitter isotope has a long half-life of 9.9 days [5,22].

Starting from ^{225}Ac to reach ^{209}Bi ($T_{1/2} = 1.9 \times 10^{19}$ y), the decay series includes six short-lived radionuclide daughters [5,23].

This radioactive cascade is represented by ^{221}Fr ($T_{1/2}$ = 4.8 min; 6.3 MeV α particle and 218 keV γ emission), ^{217}At ($T_{1/2}$ = 32.3 ms; 7.1 MeV α particle), ^{213}Bi ($T_{1/2}$ = 45.6 min; 5.9 MeV α particle, 492 keV β− particle and 440 keV γ emission), ^{213}Po ($T_{1/2}$ = 3.72 μs; 8.4 MeV α particle), ^{209}Tl ($T_{1/2}$ = 2.2 min; 178 keV β− particle), ^{209}Pb ($T_{1/2}$ = 3.23 h; 198 keV β− particle) [24] (Figure 2) [14].

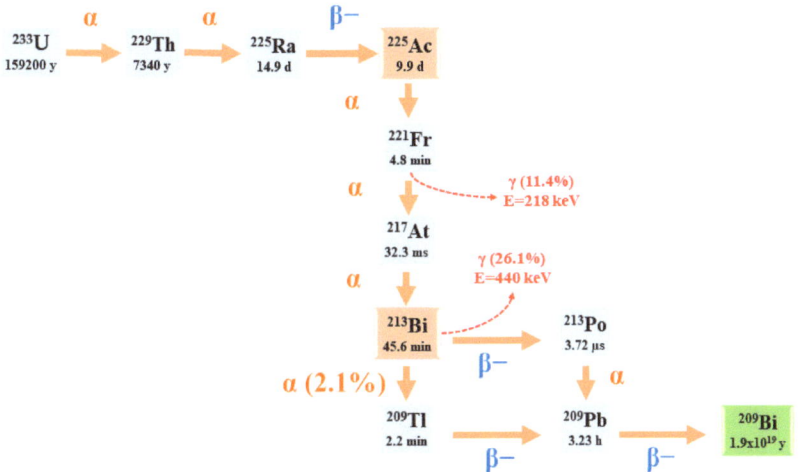

Figure 2. The decay chain of ^{233}U to ^{225}Ac and ^{213}Bi.

3. ^{225}Ac and Its Potential Theranostic Use

^{225}Ac is considered a "nanogenerator", since one decay of this element produces a total of four α and three β particles, in addition to two γ emissions [24]. Taking into account its α particle emissions, along with the fact that the non-tumour binding activity can be eliminated before most of its dose is deposited in organs, ^{225}Ac is considered an appealing choice for TAT [24,25]. However, it is important to give attention to the notable ^{225}Ac cytotoxicity, including renal toxicity [26], due to its extended half-life and the various α particles produced throughout its decay chain [5].

A theranostic-based approach, characterised by the imaging–therapeutic duality, is the process of obtaining positron emission tomography (PET) and SPECT scans by exchanging the therapeutic α-emitting radionuclide with a positron or gamma diagnostic imaging radionuclide. Significant information on dosimetry and TAT reactions is obtained from these relevant nuclear medicine images.

Chemical characteristics, half-life, radioactive emission type and intensity, related dosimetry, ease and scalability of production, radionuclidic purity, economics, and radionuclide progeny considerations are the factors that determine "the ideal" imaging surrogates for targeted alpha therapy [27,28].

Therapeutic use of ^{225}Ac is often paired with imperfect PET imaging surrogates, such as ^{68}Ga, ^{89}Zr, or ^{111}In, despite significant differences in their half-lives or chelation chemistry [29]. Studies are being conducted to address the limitations of imaging radionuclides by utilising lanthanum (La) as a potential alternative, especially ^{132}La ($T_{1/2}$ = 4.8 h, 42% β+) and ^{133}La ($T_{1/2}$ = 3.9 h, 7% β+) [30,31]. However, the half-lives of these isotopes are much shorter than that of ^{225}Ac, limiting their applicability in PET imaging [29]. In this regard, the production of ^{134}Ce ($T_{1/2}$ = 3.2 d) has recently been started by the U.S. Department of Energy (DOE) Isotope Program [32]. The long ^{134}Ce $T_{1/2}$ and the similar chemical properties of ^{225}Ac and ^{134}Ce were considered potential benefits for monitoring in vivo pharmacokinetics. For PET imaging of the chelate and the antibody trastuzumab, ^{134}Ce has been demonstrated to bind with diethylenetriamine pentaacetate (DTPA) [32] and dodecane tetraacetic acid (DOTA) [33]. On the other hand, greater molar ratios and higher temperatures are needed for isotope combinations with DOTA and DTPA [29]. In contrast, N, N'-bis[(6-carboxy-2-pyridyl)methyl]-4,13-diaza-18-crown-6 (macropa) has shown great stability for nonradioactive cerium and better chelate characteristics for ^{225}Ac [34], indicating that it might be useful for the theranostic development of ^{134}Ce/^{225}Ac [35].

The potential use of γ disintegrations, obtained by the decay of the intermediate ^{221}Fr (218 keV, 11.6% emission probability) and ^{213}Bi (440 keV, 26.1% emission probability) [5], in SPECT in vivo imaging could lead the ^{225}Ac radioactive cascade to a possible theranostic prospective in nuclear medicine applications. Nonetheless, planar SPECT imaging would be challenging because of the effectiveness of ^{225}Ac, which results in modest administered doses (~50–200 kBq/kg [5]), along with low γ emissions [24,25]. As a possible solution to this limitation, we can notice the suitable use of ^{213}Bi, which can be isolated from the ^{225}Ac decay cascades [24]. Nevertheless, it is mandatory to consider the short half-life of ^{213}Bi (45.6 min), which poses difficulties for processing, radiolabelling, and radiopharmaceutical delivery [24]. In addition, it is necessary to point out that these radiations make reaction monitoring complicated. Moreover, the secular equilibrium must be attained (for at least 6 h) before measuring a trustworthy radiochemical yield (RCY) [21]. Actinium's chemistry lacks advancement because of its restricted availability; all Ac isotopes need specific management and facilities [20].

4. Radiochemistry

During the production of radionuclides, it is mandatory to take into consideration a set of important aspects, such as safety, the co-generation of a few long-lived radionuclidic impurities, and adjustability, to enable delivery through clinical sites [27]. Once the target material has been irradiated, potent chemical purification methods are required to isolate the radioisotope [27,36–38]. Furthermore, the alpha particle may radiolytically damage the radiopharmaceutical itself, reducing in vivo targeting and producing more radioactive deposits in nontarget tissue. [27].

Since radiopharmaceuticals are considered typical pharmaceuticals, special manuals have been developed in the *European Pharmacopoeia* to deal with quality control issues [39]. Additionally, optimised protocols for preparing ^{225}Ac agents in therapeutic doses have been established [40] (Table 1).

Table 1. Research on ^{225}Ac chemistry. RCY = Radiochemical yield, RCP = Radiochemical purity, TLC = Thin-layer chromatography, ITLC = Instant thin-layer chromatography.

Study	Preparation Method	Radiopharmaceutical	RCY/RCP
Abou. et al., 2022 [41]	❖ The labelling of the DOTA-conjugated peptide was carried out under good manufacturing practice within a shielded hot cell using a multifunctional automated radiosynthesis module (Trasis, AllinOne mini). ❖ 46.6 MBq of the ^{225}Ac source dissolved in 0.2 M HCl was loaded under vacuum in the initial vial for radiolabelling with the DOTA-conjugated precursor (200 µg) on day 5 postsource purification. The source was transferred to the one-pot radiolabelling reactor cassette, in which the reaction occurred in Tris buffer (1 M, pH 7.2) at 85 °C for 70 min in the presence of 20% v/v L-ascorbic acid at pH 6–8. The radiolabelled peptide was transferred in saline and passed through a 0.2 µm sterilizing filter, resulting in a final volume of 9.7 mL. ❖ The radiolabelled products were characterised using thin-layer chromatography, high-pressure liquid chromatography, gamma counting, and high-energy resolution gamma spectroscopy.	^{225}Ac-DOTA-conjugated peptide	>99%/>95%
Dumond. et al., 2022 [42]	❖ PSMA-617 precursor was dissolved in 25 µL metal-free water (0.67 mg/mL) and combined with 500 µL 0.05M Tris buffer, pH 9. ^{225}Ac solution (~65 µCi in 15 µL) was added and the reaction was heated at 120 °C for 40–50 min. The resulting reaction was cooled and 0.6 mL gentisic acid solution (4 mg/mL in 0.2 M NH$_4$OAc) was added. To formulate the dose for injection, sterile saline (8 mL) was added and the pH was adjusted by the addition of 100 µL 0.05 M Tris buffer (pH 9) to give a final pH of ~7.2. The final solution was filtered using a 0.22 µm GV sterile filter into a sterile dose vial. ❖ Radiochemical purity was determined by radio-TLC (eluent: 50mM sodium citrate, pH 5), and plates were analysed using an AR2000 scanner.	^{225}Ac-PSMA-617	>99%/98 ± 1%
Thakral. et al., 2021 [43]	❖ ^{225}Ac-PSMA-617 was prepared by adding the peptidic precursor-PSMA-617 (molar ratios, ^{225}Ac: PSMA-617 = 30:1) in 1 mL ascorbate buffer to ^{225}Ac and heating the reaction mixture at 90 °C for 25 min. ❖ pH was determined using pH paper. ❖ RCP of ^{225}Ac-PSMA-617 was determined by ITLC.	^{225}Ac-PSMA-617	85–87%/97–99%
Kelly. et al., 2021 [44]	❖ ^{225}Ac (9.25 MBq) was obtained from a thorium generator at Canadian Nuclear Laboratories and supplied as the dried [^{225}Ac]AcCl$_3$ salt. The [^{225}Ac]AcCl$_3$ was dissolved in 1 mL 1 M NH$_4$OAc, pH 7.0, transferred by pipette to a 50 mL centrifuge tube, and diluted to 45 mL in 1 M NH$_4$OAc. Stock solution (1 mL), containing approximately 205 kBq [^{225}Ac]Ac(OAc)$_3$, was transferred by pipette to a plastic Eppendorf tube placed on a digital TermoMixer heating block. Then, 20 µL of the ligand stock solution (0.01–1 mg/mL of PSMA or DOTA or macropa) was added and the reaction was shaken at 300 rpm at either 25 °C or 95 °C. A 3 µL aliquot of the reaction mixture was withdrawn and deposited on the origin of a silica-gel-60-coated aluminium plate (Sigma Aldrich) after incubating the reaction for 1 min, 5 min, and 15 min.	^{225}Ac-PSMA conjugated peptide/ ^{225}Ac-DOTA conjugated peptide/ ^{225}Ac-macropa conjugated peptide	2.7 ± 0.55%– 98.8 ± 0.09%/ 1.8–99.5%

Table 1. Cont.

Study	Preparation Method	Radiopharmaceutical	RCY/RCP
	❖ A TLC method was developed to separate the metal complexed ligand from uncomplexed ^{225}Ac and its daughter radionuclides.		1.8–99.5%
Hooijman. et al., 2021 [45]	❖ ^{225}Ac was diluted into 0.1 M HCl. Stock solutions (10 mL) were proceeded in quartz-coated sterile vials. All purchased chemicals were prepared with Milli-Q water. Stock solutions prepared the day before labelling were 1 M HCl (from 37% HCl), 10 M NaOH, and 0.1 M TRIS-buffer pH 9. Two stock solutions were prepared on the day of labelling: First, 20% ascorbic acid was prepared; the ascorbic acid solution was transformed to ascorbate by the addition of 10 M NaOH to a pH 5.8. Secondly, PSMA-I&T (250 µg) was dissolved in 0.1 M TRIS buffer (pH 9) to a concentration of 600 µg/mL. Directly after labelling, 4 mg/mL diethylenetriaminepentaacetic acid (DTPA) was added to the labelling mixture. A solution for injection was prepared by the addition of ascorbate (50% v/v) and ethanol (6% v/v, 96%) into saline.	^{225}Ac-PSMA-I&T	>95%/>90%

5. ^{225}Ac Radiopharmaceuticals and Clinical Applications

The delivery of the radiopharmaceutical via the circulatory system enables the targeting of both the main tumour and its metastases. Whether a radiopharmaceutical is intended for therapeutic or diagnostic purposes depends on the decay properties of the linked radioisotope. For the purpose of curing, controlling, or palliating symptoms, TAT aims to provide an adequate amount of ionising radiation to intended malignities areas [27]. This means that any TAT agent must have a thorough understanding of its stability, pharmacokinetics, and dosimetry.

Investigations on ^{225}Ac have shown potential in treating neuroendocrine tumours, acute myeloid leukaemia, and metastatic prostate cancer, and more radiopharmaceuticals are being developed for other cancer types [46–52] (Table 2).

Table 2. Clinical research based on ^{225}Ac.

Disease	Study	Radiopharmaceutical
Prostate cancer	Parida et al., 2023 [53]	^{225}Ac-PSMA RLT
	Ma et al., 2022 [54]	^{225}Ac-PSMA-617
	Sanli et al., 2021 [55]	^{225}Ac-PSMA-617
	Sen et al., 2021 [56]	^{225}Ac-PSMA-617
	Zacherl et al., 2021 [50]	^{225}Ac-PSMA-I&T
	Feuerecker et al., 2021 [57]	^{225}Ac-PSMA-617
	Van Der Doelen et al., 2021 [58]	^{225}Ac-PSMA-617
	Sathekge et al., 2020 [51]	^{225}Ac-PSMA-617
	Yadav et al., 2020 [59]	^{225}Ac-PSMA-617
	Satapathy et al., 2020 [60]	^{225}Ac-PSMA-617
	Sathekge et al., 2019 [61]	^{225}Ac-PSMA-617
	Kratochwil et al., 2018 [62]	^{225}Ac-PSMA-617
Neuroendocrine tumours	Ballal et al., 2022 [63]	^{225}Ac-DOTATATE
	Yadav et al., 2022 [48]	^{225}Ac-DOTATATE
	Kratochwil et al., 2021 [64]	^{225}Ac-DOTATATE

Table 2. Cont.

Disease	Study	Radiopharmaceutical
	Ballal et al., 2020 [65]	^{225}Ac-DOTATATE
	Kratochwil et al., 2015 [66]	^{225}Ac-DOTATOC
Acute myeloid leukaemia	Rosenblat et al., 2022 [67]	^{225}Ac-lintuzumab
	Jurcic, 2018 [68]	^{225}Ac-lintuzumab
	Jurcic et al., 2016 [69]	^{225}Ac-lintuzumab
	Jurcic et al., 2011 [70]	^{225}Ac-lintuzumab

The use of ^{225}Ac in clinical practice is limited by its low availability. Breaking through this barrier would allow ^{225}Ac therapy to spread widely. Automated synthesis and consistent patient doses are essential, regardless of the production route chosen for this α-isotope acquisition. ^{225}Ac can be adapted for the commonly accessible DOTA-conjugated peptides for therapy [41], which are already capable of labelling ^{177}Lu or ^{90}Y. Marc Pretze et al. [71] studied the effectiveness and consistency of the radiosynthesis process for creating ^{225}Ac-labelled DOTA-conjugated peptides. Additionally, the research aimed to establish whether this process could be adapted for clinical production purposes through an automated synthesis platform (cassette-based module—Modular-Lab EAZY, Eckert & Ziegler) [72]. After comparing two purification methods, the researchers obtained ^{225}Ac-labelled peptides in an RCY of 80–90% for tumour therapy in patients [71]. Thus, the whole process was meticulously validated in accordance with the regulations of the German Pharmaceuticals Act §13.2b, knowing that the estimated costs for the automated synthesis of 1 MBq ^{225}Ac is around EUR 300–390, taking into account that the peptides would cost EUR 600–1000, the cassettes would cost EUR 180–200, and the ML EAZY would cost EUR ~30,000 [71].

6. The Production Routes of ^{225}Ac

As already mentioned, ^{225}Ac is part of the ^{237}Np disintegration family that has vanished in nature. This radioactive element could be artificially reproduced [21]. In addition to direct production paths, ^{225}Ac is conveniently reachable at numerous points along the decay chain, in particular via ^{233}U ($T_{1/2}$ = 159200 y, 100% α), ^{229}Th ($T_{1/2}$ = 7340 y, 100% α), and ^{225}Ra ($T_{1/2}$ = 14.9 d, 100% β−) [19]. ^{225}Ac possesses many fewer nucleons than other actinide nuclei that are more stable to be employed as production targets, such as ^{232}Th and ^{226}Ra [19]. Thus, production methods should, with rare exceptions, rely on radioactive decay or greater energy bombardments.

The available production routes of ^{225}Ac and its parents are listed below (Figure 3) [14]:

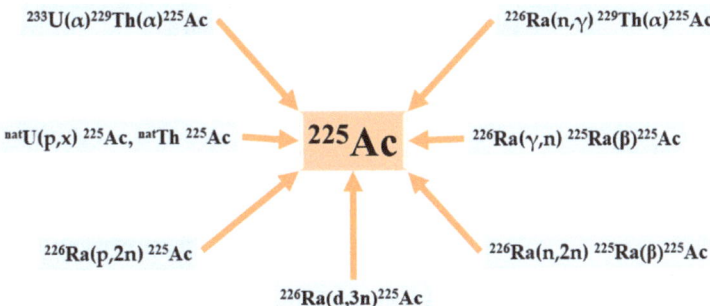

Figure 3. The principal production routes for ^{225}Ac.

6.1. Radiochemical Extraction from ^{229}Th

For more than two decades, the main source of ^{225}Ac has been the accumulation of ^{229}Th ($T_{1/2}$ = 7340 y) from the disintegration of ^{233}U ($T_{1/2}$ = 160,000 y) reserves. At this time, all clinical trials and a large number of pre-clinical studies involving ^{225}Ac and ^{213}Bi have so far used this type of generation route [5].

A large portion of ^{233}U was created between 1954 and 1970 by neutron irradiating ^{232}Th when it was being researched for use in nuclear weapons and reactors that were never completely implemented [73,74]. A significant stockpile of ^{233}U was kept after the thorium fuel cycle was abandoned in favour of fast reactors powered by plutonium at the end of the 1970s [21]. From supplies kept at the Oak Ridge National Laboratory (ORNL, Oak Ridge, TN, USA), ^{229}Th produced via ^{233}U disintegration was recovered between 1995 and 2005 [74]. Currently, there are three principal sources for this ^{229}Th: at ORNL (5.55 GBq (150 mCi), or 704 mg) [74,75], at the Directorate for Nuclear Safety and Security of the Joint Research Centre (JRC) of the European Commission (JRC, Karlsruhe, Germany) (1.7 GBq (46 mCi), or 215 mg), formerly known as the Institute for Transuranium Elements (ITU) [74,76], and at the Leipunskii Institute for Physics and Power Engineering (IPPE, Obninsk, Russia) (5.55 GBq (150 mCi), or 704 mg) [74,77]. Canadian Nuclear Laboratories (CNL) has more recently announced the isolation of an important ^{229}Th source [5]. Very pure sources of ^{229}Th were also discovered, prepared, and used for pre-clinical research at the Belgian Nuclear Research Centre (SCK CEN) in Mol, Belgium [14].

By producing approximately 33 GBq (893,23 mCi) (ORNL) [78] and 13.1 GBq (350 mCi) (JRC) [74,76] of ^{225}Ac annually, the ORNL and JRC represent, up to now, the principal worldwide providers of ^{225}Ac and its parent ^{225}Ra ($T_{1/2}$ = 14.9 d). Anion exchange and extraction chromatography are combined to produce ^{225}Ac from ^{229}Th at JRC Karlsruhe, whereas anion [52] and cation exchange are used in the process at ORNL [78]. Even though the IPPE source has the same amount of ^{229}Th as the ORNL source, the recorded values show that the IPPE source intermittently produces ^{225}Ac [74,77,79]. According to Samsonov MD et al., IPPE ^{225}Ac production could reach 22 GBq per year [80].

Additionally, it has been noted that starting from 2019, a very considerable rise in the availability of ^{229}Th will be produced through the extraction of ^{229}Th from historical wastes kept by the US DOE [4,52,78]. According to estimations, there could be up to 45 g of total ^{229}Th available, which could result in a 40-fold boost in the supply of ^{225}Ac above current levels [78].

The ^{225}Ac developed at JRC Karlsruhe and ORNL is considered safe for human use and has been significantly utilised for patient treatment [5], although there have been no reports to date about the direct clinical application of ^{225}Ac made at IPPE [5].

Approximately 68 GBq of ^{225}Ac from ^{229}Th are generated per year on a global scale [5]. Knowing that the ^{225}Ac-labelled ligands' given activities typically range from 4 to 50 MBq per therapeutic dosage [5], the amount of this isotope's supply is sufficient to treat several hundred patients annually and permits the performance of pre-clinical research. Although a major benefit of this production method is that the resulting ^{225}Ac is free of other actinium isotopes, the globally generated ^{229}Th is not enough to satisfy the extensive use and implementation in healthcare applications across the world [74,81]. Therefore, the development of ^{225}Ac radiopharmaceuticals is hindered by the limited supply and high cost that make ^{225}Ac inaccessible to many researchers [74]. In addition, the production of ^{233}U ($T_{1/2}$ = 160,000 y) is not viewed as a realistic solution for addressing expected short-term ^{225}Ac demand, because decades of steady growth are necessary to boost ^{229}Th ($T_{1/2}$ = 7340 y) supply [19,82,83]. As a result, numerous other techniques for generating ^{225}Ac on a wide scale have been researched.

Exposing radium targets to high fluxes of thermal neutrons is considered an effective procedure to induce ^{229}Th production [19]. This approach has been carefully investigated by ORNL researchers with access to the High Flux Isotope Reactor's (HFIR) > 10^{15} n cm^{-2} s thermal fluxes, noticing the production of ^{229}Th from ^{226}Ra, ^{228}Ra, and ^{227}Ac [19]. An HFIR cycle of 26 days generated ^{229}Th yields at 74 ± 7.4 MBq g^{-1} from ^{226}Ra, 260 ± 10 Bq g^{-1} ^{229}Th from ^{228}Ra, and 1200 ± 50 MBq g^{-1} from ^{227}Ac [19,84].

^{226}Ra(n,γ)^{227}Ra($\beta-$)^{227}Ac(n,γ)^{228}Ac($\beta-$)^{228}Th(n,γ)^{229}Th is the predominant generation pathway from ^{226}Ra targets and is driven by a combination of neutron capture probability and decay kinetics [19]. The short half-lives of ^{227}Ra ($T_{1/2}$ = 42.2 min, 100% β−) and ^{228}Ac ($T_{1/2}$ = 6.15 h, 100% β−) represent the important restrictions for these possible ^{229}Th generation routes [19]. The magnitude of the ^{226}Ra(n, γ) ^{229}Th cross section has the biggest impact on the amount of ^{229}Th that can be produced [19]. Unfortunately, this predominant pathway passes through ^{228}Th. This Th isotope is a dosimetrically undesirable contaminant that can only be eliminated from ^{229}Th by mass isolation or burnup and lowers the yield of ^{229}Th that may be produced [19]. The handling of the radium target and the generation of ^{228}Th ($T_{1/2}$ = 1.9 y) intermediate represent important challenges of this process [14,52,85]. In addition, there is still a sizable gap between the theoretically predicted yields and the measured ones. In HFIR, ideal 5-cycle activations are expected to provide approximately 0.8 GBq (20 mCi g^{-1}) of ^{229}Th for every gram of ^{226}Ra [19].

Whereas pure ^{227}Ac or ^{228}Ra targets are projected to generate somewhat more ^{229}Th, the current supply of these radionuclides is substantially less than that of ^{226}Ra [19]. Although improving the cost effectiveness of centralised recovery and distribution from ^{229}Th stocks, the dedication of even relatively small quantities of ^{226}Ra to such irradiations will significantly help to ease the current ^{225}Ac shortages. Yet, the full scope of the predicted need cannot be promptly met using this production technique. Thus, other production methods will undoubtedly be pursued simultaneously.

6.2. Accelerator-Based Routes

6.2.1. The Spallation of ^{232}Th

This method is based on the spallation of ^{232}Th to produce ^{225}Ac. As a target material, ^{232}Th (4.1103 Bq/g, 110 nCi/g) is widely accessible, not excessively radioactive, and presents fewer radiation risks [74]. Many countries are known to have stocks of tens of kilograms of thorium metal and hundreds of tonnes of thorium oxide or thorium nitrate, which are created every year as a byproduct of rare-earth mining and used to make more thorium metal in large amounts [74,86].

Waste recycling of the irradiated ^{232}Th target material might not be necessary because of its important accessibility [74].

The irradiation of ^{232}Th with highly energetic protons (0.6–2 GeV) accessible at large accelerators has been shown to produce considerable amounts of ^{225}Ac [5,87,88]. Production yields of several GBq have been recorded for 10-day irradiations utilising highly energetic proton beams [5,89,90]. From the irradiations of 5 g cm^{-2} targets throughout their roughly 8-month annual running durations, Los Alamos National Laboratory (LANL) can create between 40 and 80 GBq (1–2 Ci) every 10 days. This method is considered to be the most developed production procedure [78] and was validated at the Institute for Nuclear Research (INR), Russian Academy of Sciences (RAS) in Troitsk, Russia, and LANL in the US [78]. Furthermore, the routine use of this technique was introduced by the US DOE Tri-Lab (ORNL, Brookhaven National Laboratory (BNL), LANL) [78]. Once the targets are being handled and the completed product is delivered from ORNL, irradiations can be carried out at BNL (200 MeV at 165 mA) and LANL (100 MeV at 275 mA) [78,91].

The co-production of long-lived ^{227}Ac ($T_{1/2}$ = 21.8 y) is the process' primary constraint [27,78]. A large amount of these radionuclidic impurities is simultaneously produced by the spallation of ^{232}Th and needs to be eliminated using the proper multi-step chemical separation methods [5,92–94]. The effects of the isotopic impurity on the therapeutic application of the produced ^{225}Ac need to be taken into account because ^{225}Ac and ^{227}Ac cannot be totally chemically separated (0.1–0.2% of the relative activity of ^{225}Ac) [21,88]. Even with this limitation, the ^{225}Ac produced from high-energy accelerators may still be perfectly suitable for the manufacturing of ^{225}Ac/^{213}Bi generators, as all actinium daughters will be kept on the generator [14]. According to preliminary research, the ^{227}Ac impurity will not significantly affect patient dosimetry [78]. Recently, new purifying techniques that enable a reduction in the ^{227}Ac level and the recovery of ^{225}Ac with better purity, such as isotope separation (isotope separation on-line (ISOL) at Canada's particle accelerator centre (TRIUMF)) or a manufacturing method using ^{225}Ra produced after the proton irradiation of ^{232}Th, have been developed [4,21,95–97]. Nonetheless, there are still challenges to be resolved regarding long-lived ^{227}Ac licensing and accessibility in medical applications. In addition, due to the 21.8-year half-life, waste management is still a serious issue and will necessitate measures with possibly high related costs.

6.2.2. The Irradiations of ^{226}Ra

The Proton Irradiation of ^{226}Ra

Compared with the ^{232}Th spallation reaction, the generation of ^{225}Ac from ^{226}Ra targets by proton irradiation in a cyclotron has several benefits. This method is based on the reaction ^{226}Ra(p,2n)^{225}Ac. In medium-sized cyclotrons, at proton energies below 20 MeV (around 16 MeV), this procedure can be carried out with excellent results and at a reasonable cost [5,78,98]. About 5 GBq ^{225}Ac, which is comparable to 500 patient doses of 10 MBq ^{225}Ac, should be produced after a 24 h exposure of 50 mg ^{226}Ra to the highest excitation function at 15–16 MeV with a current of 100 mA protons [78]. It is noteworthy that research, both fundamental and applied, is believed to have relevance to medical cyclotrons that produce radioisotopes at energies between 15 and 25 MeV [14,99].

Since no other long-lived actinium isotopes, such as ^{227}Ac, are created during the chemical purification of the irradiation targets, ^{225}Ac with high isotopic purity is obtained. By choosing the right proton energies, it is possible to reduce the co-production of the short-lived ^{226}Ac ($T_{1/2}$ = 29 h) and ^{224}Ac ($T_{1/2}$ = 2.9 h) impurities produced by the reactions ^{226}Ra(p,n)^{226}Ac and ^{226}Ra(p,3n)^{224}Ac [5,78]. Furthermore, during the time needed for target cooling and reprocessing, their activity will continue to decrease to low levels. Handling targets that contain milligram amounts of radioactive ^{226}Ra ($T_{1/2}$ = 1600 y) and controlling its highly radiotoxic gaseous decay product ^{222}Rn ($T_{1/2}$ = 3.8 d) [5,14,98,100] pose significant challenges in the production, processing, and control procedures [5,78]. In addition, due to the limited availability of the target material, it is necessary to consider its recycling process [20]. Currently, facilities in North and South America, Europe, and Asia are researching how to utilise this production strategy. For instance, work on the investigation and development of ^{225}Ac generation using ^{226}Ra (stored as radioactive waste) has started at the National Institutes for Quantum Science and Technology (QST), Chiba, Japan [100]. These amounts of ^{226}Ra have previously been used as a sealed source for brachytherapy. Even in this resource-constrained country, some ^{226}Ra was accessible as a target for proton irradiation thanks to the national waste management program [100].

The Deuterons' Irradiation of ^{226}Ra

An improved method for producing ^{225}Ac, which involves irradiating ^{226}Ra with deuterons through the reaction ^{226}Ra(d,3n)^{225}Ac, has been proposed [101]. Although experimental measurements of the reaction's cross sections are still in development, simulations indicate that the process will have a greater production yield than the ^{226}Ra(p,2n)^{225}Ac reaction and a maximum cross section of 864 mb at 18.5 MeV [78]. It is important to consider the prolonged cooling period by the ^{226}Ac decay, since deuteron irradiation might result in an increased co-production of ^{226}Ac ($T_{1/2}$ = 29 h) [78]. Moreover, there are only a few accelerators that can produce deuteron beams with enough energy.

The photonuclear reaction ^{226}Ra(γ,n)^{225}Ra

The photonuclear reaction ^{226}Ra(γ,n)^{225}Ra, followed by the beta decay of ^{225}Ra to ^{225}Ac is a different method for producing ^{225}Ac by irradiating ^{226}Ra. It is noticed that the photon energy cutoff for the reaction is 6.4 MeV. However, experimentally established cross-section data are not yet available [78]. Modelling data predict modest reaction yields and high-intensity electron beams from modern accelerators are required for commercially viable production. At JRC Karlsruhe, the process's fundamentals have been experimentally verified [78]. A zircaloy capsule containing 1 mg of ^{226}Ra embedded in 800 mg of a BaCl^2 matrix underwent 3.5 h of 52 MeV betatron irradiation to generate 0.24 mCi of ^{225}Ac [78]. At the INR in Dubna, Russia [102], as well as the Illawarra Cancer Centre (ICC) in Wollongong, Australia [103], the procedure's viability has also been effectively validated. At a maximum photon energy of 24 MeV, a radiation yield of 550 Bq/(mAh mg ^{226}Ra) was recorded [102]. For a more precise estimate of production yields, it is extremely important to quantify the cross-section data in detail in this reaction.

The main challenges in this method are the recycling requirement of the ^{226}Ra target and some handling issues with the ^{222}Rn daughter [20]. However, large-scale ^{225}Ac manufacturing using this procedure is already being implemented at several plants [104]. It was reported that SCK CEN is capable of generating high-grade GMP-grade ^{225}Ac and also continually supplying it using a backup system [18,100]. During the creation of GMP-grade ^{225}Ac, SCK CEN has been collaborating with the Institute of Radioelements Environment & Lifescience Technology (IRE Elit) and Global Morpho Pharma (GMP) (France) [100]. Starting in 2019, SCK-CEN began irradiating their stock of several hundred grammes of ^{226}Ra. This Belgian research centre is also equipped with a BR2 reactor and an accelerator-driven subcritical reactor named Multi-purpose hYbrid Research Reactor for High-tech Application (MYRRHA) that are used in this approach [100]. Additionally, utilising an IBA (Ion Beam Applications S.A., EURONEXT) Rhodotron, SCK CEN could produce GMP-grade ^{225}Ac at a weekly rate of 37 GBq (1000 mCi) by irradiating with 40 MeV electrons at 125 kW [100]. The prospects should be kept an eye on, as SCK CEN and IBA established a research and development partnership agreement for the joint production of ^{225}Ac in 2021 [105] (Table 3).

Table 3. Advantages and disadvantages of the potential ^{225}Ac production methods.

Production Methods	Advantages	Disadvantages
Radiochemical extraction of ^{225}Ac from ^{229}Th	❖ A large portion of ^{233}U was created by neutron irradiating ^{232}Th ❖ A significant stockpile of ^{233}U was kept after the thorium fuel cycle was abandoned in favour of fast reactors powered by plutonium ❖ The CNL has more recently announced the isolation of an important ^{229}Th source ❖ Very pure sources of ^{229}Th were discovered, prepared, and used for pre-clinical research at the SCK CEN ❖ Starting from 2019, a considerable rise in the availability of ^{229}Th will be produced through the extraction of ^{229}Th from historical wastes kept by the US DOE ❖ The resulting ^{225}Ac is free of other actinium isotopes ❖ Exposing radium targets to high fluxes of thermal neutrons is considered an effective procedure to induce ^{229}Th production	❖ ^{229}Th and ^{233}U have long $T_{1/2}$ values ❖ The globally generated ^{229}Th is not enough to satisfy the extensive use and implementation in healthcare applications across the world ❖ The development of ^{225}Ac radiopharmaceuticals is hindered by the limited supply and high cost that make ^{225}Ac inaccessible to many researchers ❖ The short half-lives of ^{227}Ra and ^{228}Ac represent important restrictions for the possible ^{226}Ra(n,γ) ^{227}Ra(β−) ^{227}Ac(n,γ) ^{228}Ac(β−) ^{228}Th(n,γ) ^{229}Th routes ❖ The cross section of ^{226}Ra(n, γ) ^{229}Th greatly impacts ^{229}Th production but is hindered by undesirable contaminant ^{228}Th ❖ There is still a sizable gap between the theoretically predicted yields and the measured ones ❖ Whereas pure ^{227}Ac or ^{228}Ra targets are projected to generate somewhat more ^{229}Th, the current supply of these radionuclides is substantially less than that of ^{226}Ra

Table 3. Cont.

Production Methods	Advantages	Disadvantages
	❖ Improving the cost effectiveness of centralised recovery and distribution from ^{229}Th stocks, the dedication of even relatively small quantities of ^{226}Ra to such irradiations will significantly help to ease the current ^{225}Ac shortages	❖ The full scope of the predicted need cannot be promptly met using this production technique
Spallation of ^{232}Th	❖ ^{232}Th is widely accessible and presents fewer radiation risks	❖ The co-production of long-lived ^{227}Ac ($T_{1/2}$ = 21.8 y) as a radionuclidic impurity
	❖ Many countries are known to have stocks of tens of kilograms of thorium metal and hundreds of tonnes of thorium oxide or thorium nitrate	❖ ^{225}Ac and ^{227}Ac cannot be totally chemically separated
	❖ Due to its important accessibility, recycling of ^{232}Th target material may not be required	❖ Long-lived ^{227}Ac licensing and accessibility in medical applications
	❖ The irradiation of ^{232}Th with highly energetic protons has been shown to produce considerable amounts of ^{225}Ac	❖ Waste management is still a serious issue and will necessitate measures with possibly high related costs
	❖ It is considered to be the most developed production procedure	
	❖ It is suitable for the manufacturing of ^{225}Ac/^{213}Bi generators, as all actinium daughters will be kept on the generator	
Proton irradiation of ^{226}Ra	❖ In medium-sized cyclotrons, at proton energies below 20 MeV (around 16 MeV), this procedure can be carried out with excellent results and at a reasonable cost	❖ Handling targets that contain milligram amounts of radioactive ^{226}Ra ($T_{1/2}$ = 1600 y) and controlling its highly radiotoxic gaseous decay product ^{222}Rn ($T_{1/2}$ = 3.8 d)
	❖ About 5 GBq ^{225}Ac (500 patient doses of 10 MBq ^{225}Ac) should be produced after 24 h exposure of 50 mg ^{226}Ra	❖ The limited availability of the target material necessitates its recycling
	❖ Fundamental and applied research is thought to apply to medical cyclotrons that generate radioisotopes	
	❖ No other long-lived actinium isotopes, such as ^{227}Ac, are created during the chemical purification of the irradiation targets, thus ^{225}Ac with high isotopic purity is obtained	
Deuterons' irradiation of ^{226}Ra	❖ Simulations indicate that the process will have a greater production yield than the ^{226}Ra(p,2n)^{225}Ac reaction	❖ Experimental measurements of the reaction's cross sections are still in development
		❖ To consider a prolonged cooling period by the ^{226}Ac decay since deuteron irradiation might result in an increased co-production of ^{226}Ac
		❖ There are a few accelerators that can produce deuteron beams with enough energy

Table 3. Cont.

Production Methods	Advantages	Disadvantages
Photonuclear reaction $^{226}Ra(\gamma,n)\,^{225}Ra$	❖ Large-scale ^{225}Ac manufacturing using this procedure is already being implemented at several plants	❖ Experimentally established cross-section data are not yet available
		❖ Modest reaction yields are predicted by modelling data
		❖ For commercially feasible production, modern accelerators with high-intensity electron beams are needed
		❖ The recycling requirement of the ^{226}Ra target
		❖ Issues with handling the ^{222}Rn daughter

6.3. $^{225}Ac/^{213}Bi$ Radionuclide Generators

In the middle of the 1990s, the JRC was the first laboratory to offer ^{225}Ac/^{213}Bi to clinical partners [5]. Ever since, the JRC has produced these radioisotopes on an annual basis for preclinical research and clinical testing carried out at JRC Karlsruhe or in partnership with a large network of healthcare partners.

In order to produce the short-lived ^{213}Bi ($T_{1/2}$ = 45.6 min) on-site, ^{225}Ac can either be utilised directly as a therapeutic nuclide [50,106] or set onto ^{225}Ac/^{213}Bi generators [78,83]. All patient investigations with ^{213}Bi up to now have utilised ^{225}Ac/^{213}Bi generators.

There are numerous generator types available, including those based on ion exchange, extraction chromatography, and inorganic sorbents [106]. The most widely used type is a single-column "direct" generator that was invented at the ITU and based on the strongly acidic cation-exchange sorbent AG MP-50 [106].

In this well-known approach, ^{213}Bi is obtained starting from ^{225}Ac, which is tightly bound to the sorbent and drowned in 0.05M HNO$_3$ solution [14,78,83]. At roughly every 3 h [14,78], ^{213}Bi (^{213}BiI$_4^-$ and ^{213}BiI$_5^{2-}$) is obtained for immediate use through elution with a mixture of 0.1 M HCl/0.1 M NaI [104] (Figure 4) [14].

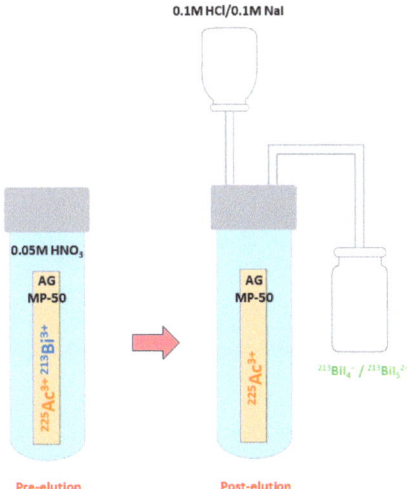

Figure 4. Schematic representation of the ^{213}Bi elution using the single-column "direct" ^{225}Ac/^{213}Bi generator.

The high-activity generator technology created at JRC Karlsruhe enables the generator to function reliably even when supplied with up to 4 GBq ^{225}Ac of activities [5,78]. Although the penetration of ^{225}Ac is less than 0.2 ppm, the yields of ^{213}Bi elution may be more than 80% [107]. The process of distributing ^{225}Ac activity uniformly over about two-thirds of the generator resin ensures stable performance over several weeks and minimises radiolytic degradation of the organic resin [5,78].

Injection-ready therapeutic dosages of ^{213}Bi-labeled peptides with activities of up to 2.3 GBq have been successfully prepared using the generator for clinical applications [78] including the locoregional therapy of brain tumours [5,13]. Due to the relatively long parent half-life, which enables the transport of the generator to radiopharmacy facilities over vast distances, these generators may be employed clinically.

7. Conclusions

Taking into account its α-particle emissions, along with the ability to eliminate the non-tumour binding activity before most of its dose is deposited in organs, ^{225}Ac is considered an appealing choice for TAT. Nevertheless, because of its long half-life and the different α particles created throughout its decay chain, it is crucial to pay attention to the considerable cytotoxicity of ^{225}Ac. Additionally, the γ disintegrations that result from the intermediate ^{221}Fr and ^{213}Bi disintegration may be used in SPECT clinical imaging. Thus, the radioactive cascade of ^{225}Ac could be used in nuclear medicine, especially in theranostic applications. However, the small ^{225}Ac doses given lead to low γ emissions, which makes planar SPECT imaging difficult. A potential alternative for this constraint is to make appropriate use of ^{213}Bi, which can be isolated from the decay cascades of ^{225}Ac. However, the brief half-life of ^{213}Bi must be taken into account since it presents challenges for radiopharmaceutical distribution, processing, and radiolabelling.

Apart from direct production pathways, ^{225}Ac can be easily accessed at many points in the decay chain, especially through ^{233}U, ^{229}Th, and ^{225}Ra. Compared with other actinide nuclei, including ^{232}Th and ^{226}Ra, which are more stable to use as production targets, ^{225}Ac has many fewer nucleons. As a result, production techniques must, for the most part, rely on radioactive decay or higher energy bombardments.

All the production techniques discussed in this paper are expensive and will all struggle to satisfy demand at the expected level if they are used separately.

It is necessary to readjust the facilities that are accessible throughout the world, to use suitable production methods that are adapted to the available infrastructure, and take into consideration the advantages and disadvantages of every used production modality. In addition, fruitful collaboration between the different centres and experienced scientific staff will pave the way for the widespread clinical use of actinium-based radiopharmaceuticals as a new standard of care.

The European medical isotope programme: Production of High-Purity Isotopes by Mass Separation Project (PRISMAP) represents an important initiative of this type of collaboration. Coordinated by the European Laboratory for Nuclear Research (CERN), the project partners come from thirteen nations: Austria, Belgium, Denmark, France, Germany, Italy, Latvia, Norway, Portugal, Poland, Sweden, Switzerland, and the United Kingdom. Nine significant EU, national, or regional infrastructures, four developing infrastructures, leader research institutes, medical facilities, the European Joint Research Centre, and one small and midsize enterprise (SME) are among the twenty-three partners that make up the PRISMAP Consortium. With the help of these considerable facilities, the programme goal is to create a sustainable source of high-purity-grade new radionuclides for medical use. It also aims to offer an accessible point of entry for all researchers working in this field, including those from SMEs, global pharmaceutical companies, nuclear centres, hospitals, and universities, by implementing standardised access procedures.

Several PRISMAP partners, including JRC Belgium, Narodowe Centrum Badań Jądrowych (NCBJ), Poland, Institut Max von Laue—Paul Langevin (ILL), France, and SCK CEN, Belgium, are additionally implicated in another promising project in the field of the sustainability of medical isotope production and its safe application in Europe, named the Strengthening the European Chain of sUpply for next-generation medical RadionuclidEs (SECURE). The project focuses on encouraging advancements in the creation of irradiation targets and manufacturing processes for both new and existing isotopes used in nuclear medicine and diagnostics. A list of crucial alpha-emitting radioisotopes in nuclear medicine was created, and ^{225}Ac was selected at the top of this list. The research aims to overcome the primary challenges to ensure the future availability of these isotopes by: (1) creating a framework of guidelines and recommendations that enable investigating the full clinical potential of alpha and beta particle therapy and its safe application; (2) offering significant insights that serve as a model for resolving challenges with upscaling and continuous isotope production; (3) removing critical obstacles along the production of specific alpha- and beta-emitting isotopes that restrict a sustainable production.

Author Contributions: Conceptualization, W.J., V.G., C.R.S. and C.S.; methodology, W.J., I.C.G. and C.S.; software, V.G., M.M., T.I. and I.C.G.; validation, W.J., T.I. and C.S.; analysis, C.R.S., I.P. and I.C.G.; data curation, V.G., C.R.S. and T.I.; writing—original draft preparation, W.J.; writing—review and editing, W.J., M.M. and C.S.; visualization, V.G., I.P. and I.C.G.; supervision, M.M., C.S. and I.P. administration, C.R.S., T.I. and I.C.G. All authors have contributed equally to this manuscript. All authors have read and agreed to the published version of the manuscript.

Funding: This work was partially supported by project SECURE (Strengthening the European Chain of sUpply for next generation medical RadionuclidEs), GA no. 101061230, a HORIZON EURATOM funded project (https://enen.eu/index.php/portfolio/secure-project/).

Institutional Review Board Statement: Not applicable.

Informed Consent Statement: Not applicable.

Data Availability Statement: Not applicable.

Acknowledgments: Thanks to the team of the North East Regional Innovative Cluster for Structural and Molecular Imaging (Imago-Mol) for the professional support.

Conflicts of Interest: The authors declare no conflict of interest.

Abbreviations

Targeted Alpha Therapy **(TAT)**, Single-Photon Emission Computed Tomography **(SPECT)**, Linear Energy Transfer **(LET)**, Reactive Oxygen Species **(ROS)**, Single-Strand Break **(SSD)**, Double-Strand Break **(DSB)**, Positron Emission Tomography **(PET)**, Department of Energy **(DOE)**, Diethylenetriamine Pentaacetate **(DTPA)**, Dodecane Tetraacetic Acid **(DOTA)**, N,N′-Bis[(6-carboxy-2-pyridyl)methyl]-4,13-diaza-18-crown-6 **(macropa)**, Radiochemical Yield **(RCY)**, Radiochemical Purity **(RCP)**, Thin-Layer Chromatography **(TLC)**, Instant Thin-Layer Chromatography **(ITLC)**, Oak Ridge National Laboratory **(ORNL)**, Directorate for Nuclear Safety and Security of the Joint Research Centre **(JRC)**, Institute for Transuranium Elements **(ITU)**, Leipunskii Institute for Physics and Power Engineering **(IPPE)**, Canadian Nuclear Laboratories **(CNL)**, Belgian Nuclear Research Centre **(SCK CEN)**, High Flux Isotope Reactor **(HFIR)**, Los Alamos National Laboratory **(LANL)**, Institute for Nuclear Research **(INR)**, Russian Academy of Sciences **(RAS)**, Brookhaven National Laboratory **(BNL)**, Isotope Separation On-Line **(ISOL)**, Canada's Particle Accelerator Centre **(TRIUMF)**, National Institutes for Quantum Science and Technology **(QST)**, Illawarra Cancer Centre **(ICC)**, Institute of Radioelements Environment & Lifescience Technology **(IRE Elit)**, Global Morpho Pharma **(GMP)**, Multi-purpose hYbrid Research Reactor for High-tech Application **(MYRRHA)**, Ion Beam Applications S.A. **(IBA)**, The European Medical Isotope Programme: Production of High-Purity Isotopes by Mass Separation **(PRISMAP)**, European Laboratory for Nuclear Research **(CERN)**, Small and Midsize Enterprise **(SME)**, Narodowe Centrum Badań Jądrowych **(NCBJ)**, Institut Max von Laue—Paul Langevin **(ILL)**, Strengthening the European Chain of sUpply for next generation medical RadionuclidEs **(SECURE)**.

References

1. McDevitt, M.R.; Sgouros, G.; Sofou, S. Targeted and Nontargeted α-Particle Therapies. *Annu. Rev. Biomed. Eng.* **2018**, *20*, 73–93. [CrossRef]
2. Parker, C.; Nilsson, S.; Heinrich, D.; Helle, S.I.; O'Sullivan, J.M.; Fosså, S.D.; Chodacki, A.; Wiechno, P.; Logue, J.; Seke, M.; et al. Alpha Emitter Radium-223 and Survival in Metastatic Prostate Cancer. *N. Engl. J. Med.* **2013**, *369*, 213–223. [CrossRef]
3. Jurcic, J.G.; Ravandi, F.; Pagel, J.M.; Park, J.H.; Smith, B.D.; Douer, D.; Estey, E.H.; Kantarjian, H.M.; Wahl, R.L.; Earle, D.; et al. Phase I Trial of Targeted Alpha-Particle Therapy Using Actinium-225 (^{225}Ac)-Lintuzumab (Anti-CD33) in Combination with Low-Dose Cytarabine (LDAC) for Older Patients with Untreated Acute Myeloid Leukemia (AML). *Blood* **2014**, *124*, 5293. [CrossRef]
4. Johnson, J.D.; Heines, M.; Bruchertseifer, F.; Chevallay, E.; Cocolios, T.E.; Dockx, K.; Duchemin, C.; Heinitz, S.; Heinke, R.; Hurier, S.; et al. Resonant Laser Ionization and Mass Separation of ^{225}Ac. *Sci. Rep.* **2023**, *13*, 1347. [CrossRef] [PubMed]
5. Morgenstern, A.; Apostolidis, C.; Kratochwil, C.; Sathekge, M.; Krolicki, L.; Bruchertseifer, F. An Overview of Targeted Alpha Therapy with ^{225}Actinium and ^{213}Bismuth. *Curr. Radiopharm.* **2018**, *11*, 200–208. [CrossRef] [PubMed]
6. Sgouros, G.; Roeske, J.C.; McDevitt, M.R.; Palm, S.; Allen, B.J.; Fisher, D.R.; Brill, A.B.; Song, H.; Howell, R.W.; Akabani, G.; et al. MIRD Pamphlet No. 22 (Abridged): Radiobiology and Dosimetry of Alpha-Particle Emitters for Targeted Radionuclide Therapy. *J. Nucl. Med.* **2010**, *51*, 311–328. [CrossRef] [PubMed]
7. Wulbrand, C.; Seidl, C.; Gaertner, F.C.; Bruchertseifer, F.; Morgenstern, A.; Essler, M.; Senekowitsch-Schmidtke, R. Alpha-Particle Emitting ^{213}Bi-Anti-EGFR Immunoconjugates Eradicate Tumor Cells Independent of Oxygenation. *PLoS ONE* **2013**, *8*, e64730. [CrossRef]
8. Elgqvist, J.; Frost, S.; Pouget, J.-P.; Albertsson, P. The Potential and Hurdles of Targeted Alpha Therapy—Clinical Trials and Beyond. *Front. Oncol.* **2014**, *3*, 324. [CrossRef] [PubMed]
9. Friesen, C.; Glatting, G.; Koop, B.; Schwarz, K.; Morgenstern, A.; Apostolidis, C.; Debatin, K.-M.; Reske, S.N. Breaking Chemoresistance and Radioresistance with [^{213}Bi]Anti-CD45 Antibodies in Leukemia Cells. *Cancer Res.* **2007**, *67*, 1950–1958. [CrossRef]
10. Kratochwil, C.; Giesel, F.L.; Bruchertseifer, F.; Mier, W.; Apostolidis, C.; Boll, R.; Murphy, K.; Haberkorn, U.; Morgenstern, A. ^{213}Bi-DOTATOC Receptor-Targeted Alpha-Radionuclide Therapy Induces Remission in Neuroendocrine Tumours Refractory to Beta Radiation: A First-in-Human Experience. *Eur. J. Nucl. Med. Mol. Imaging* **2014**, *41*, 2106–2119. [CrossRef]
11. Kratochwil, C.; Bruchertseifer, F.; Giesel, F.L.; Weis, M.; Verburg, F.A.; Mottaghy, F.; Kopka, K.; Apostolidis, C.; Haberkorn, U.; Morgenstern, A. ^{225}Ac-PSMA-617 for PSMA-Targeted α-Radiation Therapy of Metastatic Castration-Resistant Prostate Cancer. *J. Nucl. Med.* **2016**, *57*, 1941–1944. [CrossRef] [PubMed]
12. Humm, J.L.; Cobb, L.M. Nonuniformity of Tumor Dose in Radioimmunotherapy. *J. Nucl. Med.* **1990**, *31*, 75–83. [PubMed]
13. Guerra Liberal, F.D.C.; O'Sullivan, J.M.; McMahon, S.J.; Prise, K.M. Targeted Alpha Therapy: Current Clinical Applications. *Cancer Biother. Radiopharm.* **2020**, *35*, 404–417. [CrossRef] [PubMed]
14. Ahenkorah, S.; Cassells, I.; Deroose, C.M.; Cardinaels, T.; Burgoyne, A.R.; Bormans, G.; Ooms, M.; Cleeren, F. Bismuth-213 for Targeted Radionuclide Therapy: From Atom to Bedside. *Pharmaceutics* **2021**, *13*, 599. [CrossRef]
15. Vermeulen, K.; Vandamme, M.; Bormans, G.; Cleeren, F. Design and Challenges of Radiopharmaceuticals. *Semin. Nucl. Med.* **2019**, *49*, 339–356. [CrossRef]
16. Beyls, C.; Haustermans, K.; Deroose, C.M.; Pans, S.; Vanbeckevoort, D.; Verslype, C.; Dekervel, J. Could Autoimmune Disease Contribute to the Abscopal Effect in Metastatic Hepatocellular Carcinoma? *Hepatology* **2020**, *72*, 1152–1154. [CrossRef] [PubMed]
17. Seidl, C. Radioimmunotherapy with α-Particle-Emitting Radionuclides. *Immunotherapy* **2014**, *6*, 431–458. [CrossRef]
18. Zimmermann, R. Is Actinium Really Happening? *J. Nucl. Med.* **2023**, *64*, 1516–1518. [CrossRef]
19. Engle, J.W. The Production of Ac-225. *Curr. Radiopharm.* **2018**, *11*, 173–179. [CrossRef]
20. Hatcher-Lamarre, J.L.; Sanders, V.A.; Rahman, M.; Cutler, C.S.; Francesconi, L.C. Alpha Emitting Nuclides for Targeted Therapy. *Nucl. Med. Biol.* **2021**, *92*, 228–240. [CrossRef]
21. Eychenne, R.; Chérel, M.; Haddad, F.; Guérard, F.; Gestin, J.-F. Overview of the Most Promising Radionuclides for Targeted Alpha Therapy: The "Hopeful Eight". *Pharmaceutics* **2021**, *13*, 906. [CrossRef]
22. Pommé, S.; Marouli, M.; Suliman, G.; Dikmen, H.; Van Ammel, R.; Jobbágy, V.; Dirican, A.; Stroh, H.; Paepen, J.; Bruchertseifer, F.; et al. Measurement of the ^{225}Ac Half-Life. *Appl. Radiat. Isot.* **2012**, *70*, 2608–2614. [CrossRef] [PubMed]
23. Suliman, G.; Pommé, S.; Marouli, M.; Van Ammel, R.; Stroh, H.; Jobbágy, V.; Paepen, J.; Dirican, A.; Bruchertseifer, F.; Apostolidis, C.; et al. Half-Lives of ^{221}Fr, ^{217}At, ^{213}Bi, ^{213}Po and ^{209}Pb from the ^{225}Ac Decay Series. *Appl. Radiat. Isot.* **2013**, *77*, 32–37. [CrossRef] [PubMed]
24. Nelson, B.J.B.; Andersson, J.D.; Wuest, F. Targeted Alpha Therapy: Progress in Radionuclide Production, Radiochemistry, and Applications. *Pharmaceutics* **2020**, *13*, 49. [CrossRef] [PubMed]
25. Scheinberg, D.A.; McDevitt, M.R. Actinium-225 in Targeted Alpha-Particle Therapeutic Applications. *Curr. Radiopharm.* **2011**, *4*, 306–320. [CrossRef]
26. Muslimov, A.R.; Antuganov, D.; Tarakanchikova, Y.V.; Karpov, T.E.; Zhukov, M.V.; Zyuzin, M.V.; Timin, A.S. An Investigation of Calcium Carbonate Core-Shell Particles for Incorporation of ^{225}Ac and Sequester of Daughter Radionuclides: In Vitro and in Vivo Studies. *J. Control Release* **2021**, *330*, 726–737. [CrossRef] [PubMed]

27. Nelson, B.J.B.; Wilson, J.; Andersson, J.D.; Wuest, F. Theranostic Imaging Surrogates for Targeted Alpha Therapy: Progress in Production, Purification, and Applications. *Pharmaceuticals* 2023, *16*, 1622. [CrossRef] [PubMed]
28. Saini, S.; Bartels, J.L.; Appiah, J.-P.K.; Rider, J.H.; Baumhover, N.; Schultz, M.K.; Lapi, S.E. Optimized Methods for the Production of High-Purity 203Pb Using Electroplated Thallium Targets. *J. Nucl. Med.* 2023, *64*, 1791–1797. [CrossRef]
29. Bobba, K.N.; Bidkar, A.P.; Meher, N.; Fong, C.; Wadhwa, A.; Dhrona, S.; Sorlin, A.; Bidlingmaier, S.; Shuere, B.; He, J.; et al. Evaluation of ^{134}Ce/^{134}La as a PET Imaging Theranostic Pair for ^{225}Ac α-Radiotherapeutics. *J. Nucl. Med.* 2023, *64*, 1076–1082. [CrossRef]
30. Aluicio-Sarduy, E.; Barnhart, T.E.; Weichert, J.; Hernandez, R.; Engle, J.W. Cyclotron-Produced 132La as a PET Imaging Surrogate for Therapeutic ^{225}Ac. *J. Nucl. Med.* 2021, *62*, 1012–1015. [CrossRef]
31. Nelson, B.J.B.; Ferguson, S.; Wuest, M.; Wilson, J.; Duke, M.J.M.; Richter, S.; Soenke-Jans, H.; Andersson, J.D.; Juengling, F.; Wuest, F. First In Vivo and Phantom Imaging of Cyclotron-Produced ^{133}La as a Theranostic Radionuclide for ^{225}Ac and ^{135}La. *J. Nucl. Med.* 2022, *63*, 584–590. [CrossRef]
32. Bailey, T.A.; Mocko, V.; Shield, K.M.; An, D.D.; Akin, A.C.; Birnbaum, E.R.; Brugh, M.; Cooley, J.C.; Engle, J.W.; Fassbender, M.E.; et al. Developing the ^{134}Ce and ^{134}La Pair as Companion Positron Emission Tomography Diagnostic Isotopes for ^{225}Ac and ^{227}Th Radiotherapeutics. *Nat. Chem.* 2021, *13*, 284–289. [CrossRef] [PubMed]
33. Bailey, T.A.; Wacker, J.N.; An, D.D.; Carter, K.P.; Davis, R.C.; Mocko, V.; Larrabee, J.; Shield, K.M.; Lam, M.N.; Booth, C.H.; et al. Evaluation of ^{134}Ce as a PET Imaging Surrogate for Antibody Drug Conjugates Incorporating ^{225}Ac. *Nucl. Med. Biol.* 2022, *110–111*, 28–36. [CrossRef] [PubMed]
34. Hu, A.; Aluicio-Sarduy, E.; Brown, V.; MacMillan, S.N.; Becker, K.V.; Barnhart, T.E.; Radchenko, V.; Ramogida, C.F.; Engle, J.W.; Wilson, J.J. Py-Macrodipa: A Janus Chelator Capable of Binding Medicinally Relevant Rare-Earth Radiometals of Disparate Sizes. *J. Am. Chem. Soc.* 2021, *143*, 10429–10440. [CrossRef]
35. Thiele, N.A.; Brown, V.; Kelly, J.M.; Amor-Coarasa, A.; Jermilova, U.; MacMillan, S.N.; Nikolopoulou, A.; Ponnala, S.; Ramogida, C.F.; Robertson, A.K.H.; et al. An Eighteen-Membered Macrocyclic Ligand for Actinium-225 Targeted Alpha Therapy. *Angew. Chem. Int. Ed. Engl.* 2017, *56*, 14712–14717. [CrossRef]
36. Rizk, H.E.; Breky, M.M.E.; Attallah, M.F. Development of Purification of No-Carrier-Added 47Sc of Theranostic Interest: Selective Separation Study from the natTi(n,p) Process. *Radiochim. Acta* 2023, *111*, 273–282. [CrossRef]
37. Mousa, A.M.; Abdel Aziz, O.A.; Al-Hagar, O.E.A.; Gizawy, M.A.; Allan, K.F.; Attallah, M.F. Biosynthetic New Composite Material Containing CuO Nanoparticles Produced by Aspergillus Terreus for 47Sc Separation of Cancer Theranostics Application from Irradiated Ca Target. *Appl. Radiat. Isot.* 2020, *166*, 109389. [CrossRef] [PubMed]
38. Attallah, M.F.; Rizk, S.E.; Shady, S.A. Separation of 152+154Eu, 90Sr from Radioactive Waste Effluent Using Liquid–Liquid Extraction by Polyglycerol Phthalate. *Nucl. Sci. Tech.* 2018, *29*, 84. [CrossRef]
39. Hooijman, E.L.; Ntihabose, C.M.; Reuvers, T.G.A.; Nonnekens, J.; Aalbersberg, E.A.; van de Merbel, J.R.J.P.; Huijmans, J.E.; Koolen, S.L.W.; Hendrikx, J.J.M.A.; de Blois, E. Radiolabeling and Quality Control of Therapeutic Radiopharmaceuticals: Optimization, Clinical Implementation and Comparison of Radio-TLC/HPLC Analysis, Demonstrated by [^{177}Lu]Lu-PSMA. *EJNMMI Radiopharm. Chem.* 2022, *7*, 29. [CrossRef]
40. Mdanda, S.; Ngema, L.M.; Mdlophane, A.; Sathekge, M.M.; Zeevaart, J.R. Recent Innovations and Nano-Delivery of Actinium-225: A Narrative Review. *Pharmaceutics* 2023, *15*, 1719. [CrossRef]
41. Abou, D.S.; Zerkel, P.; Robben, J.; McLaughlin, M.; Hazlehurst, T.; Morse, D.; Wadas, T.J.; Pandya, D.N.; Oyama, R.; Gaehle, G.; et al. Radiopharmaceutical Quality Control Considerations for Accelerator-Produced Actinium Therapies. *Cancer Biother. Radiopharm.* 2022, *37*, 355–363. [CrossRef] [PubMed]
42. Dumond, A.R.S.; Rodnick, M.E.; Piert, M.R.; Scott, P.J.H. Synthesis of ^{225}Ac-PSMA-617 for Preclinical Use. *Curr. Radiopharm.* 2022, *15*, 96–103. [CrossRef] [PubMed]
43. Thakral, P.; Simecek, J.; Marx, S.; Kumari, J.; Pant, V.; Sen, I.B. In-House Preparation and Quality Control of Ac-225 Prostate-Specific Membrane Antigen-617 for the Targeted Alpha Therapy of Castration-Resistant Prostate Carcinoma. *Indian. J. Nucl. Med.* 2021, *36*, 114–119. [CrossRef] [PubMed]
44. Kelly, J.M.; Amor-Coarasa, A.; Sweeney, E.; Wilson, J.J.; Causey, P.W.; Babich, J.W. A Suitable Time Point for Quantifying the Radiochemical Purity of ^{225}Ac-Labeled Radiopharmaceuticals. *EJNMMI Radiopharm. Chem.* 2021, *6*, 38. [CrossRef] [PubMed]
45. Hooijman, E.L.; Chalashkan, Y.; Ling, S.W.; Kahyargil, F.F.; Segbers, M.; Bruchertseifer, F.; Morgenstern, A.; Seimbille, Y.; Koolen, S.L.W.; Brabander, T.; et al. Development of [^{225}Ac]Ac-PSMA-I&T for Targeted Alpha Therapy According to GMP Guidelines for Treatment of mCRPC. *Pharmaceutics* 2021, *13*, 715. [CrossRef] [PubMed]
46. Busslinger, S.D.; Tschan, V.J.; Richard, O.K.; Talip, Z.; Schibli, R.; Müller, C. [^{225}Ac]Ac-SibuDAB for Targeted Alpha Therapy of Prostate Cancer: Preclinical Evaluation and Comparison with [^{225}Ac]Ac-PSMA-617. *Cancers* 2022, *14*, 5651. [CrossRef] [PubMed]
47. King, A.P.; Gutsche, N.T.; Raju, N.; Fayn, S.; Baidoo, K.E.; Bell, M.M.; Olkowski, C.S.; Swenson, R.E.; Lin, F.I.; Sadowski, S.M.; et al. ^{225}Ac-MACROPATATE: A Novel α-Particle Peptide Receptor Radionuclide Therapy for Neuroendocrine Tumors. *J. Nucl. Med.* 2023, *64*, 549–554. [CrossRef]
48. Yadav, M.P.; Ballal, S.; Sahoo, R.K.; Bal, C. Efficacy and Safety of ^{225}Ac-DOTATATE Targeted Alpha Therapy in Metastatic Paragangliomas: A Pilot Study. *Eur. J. Nucl. Med. Mol. Imaging* 2022, *49*, 1595–1606. [CrossRef]
49. Rathke, H.; Bruchertseifer, F.; Kratochwil, C.; Keller, H.; Giesel, F.L.; Apostolidis, C.; Haberkorn, U.; Morgenstern, A. First Patient Exceeding 5-Year Complete Remission after ^{225}Ac-PSMA-TAT. *Eur. J. Nucl. Med. Mol. Imaging* 2021, *48*, 311–312. [CrossRef]

50. Zacherl, M.J.; Gildehaus, F.J.; Mittlmeier, L.; Böning, G.; Gosewisch, A.; Wenter, V.; Unterrainer, M.; Schmidt-Hegemann, N.; Belka, C.; Kretschmer, A.; et al. First Clinical Results for PSMA-Targeted α-Therapy Using ^{225}Ac-PSMA-I&T in Advanced-mCRPC Patients. *J. Nucl. Med.* **2021**, *62*, 669–674. [CrossRef]
51. Sathekge, M.; Bruchertseifer, F.; Vorster, M.; Lawal, I.O.; Knoesen, O.; Mahapane, J.; Davis, C.; Reyneke, F.; Maes, A.; Kratochwil, C.; et al. Predictors of Overall and Disease-Free Survival in Metastatic Castration-Resistant Prostate Cancer Patients Receiving ^{225}Ac-PSMA-617 Radioligand Therapy. *J. Nucl. Med.* **2020**, *61*, 62–69. [CrossRef] [PubMed]
52. Camacaro, J.F.; Dunckley, C.P.; Harman, S.E.; Fitzgerald, H.A.; Lakes, A.L.; Liao, Z.; Ludwig, R.C.; McBride, K.M.; Yalcintas Bethune, E.; Younes, A.; et al. Development of ^{225}Ac Production from Low Isotopic Dilution 229Th. *ACS Omega* **2023**, *8*, 38822–38827. [CrossRef]
53. Parida, G.K.; Panda, R.A.; Bishnoi, K.; Agrawal, K. Efficacy and Safety of Actinium-225 Prostate-Specific Membrane Antigen Radioligand Therapy in Metastatic Prostate Cancer: A Systematic Review and Metanalysis. *Med. Princ. Pract.* **2023**, *32*, 178–191. [CrossRef] [PubMed]
54. Ma, J.; Li, L.; Liao, T.; Gong, W.; Zhang, C. Efficacy and Safety of ^{225}Ac-PSMA-617-Targeted Alpha Therapy in Metastatic Castration-Resistant Prostate Cancer: A Systematic Review and Meta-Analysis. *Front. Oncol.* **2022**, *12*, 796657. [CrossRef]
55. Sanli, Y.; Kuyumcu, S.; Simsek, D.H.; Büyükkaya, F.; Civan, C.; Isik, E.G.; Ozkan, Z.G.; Basaran, M.; Sanli, O. ^{225}Ac-Prostate-Specific Membrane Antigen Therapy for Castration-Resistant Prostate Cancer: A Single-Center Experience. *Clin. Nucl. Med.* **2021**, *46*, 943–951. [CrossRef] [PubMed]
56. Sen, I.; Thakral, P.; Tiwari, P.; Pant, V.; Das, S.S.; Manda, D.; Raina, V. Therapeutic Efficacy of ^{225}Ac-PSMA-617 Targeted Alpha Therapy in Patients of Metastatic Castrate Resistant Prostate Cancer after Taxane-Based Chemotherapy. *Ann. Nucl. Med.* **2021**, *35*, 794–810. [CrossRef]
57. Feuerecker, B.; Tauber, R.; Knorr, K.; Heck, M.; Beheshti, A.; Seidl, C.; Bruchertseifer, F.; Pickhard, A.; Gafita, A.; Kratochwil, C.; et al. Activity and Adverse Events of Actinium-225-PSMA-617 in Advanced Metastatic Castration-Resistant Prostate Cancer After Failure of Lutetium-177-PSMA. *Eur. Urol.* **2021**, *79*, 343–350. [CrossRef]
58. Van der Doelen, M.J.; Mehra, N.; van Oort, I.M.; Looijen-Salamon, M.G.; Janssen, M.J.R.; Custers, J.A.E.; Slootbeek, P.H.J.; Kroeze, L.I.; Bruchertseifer, F.; Morgenstern, A.; et al. Clinical Outcomes and Molecular Profiling of Advanced Metastatic Castration-Resistant Prostate Cancer Patients Treated with ^{225}Ac-PSMA-617 Targeted Alpha-Radiation Therapy. *Urol. Oncol.* **2021**, *39*, 729.e7–729.e16. [CrossRef]
59. Yadav, M.P.; Ballal, S.; Sahoo, R.K.; Tripathi, M.; Seth, A.; Bal, C. Efficacy and Safety of ^{225}Ac-PSMA-617 Targeted Alpha Therapy in Metastatic Castration-Resistant Prostate Cancer Patients. *Theranostics* **2020**, *10*, 9364–9377. [CrossRef]
60. Satapathy, S.; Mittal, B.R.; Sood, A.; Das, C.K.; Singh, S.K.; Mavuduru, R.S.; Bora, G.S. Health-Related Quality-of-Life Outcomes with Actinium-225-Prostate-Specific Membrane Antigen-617 Therapy in Patients with Heavily Pretreated Metastatic Castration-Resistant Prostate Cancer. *Indian. J. Nucl. Med.* **2020**, *35*, 299–304. [CrossRef]
61. Sathekge, M.; Bruchertseifer, F.; Knoesen, O.; Reyneke, F.; Lawal, I.; Lengana, T.; Davis, C.; Mahapane, J.; Corbett, C.; Vorster, M.; et al. ^{225}Ac-PSMA-617 in Chemotherapy-Naive Patients with Advanced Prostate Cancer: A Pilot Study. *Eur. J. Nucl. Med. Mol. Imaging* **2019**, *46*, 129–138. [CrossRef] [PubMed]
62. Kratochwil, C.; Bruchertseifer, F.; Rathke, H.; Hohenfellner, M.; Giesel, F.L.; Haberkorn, U.; Morgenstern, A. Targeted α-Therapy of Metastatic Castration-Resistant Prostate Cancer with ^{225}Ac-PSMA-617: Swimmer-Plot Analysis Suggests Efficacy Regarding Duration of Tumor Control. *J. Nucl. Med.* **2018**, *59*, 795–802. [CrossRef]
63. Ballal, S.; Yadav, M.P.; Tripathi, M.; Sahoo, R.K.; Bal, C. Survival Outcomes in Metastatic Gastroenteropancreatic Neuroendocrine Tumor Patients Receiving Concomitant ^{225}Ac-DOTATATE Targeted Alpha Therapy and Capecitabine: A Real-World Scenario Management Based Long-Term Outcome Study. *J. Nucl. Med.* **2022**, *64*, 211–218. [CrossRef]
64. Kratochwil, C.; Apostolidis, L.; Rathke, H.; Apostolidis, C.; Bicu, F.; Bruchertseifer, F.; Choyke, P.L.; Haberkorn, U.; Giesel, F.L.; Morgenstern, A. Dosing ^{225}Ac-DOTATOC in Patients with Somatostatin-Receptor-Positive Solid Tumors: 5-Year Follow-up of Hematological and Renal Toxicity. *Eur. J. Nucl. Med. Mol. Imaging* **2021**, *49*, 54–63. [CrossRef]
65. Ballal, S.; Yadav, M.P.; Bal, C.; Sahoo, R.K.; Tripathi, M. Broadening Horizons with ^{225}Ac-DOTATATE Targeted Alpha Therapy for Gastroenteropancreatic Neuroendocrine Tumour Patients Stable or Refractory to ^{177}Lu-DOTATATE PRRT: First Clinical Experience on the Efficacy and Safety. *Eur. J. Nucl. Med. Mol. Imaging* **2020**, *47*, 934–946. [CrossRef]
66. Kratochwil, C.; Bruchertseifer, F.; Giesel, F.; Apostolidis, C.; Haberkorn, U.; Morgenstern, A. Ac-225-DOTATOC—An Empiric Dose Finding for Alpha Particle Emitter Based Radionuclide Therapy of Neuroendocrine Tumors. *J. Nucl. Med.* **2015**, *56*, 1232.
67. Rosenblat, T.L.; McDevitt, M.R.; Carrasquillo, J.A.; Pandit-Taskar, N.; Frattini, M.G.; Maslak, P.G.; Park, J.H.; Douer, D.; Cicic, D.; Larson, S.M.; et al. Treatment of Patients with Acute Myeloid Leukemia with the Targeted Alpha-Particle Nanogenerator Actinium-225-Lintuzumab. *Clin. Cancer Res.* **2022**, *28*, 2030–2037. [CrossRef] [PubMed]
68. Jurcic, J.G. Clinical Studies with Bismuth-213 and Actinium-225 for Hematologic Malignancies. *Curr. Radiopharm.* **2018**, *11*, 192–199. [CrossRef] [PubMed]
69. Jurcic, J.G.; Levy, M.Y.; Park, J.H.; Ravandi, F.; Perl, A.E.; Pagel, J.M.; Smith, B.D.; Estey, E.H.; Kantarjian, H.; Cicic, D.; et al. Phase I Trial of Targeted Alpha-Particle Therapy with Actinium-225 (^{225}Ac)-Lintuzumab and Low-Dose Cytarabine (LDAC) in Patients Age 60 or Older with Untreated Acute Myeloid Leukemia (AML). *Blood* **2016**, *128*, 4050. [CrossRef]

70. Jurcic, J.G.; Rosenblat, T.L.; McDevitt, M.R.; Pandit-Taskar, N.; Carrasquillo, J.A.; Chanel, S.M.; Zikaras, K.; Frattini, M.G.; Maslak, P.G.; Cicic, D.; et al. Phase I Trial of the Targeted Alpha-Particle Nano-Generator Actinium-225 (^{225}Ac)-Lintuzumab (Anti-CD33; HuM195) in Acute Myeloid Leukemia (AML). *Blood* **2011**, *118*, 768. [CrossRef]
71. Pretze, M.; Kunkel, F.; Runge, R.; Freudenberg, R.; Braune, A.; Hartmann, H.; Schwarz, U.; Brogsitter, C.; Kotzerke, J. Ac-EAZY! Towards GMP-Compliant Module Syntheses of ^{225}Ac-Labeled Peptides for Clinical Application. *Pharmaceuticals* **2021**, *14*, 652. [CrossRef]
72. Eryilmaz, K.; Kilbas, B. Fully-Automated Synthesis of ^{177}Lu Labelled FAPI Derivatives on the Module Modular Lab-Eazy. *EJNMMI Radiopharm. Chem.* **2021**, *6*, 16. [CrossRef] [PubMed]
73. Alvarez, R. Managing the Uranium-233 Stockpile of the United States. *Sci. Glob. Secur.* **2013**, *21*, 53–69. [CrossRef]
74. Robertson, A.K.H.; Ramogida, C.F.; Schaffer, P.; Radchenko, V. Development of ^{225}Ac Radiopharmaceuticals: TRIUMF Perspectives and Experiences. *Curr. Radiopharm.* **2018**, *11*, 156–172. [CrossRef] [PubMed]
75. Boll, R.A.; Malkemus, D.; Mirzadeh, S. Production of Actinium-225 for Alpha Particle Mediated Radioimmunotherapy. *Appl. Radiat. Isot.* **2005**, *62*, 667–679. [CrossRef] [PubMed]
76. Apostolidis, C.; Molinet, R.; Rasmussen, G.; Morgenstern, A. Production of Ac-225 from Th-229 for Targeted Alpha Therapy. *Anal. Chem.* **2005**, *77*, 6288–6291. [CrossRef]
77. Kotovskii, A.A.; Nerozin, N.A.; Prokof'ev, I.V.; Shapovalov, V.V.; Yakovshchits, Y.A.; Bolonkin, A.S.; Dunin, A.V. Isolation of Actinium-225 for Medical Purposes. *Radiochemistry* **2015**, *57*, 285–291. [CrossRef]
78. Morgenstern, A.; Apostolidis, C.; Bruchertseifer, F. Supply and Clinical Application of Actinium-225 and Bismuth-213. *Semin. Nucl. Med.* **2020**, *50*, 119–123. [CrossRef]
79. Harvey, J.T.; Nolen, J.; Vandergrift, G.; Gomes, I.; Kroc, T.; Horwitz, P.; McAlister, D.; Bowers, D.; Sullivan, V.; Greene, J. *Production of Actinium-225 via High Energy Proton Induced Spallation of Thorium-232*; NorthStar Medical Radioisotopes, LLC.: Madison, WI, USA, 2011.
80. Samsonov, M.D.; Nerozin, N.A.; Podsoblyaev, D.A.; Prokof'ev, I.V.; Tkachev, S.V.; Khamianov, S.V.; Shapovalov, V.V. Isolation of Alpha-Emitting Radionuclides for Nuclear Medicine in JSC "SSC RF–IPPE. In Proceedings of the 10th International Symposium on Targeted Alpha Therapy, Kanazawa, Japan, 30 May–1 June 2017.
81. USDOE Office of Science (SC). *Meeting Isotope Needs and Capturing Opportunities for the Future: The 2015 Long. Range Plan. for the DOE-NP Isotope Progarm, NSAC Isotopes Subcommittee, July 2015*; USDOE Office of Science (SC): Bethesda, MD, USA, 2015.
82. Makvandi, M.; Dupis, E.; Engle, J.W.; Nortier, F.M.; Fassbender, M.E.; Simon, S.; Birnbaum, E.R.; Atcher, R.W.; John, K.D.; Rixe, O.; et al. Alpha-Emitters and Targeted Alpha Therapy in Oncology: From Basic Science to Clinical Investigations. *Target. Oncol.* **2018**, *13*, 189–203. [CrossRef]
83. Morgenstern, A.; Bruchertseifer, F.; Apostolidis, C. Bismuth-213 and Actinium-225—Generator Performance and Evolving Therapeutic Applications of Two Generator-Derived Alpha-Emitting Radioisotopes. *Curr. Radiopharm.* **2012**, *5*, 221–227. [CrossRef]
84. Hogle, S.; Boll, R.A.; Murphy, K.; Denton, D.; Owens, A.; Haverlock, T.J.; Garland, M.; Mirzadeh, S. Reactor Production of Thorium-229. *Appl. Radiat. Isot.* **2016**, *114*, 19–27. [CrossRef]
85. Kratochwil, C.; Bruchertseifer, F.; Rathke, H.; Bronzel, M.; Apostolidis, C.; Weichert, W.; Haberkorn, U.; Giesel, F.L.; Morgenstern, A. Targeted α-Therapy of Metastatic Castration-Resistant Prostate Cancer with ^{225}Ac-PSMA-617: Dosimetry Estimate and Empiric Dose Finding. *J. Nucl. Med.* **2017**, *58*, 1624–1631. [CrossRef] [PubMed]
86. Englert, M.; Krall, L.; Ewing, R.C. Is Nuclear Fission a Sustainable Source of Energy? *MRS Bull.* **2012**, *37*, 417–424. [CrossRef]
87. Hoehr, C.; Bénard, F.; Buckley, K.; Crawford, J.; Gottberg, A.; Hanemaayer, V.; Kunz, P.; Ladouceur, K.; Radchenko, V.; Ramogida, C.; et al. Medical Isotope Production at TRIUMF—From Imaging to Treatment. *Phys. Procedia* **2017**, *90*, 200–208. [CrossRef]
88. Griswold, J.R.; Medvedev, D.G.; Engle, J.W.; Copping, R.; Fitzsimmons, J.M.; Radchenko, V.; Cooley, J.C.; Fassbender, M.E.; Denton, D.L.; Murphy, K.E.; et al. Large Scale Accelerator Production of ^{225}Ac: Effective Cross Sections for 78-192MeV Protons Incident on ^{232}Th Targets. *Appl. Radiat. Isot.* **2016**, *118*, 366–374. [CrossRef] [PubMed]
89. Weidner, J.W.; Mashnik, S.G.; John, K.D.; Ballard, B.; Birnbaum, E.R.; Bitteker, L.J.; Couture, A.; Fassbender, M.E.; Goff, G.S.; Gritzo, R.; et al. ^{225}Ac and ^{223}Ra Production via 800 MeV Proton Irradiation of Natural Thorium Targets. *Appl. Radiat. Isot.* **2012**, *70*, 2590–2595. [CrossRef] [PubMed]
90. Weidner, J.W.; Mashnik, S.G.; John, K.D.; Hemez, F.; Ballard, B.; Bach, H.; Birnbaum, E.R.; Bitteker, L.J.; Couture, A.; Dry, D.; et al. Proton-Induced Cross Sections Relevant to Production of ^{225}Ac and ^{223}Ra in Natural Thorium Targets below 200 MeV. *Appl. Radiat. Isot.* **2012**, *70*, 2602–2607. [CrossRef]
91. Cutler, C.S. *US DOE Tri-Lab Effort to Produce Ac-225*; International Atomic Energy Agency (IAEA): Vienna, Austria, 2020.
92. Aliev, R.A.; Ermolaev, S.V.; Vasiliev, A.N.; Ostapenko, V.S.; Lapshina, E.V.; Zhuikov, B.L.; Zakharov, N.V.; Pozdeev, V.V.; Kokhanyuk, V.M.; Myasoedov, B.F.; et al. Isolation of Medicine-Applicable Actinium-225 from Thorium Targets Irradiated by Medium-Energy Protons. *Solvent Extr. Ion Exch.* **2014**, *32*, 468–477. [CrossRef]
93. Mastren, T.; Radchenko, V.; Owens, A.; Copping, R.; Boll, R.; Griswold, J.R.; Mirzadeh, S.; Wyant, L.E.; Brugh, M.; Engle, J.W.; et al. Simultaneous Separation of Actinium and Radium Isotopes from a Proton Irradiated Thorium Matrix. *Sci. Rep.* **2017**, *7*, 8216. [CrossRef]

94. Radchenko, V.; Engle, J.W.; Wilson, J.J.; Maassen, J.R.; Nortier, F.M.; Taylor, W.A.; Birnbaum, E.R.; Hudston, L.A.; John, K.D.; Fassbender, M.E. Application of Ion Exchange and Extraction Chromatography to the Separation of Actinium from Proton-Irradiated Thorium Metal for Analytical Purposes. *J. Chromatogr. A* **2015**, *1380*, 55–63. [CrossRef]
95. Ramogida, C.F.; Robertson, A.K.H.; Jermilova, U.; Zhang, C.; Yang, H.; Kunz, P.; Lassen, J.; Bratanovic, I.; Brown, V.; Southcott, L.; et al. Evaluation of Polydentate Picolinic Acid Chelating Ligands and an α-Melanocyte-Stimulating Hormone Derivative for Targeted Alpha Therapy Using ISOL-Produced ^{225}Ac. *EJNMMI Radiopharm. Chem.* **2019**, *4*, 21. [CrossRef]
96. Robertson, A.K.H.; McNeil, B.L.; Yang, H.; Gendron, D.; Perron, R.; Radchenko, V.; Zeisler, S.; Causey, P.; Schaffer, P. ^{232}Th-Spallation-Produced ^{225}Ac with Reduced ^{227}Ac Content. *Inorg. Chem.* **2020**, *59*, 12156–12165. [CrossRef] [PubMed]
97. Augusto, R.S.; Smith, J.; Varah, S.; Paley, W.; Egoriti, L.; McEwen, S.; Goodacre, T.D.; Mildenberger, J.; Gottberg, A.; Trudel, A.; et al. Design and Radiological Study of the ^{225}Ac Medical Target at the TRIUMF-ARIEL Proton-Target Station. *Radiat. Phys. Chem.* **2022**, *201*, 110491. [CrossRef]
98. Apostolidis, C.; Molinet, R.; McGinley, J.; Abbas, K.; Möllenbeck, J.; Morgenstern, A. Cyclotron Production of Ac-225 for Targeted Alpha Therapy. *Appl. Radiat. Isot.* **2005**, *62*, 383–387. [CrossRef] [PubMed]
99. Nesteruk, K.P.; Ramseyer, L.; Carzaniga, T.S.; Braccini, S. Measurement of the Beam Energy Distribution of a Medical Cyclotron with a Multi-Leaf Faraday Cup. *Instruments* **2019**, *3*, 4. [CrossRef]
100. Higashi, T.; Nagatsu, K.; Tsuji, A.B.; Zhang, M.-R. Research and Development for Cyclotron Production of ^{225}Ac from ^{226}Ra—The Challenges in a Country Lacking Natural Resources for Medical Applications. *Processes* **2022**, *10*, 1215. [CrossRef]
101. Morgenstern, A.; Abbas, K.; Bruchertseifer, F.; Apostolidis, C. Production of Alpha Emitters for Targeted Alpha Therapy. *Curr. Radiopharm.* **2008**, *1*, 135–143. [CrossRef]
102. Maslov, O.D.; Sabel'nikov, A.V.; Dmitriev, S.N. Preparation of ^{225}Ac by ^{226}Ra(γ, n) Photonuclear Reaction on an Electron Accelerator, MT-25 Microtron. *Radiochemistry* **2006**, *48*, 195–197. [CrossRef]
103. Melville, G.; Meriarty, H.; Metcalfe, P.; Knittel, T.; Allen, B.J. Production of Ac-225 for Cancer Therapy by Photon-Induced Transmutation of Ra-226. *Appl. Radiat. Isot.* **2007**, *65*, 1014–1022. [CrossRef]
104. Bruchertseifer, F.; Kellerbauer, A.; Malmbeck, R.; Morgenstern, A. Targeted Alpha Therapy with Bismuth-213 and Actinium-225: Meeting Future Demand. *J. Labelled Comp. Radiopharm.* **2019**, *62*, 794–802. [CrossRef]
105. IBA and SCK CEN Join Forces to Enable Production of Actinium-225 I SCK CEN. Available online: https://www.sckcen.be/en/news/iba-and-sck-cen-join-forces-enable-production-actinium-225 (accessed on 5 June 2023).
106. Ermolaev, S.; Skasyrskaya, A.; Vasiliev, A. A Radionuclide Generator of High-Purity Bi-213 for Instant Labeling. *Pharmaceutics* **2021**, *13*, 914. [CrossRef] [PubMed]
107. Bruchertseifer, F.; Apostolidis, C.; Mirzadeh, S.; Boll, R.; Murphy, K.; Morgenstern, A. Development of a High-Activity ^{225}Ac/^{213}Bi Radionuclide Generator for Synthesis of Clinical Doses of ^{213}Bi-Labelled Biomolecules. Available online: https://publications.jrc.ec.europa.eu/repository/handle/JRC82742 (accessed on 4 June 2023).

Disclaimer/Publisher's Note: The statements, opinions and data contained in all publications are solely those of the individual author(s) and contributor(s) and not of MDPI and/or the editor(s). MDPI and/or the editor(s) disclaim responsibility for any injury to people or property resulting from any ideas, methods, instructions or products referred to in the content.

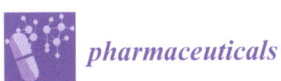

Review

Theranostic Imaging Surrogates for Targeted Alpha Therapy: Progress in Production, Purification, and Applications

Bryce J. B. Nelson [1], John Wilson [1], Jan D. Andersson [1,2] and Frank Wuest [1,3,*]

1. Department of Oncology, University of Alberta, 11560 University Ave., Edmonton, AB T6G 1Z2, Canada; bjnelson@ualberta.ca (B.J.B.N.); john.wilson2@albertahealthservices.ca (J.W.); jan.andersson@albertahealthservices.ca (J.D.A.)
2. Edmonton Radiopharmaceutical Center, Alberta Health Services, 11560 University Ave., Edmonton, AB T6G 1Z2, Canada
3. Cancer Research Institute of Northern Alberta, University of Alberta, Edmonton, AB T6G 2E1, Canada
* Correspondence: wuest@ualberta.ca; Tel.: +1-780-391-7666; Fax: +1-780-432-8483

Abstract: This article highlights recent developments of SPECT and PET diagnostic imaging surrogates for targeted alpha particle therapy (TAT) radiopharmaceuticals. It outlines the rationale for using imaging surrogates to improve diagnostic-scan accuracy and facilitate research, and the properties an imaging-surrogate candidate should possess. It evaluates the strengths and limitations of each potential imaging surrogate. Thirteen surrogates for TAT are explored: ^{133}La, ^{132}La, ^{134}Ce/^{134}La, and ^{226}Ac for ^{225}Ac TAT; ^{203}Pb for ^{212}Pb TAT; ^{131}Ba for ^{223}Ra and ^{224}Ra TAT; ^{123}I, ^{124}I, ^{131}I and ^{209}At for ^{211}At TAT; ^{134}Ce/^{134}La for ^{227}Th TAT; and ^{155}Tb and ^{152}Tb for ^{149}Tb TAT.

Keywords: targeted alpha therapy; alpha particle therapy; PET imaging; SPECT imaging; targeted radionuclide therapy; theranostics; actinium-225; lanthanum-133; lead-212; lead-203

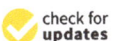

Citation: Nelson, B.J.B.; Wilson, J.; Andersson, J.D.; Wuest, F. Theranostic Imaging Surrogates for Targeted Alpha Therapy: Progress in Production, Purification, and Applications. *Pharmaceuticals* **2023**, *16*, 1622. https://doi.org/10.3390/ph16111622

Academic Editors: Marc Pretze and Jörg Kotzerke

Received: 11 October 2023
Revised: 8 November 2023
Accepted: 14 November 2023
Published: 17 November 2023

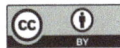

Copyright: © 2023 by the authors. Licensee MDPI, Basel, Switzerland. This article is an open access article distributed under the terms and conditions of the Creative Commons Attribution (CC BY) license (https:// creativecommons.org/licenses/by/ 4.0/).

1. Introduction

Targeted alpha therapy (TAT) involves utilizing radiopharmaceuticals to precisely eliminate malignancies with alpha particle emissions, while sparing surrounding healthy tissues. These radiopharmaceuticals consist of alpha (α)-emitting radionuclides conjugated to a biological-targeting vector such as monoclonal antibodies, peptides, and nanocarriers [1]. Key advantages of TAT include highly selective radiation delivery to the target, reduced patient side effects, and the ability to assess radiopharmaceutical uptake and, therefore, patient eligibility using a diagnostic radionuclide before therapy [2].

While beta minus (β^-) radiopharmaceuticals employing radionuclides such as ^{177}Lu have made significant advances in clinical care of advanced prostate and neuroendocrine tumors [3,4], alpha particle emissions are significantly more precise and cytotoxic than β^- emissions. This is attributed to the much larger size of alpha particles (7300 times the mass of electrons), their 2+ charge resulting in a highly ionized emission path, and high linear energy transfer that deposits their energy over a path length of only several cell diameters. These properties make alpha emitters ideal for combatting metastatic cancers and other systemic malignancies where traditional treatment avenues have failed [2,5–7].

Approximately 400 alpha-emitting radionuclides (5–100% emission intensity) are known; however, only radionuclides that possess a sufficiently long half-life, absence of long-lived toxic progeny, and feasible high-yield production routes are suitable for TAT consideration [8,9]. Radionuclides that have shown potential for TAT include ^{227}Th, ^{225}Ac, ^{224}Ra, ^{223}Ra, ^{212}Pb, ^{211}At, and ^{149}Tb [1,2,10–20].

While the potency of TAT offers significantly enhanced therapeutic efficacy, TAT must be treated as a double-edged sword with the possibility of severe off-target toxicity to nontarget organs and tissues. This mandates a comprehensive understanding of the stability, pharmacokinetics, and dosimetry of any TAT radiopharmaceutical. During preclinical development, these data can be acquired from biodistribution studies in mice, where mice are sacrificed at multiple time points, and gamma-ray co-emissions are counted in the dissected organs and tissues.

Additionally, positron emission tomography (PET) and single-photon emission computed tomography (SPECT) scans can be acquired by exchanging the alpha-emitting radionuclide with a positron or gamma-ray-emitting diagnostic imaging radionuclide. This imaging–therapeutic duality is termed "theranostics", and these PET and SPECT scans provide crucial information on dosimetry and monitor response to TAT.

Most TAT radionuclides lack or possess insufficient co-emitted positrons or gamma rays for acquiring higher-quality PET or SPECT scans. This motivated the development of chemically similar diagnostic imaging surrogates for TAT radionuclides. As the current supply of alpha-emitting radionuclides is scarce, utilizing imaging surrogates also has the potential to open more opportunities for TAT research to facilities without access to alpha-emitting radionuclides and serve as a bridge for centers planning to introduce TAT radiopharmaceuticals. Since many of these surrogates can be synthesized in existing cyclotron facilities, this can facilitate radiopharmaceutical developments. Additionally, imaging surrogates fit well into the existing research and clinical setup. As such, TAT imaging surrogates have the potential to assist the deployment of TAT radiopharmaceuticals in the clinic and accelerate the development of new TAT targeting vectors.

2. Properties of Ideal Imaging Surrogates for Alpha Emitters

Multiple factors determine what makes a suitable imaging surrogate for targeted alpha therapy. These include chemical properties, half-life, radioactive emission type and intensity, associated dosimetry, production ease and scalability, radionuclidic purity, economics, and radionuclide progeny considerations.

PET and SPECT scans that evaluate the pharmacokinetics and dosimetry of TAT radiopharmaceuticals are often performed with ^{68}Ga and ^{18}F. However, ^{68}Ga, ^{18}F, and other common imaging radionuclides often have substantially different chemical properties than alpha-emitting radionuclides. For some targeting vectors, this can result in differing biodistributions between the TAT radiopharmaceutical and its diagnostic counterpart [21–23]. Potential inconsistencies observed in diagnostic imaging scans and subsequent biodistribution of the therapeutic radiopharmaceutical could result in sub-optimal tumor dosing or unintended and destructive alpha-irradiation of healthy tissues.

Imaging surrogates should, therefore, possess a similar chemistry and half-life to ensure their biodistribution and dosimetry are similar to their paired alpha emitters. These surrogates are ideally isotopes of the same element possessing identical chemistries, such as ^{226}Ac paired with ^{225}Ac TAT, ^{203}Pb paired with ^{212}Pb TAT, ^{209}At paired with ^{211}At, and ^{155}Tb or ^{152}Tb paired with ^{149}Tb TAT.

However, if suitable isotopes of the same element are not available, chemically similar elements in the same chemical group can be employed. These include ^{133}La, ^{132}La, or ^{134}Ce/^{134}La paired with ^{225}Ac, ^{134}Ce/^{134}La, paired with ^{227}Th, and ^{123}I, ^{124}I, or ^{131}I, paired with ^{211}At.

It is also preferable that the physical half-life of the imaging surrogate is similar to its TAT counterpart. This permits the acquisition of biodistribution data for the full in vivo residence of the TAT radiopharmaceutical to assist preclinical development and initial clinical validation. For TAT employing radionuclides with long physical half-lives (^{225}Ac, ^{223}Ra, ^{224}Ra, ^{227}Th) and targeting vectors with long biological half-lives, using a long-lived imaging surrogate is crucial to confirm that the radiopharmaceutical remains at the target site for the extended duration without redistributing to and irradiating healthy tissues. While additional patient radiation dose might result from using a diagnostic radionuclide with a longer half-life, some targeting vectors such as antibodies may require longer circulation times to acquire sufficient quality images. For TAT employing long-lived radionuclides and targeting vectors with short biological half-lives, a radionuclide imaging surrogate with a shorter physical half-life may be used in certain situations. This can be a valuable tool for evaluating patient dosimetry, provided that the targeting vector exhibits rapid in vivo clearance, minimal off-target binding, and the radionuclide is stably incorporated within the radiopharmaceutical. Radiopharmaceutical pretargeting approaches may reduce the advantage of selecting diagnostic and therapeutic TAT radionuclides with similar half-lives; however, it is uncertain whether most theranostic targeting vectors will employ a pretargeting approach.

Regarding radioactive emissions, it is preferable that PET imaging surrogates possess a high positron branching ratio and low positron emission energy to facilitate high-resolution PET imaging and minimal co-emitted electrons and gamma/X-rays to reduce the radioactive dose. Radionuclides with lower positron branching ratios may require additional injected activity to resolve the same quality image. For SPECT imaging, radionuclides should possess lower energy gamma rays within the optimal energy window of scanners and minimal co-emitted electrons and gamma/X-rays.

To produce imaging surrogates, sufficient cyclotron or nuclear reactor facilities are required to synthesize the radionuclide. Target material (natural or isotopically enriched) should be available in adequate quantity and enrichment to support routine production, and a favorable nuclear cross-section must exist within the capabilities of production facilities. Radionuclide production should be performed safely, create few long-lived radionuclidic impurities, and be scalable to sufficient activities that allow distribution to clinical sites. Robust chemical-purification techniques must separate the imaging surrogate from potentially hazardous target material post-irradiation. Finally, the radionuclide progeny of the imaging surrogate should be considered since this can influence imaging quality and impact radioactive waste management.

Most radionuclides used in TAT are part of decay chains where each decay results in the recoil of the daughter nucleus with energy sufficient to liberate the daughter nucleus from the chelator into solution. Additionally, the alpha particle itself may induce radiolytic damage to the radiopharmaceutical, reducing the in vivo targeting and leading to further accumulation of radioactivity in nontarget tissue. These inherent physical properties are not easily covered by the surrogates in question, so they should be considered in experimental methods and conclusions.

In this article, a selection of 13 diagnostic imaging surrogates for promising alpha-emitting radionuclides have been highlighted for their production, purification, applications, and overall strengths and limitations.

3. Theranostic Imaging Surrogates Proposed for Actinium-225

Actinium-225 ($t_{1/2}$ = 9.9 d) has been explored extensively for TAT. Its long half-life permits extended dose delivery and decay via a cascade of six short-lived radionuclide progeny with four alpha particle emissions to near-stable ^{209}Bi, making ^{225}Ac particularly attractive for TAT. ^{225}Ac studies have demonstrated efficacy in metastatic prostate cancer and neuroendocrine tumors, and additional radiopharmaceuticals are under development for other cancers [11,24–30] There are considerable efforts underway to significantly increase the ^{225}Ac supply to meet the significant anticipated clinical demand [31–34].

However, ^{225}Ac does not emit gamma rays of sufficient intensity for imaging. Although its ^{213}Bi and ^{221}Fr progeny possess gamma rays of suitable energy and intensity for SPECT imaging [9], the ^{225}Ac activities injected into patients (~50–200 kBq/kg [11]) would be insufficient to resolve a high-quality image within a reasonable scan duration. Additionally, the supply of high-purity ^{225}Ac from ^{225}Ra/^{225}Ac generators is limited, constraining AT development efforts [31]. While other sources of ^{225}Ac from high-energy spallation reactions are available [32,35,36], these often contain a small activity of co-produced and inseparable ^{227}Ac ($t_{1/2}$ = 21 y), which complicates radioactive waste management. Therefore, the desire to enable ^{225}Ac imaging and enhance research throughput motivates the development of imaging surrogates.

For SPECT imaging, ^{226}Ac is an elementally matched surrogate for ^{225}Ac. Radiolanthanum isotopes ^{133}La, ^{132}La, and ^{134}La are particularly attractive for PET imaging of ^{225}Ac due to the similar ionic radii of La^{3+} and Ac^{3+} (~1.03 and ~1.12 Å, respectively [37,38]) and their resulting similar chemistries. Both lanthanum and actinium possess similar chelation chemistry with chelators such as DOTA, macropa, and crown ethers, and exhibit similar in vivo biodistributions [39–44]. The subsequent sections will outline the properties, strengths, and limitations of ^{133}La, ^{132}La, ^{134}Ce/^{134}La, and ^{226}Ac.

3.1. Lanthanum-133 (PET)

Lanthanum-133 ($t_{1/2}$ = 3.9 h) has been synthesized via the ^{135}Ba(p,3n)^{133}La and ^{135}Ba(p,2n)^{133}La nuclear reactions on medical cyclotrons [45]. Natural Ba metal can be used as a target material, with one study producing 231 MBq ^{133}La and 166 MBq ^{135}La for 500 µA·min cyclotron irradiations at 22 MeV. Subsequent chemical processing using a diglycolamide (DGA) resin produced a highly pure [^{133}La]LaCl$_3$ product that, when used to radiolabel DOTA and macropa chelators, achieved molar activities sufficient for preclinical and clinical application [40]. Co-production of ^{135}La ($t_{1/2}$ = 18.9 h (44)) is unavoidable using natural barium target material. While ^{135}La has potential applications for Auger-Meitner electron therapy, it would add additional patient radioactive dose and is undesirable for ^{133}La PET imaging applications.

Alternatively, natural or isotopically enriched $BaCO_3$ can be employed to simplify target preparation to boost ^{133}La yields and selectivity from co-produced ^{135}La. Another study irradiated [^{135}Ba]BaCO$_3$ at a 23.3 MeV proton energy, significantly improving ^{133}La/^{135}La selectivity relative to natural Ba target material, producing 214 MBq ^{133}La with 28 MBq ^{135}La using [^{135}Ba]BaCO$_3$, versus 59 MBq ^{133}La with 35 MBq ^{135}La using [^{nat}Ba]BaCO$_3$ [41]. Another approach involved irradiating isotopically enriched [^{134}Ba]BaCO$_3$ at a proton energy of 22 MeV, with subsequent purification yielding up to 1.2–1.8 GBq [^{133}La]LaCl$_3$ with 0.4% co-produced ^{135}La and a radionuclidic purity of >99.5%. The decay of ^{133}La into its long-lived daughter ^{133}Ba ($t_{1/2}$ = 10.6 y) resulted in 4 kBq ^{133}Ba per 100 MBq ^{133}La, which was deemed uncritical concerning dose and waste management [42].

As shown in Figure 1, ^{133}La PET imaging analysis was performed in Derenzo phantoms and compared with other common PET radionuclides, with ^{133}La found to have superior spatial resolution compared to ^{44}Sc, ^{68}Ga, and another radiolanthanum positron emitter, ^{132}La [41].

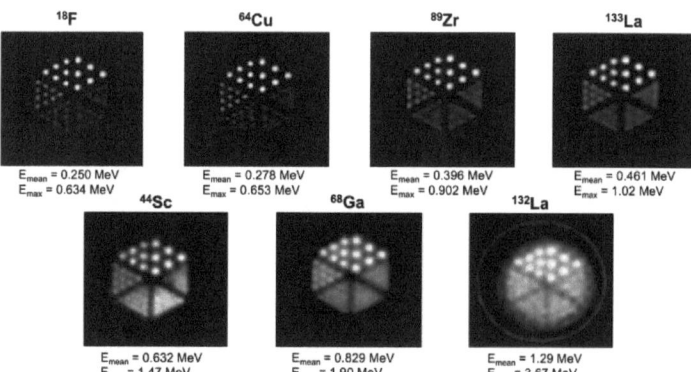

Figure 1. Derenzo phantom PET images reconstructed with MAP for different PET radionuclides, listed in order of increasing positron emission energy. Figure from Nelson et al. [41], with ^{18}F, ^{64}Cu, ^{44}Sc, and ^{68}Ga data from Ferguson et al. [46].

As depicted in Figure 2, PET imaging was performed with [^{133}La]La-PSMA I&T in a prostate cancer mouse model. The LNCaP prostate cancer tumors were delineated with high spatial resolution and minimal off-target uptake, demonstrating the potential for further ^{133}La PET imaging applications [41].

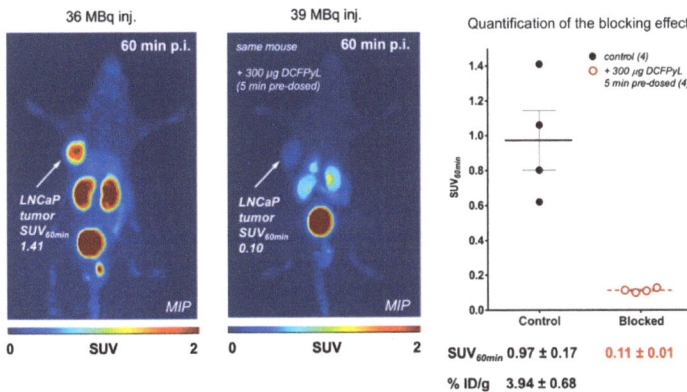

Figure 2. Representative PET images (MIP—maximum intensity projection) at 60 min of [^{133}La]La-PSMA-I&T with and without pre-dose of DCFPyL in LNCaP tumor-bearing mice. Figure from Nelson et al. [41].

Strengths of ^{133}La include its 3.9 h half-life that allows sufficient time for separation and distribution to external clinics; a lower positron emission energy compared to ^{68}Ga, ^{44}Sc, and ^{132}La that results in a higher PET imaging spatial resolution [47]; and low energy and intensity co-emitted gamma rays that reduce the radioactive dose. Limitations include the production requirement of medium-energy cyclotron facilities; its lower positron branching ratio of 7.2% that may require additional injected activity relative to other PET radionuclides such as ^{18}F; and its decay into relatively long-lived ^{133}Ba.

3.2. Lanthanum-132 (PET)

Lanthanum-132 ($t_{1/2}$ = 4.6 h) can be produced via the ^{132}Ba(p,n)^{132}La nuclear reaction using natural Ba metal target material [48–51]. This beam energy co-produces significant activities of ^{135}La and is just below the threshold of the ^{133}La production. One study reported yields of 0.26 ± 0.05 MBq·µA^{-1}·h^{-1} ^{132}La and 5.6 ± 1.1 MBq·µA^{-1}·h^{-1} ^{135}La for irradiation with 11.9 MeV protons, with ^{132}La activity approximately 5% relative to ^{135}La activity at the end of bombardment [48,49]. Another study reported yields of 0.8 MBq ^{132}La and 17.9 MBq ^{135}La for 500 µA·min runs at 11.9 MeV [40]. ^{132}La can be purified using DGA resin and complexed with chelators at molar activities suitable for radiopharmaceutical application [49]. A study using a tumor-targeting alkylphosphocholine, NM600, demonstrated significant tumor uptake of [^{132}La]La-NM600 and a similar biodistribution to [^{225}Ac]Ac-NM600 using PET/CT imaging and ex vivo analysis [48].

Strengths of ^{132}La include its 4.6 h half-life, which allows ease of radiopharmaceutical preparation and distribution compared to shorter-lived PET emitters such as ^{68}Ga; its stable ^{132}Ba decay daughter; and its significant 41.2% positron branching ratio [9]. Limitations include severe cyclotron production constraints owing to the 0.1% natural isotopic abundance of ^{132}Ba target material; high energy and intensity co-emitted gamma rays that contribute to excess radioactive dose; and the high maximum positron emission energy of 3.67 MeV, which leads to a low PET spatial resolution and image blurring as shown in Figure 1.

3.3. Lanthanum-134/Cerium-134 (PET)

Lanthanum-134 ($t_{1/2}$ = 6.5 min) can be produced via irradiation of natural barium target material; however, its short half-life precludes its direct use for PET imaging. Cerium-134 ($t_{1/2}$ = 3.2 d) decays into ^{134}La, permitting an in vivo generator configuration where ^{134}Ce can be labelled to a targeting vector, with ^{134}La progeny used for PET imaging. Production involves irradiating ^{nat}La metal, with yields of 59 MBq·µA^{-1}·h^{-1} at proton energies of 62.1–72.1 MeV [52]. A subsequent production route utilized 100 MeV protons to irradiate ^{nat}La metal, producing over 3 Ci of ^{134}Ce with a 100 µA irradiation for 30 h.

Chemical purification can be performed with Bio-Rad AGMP-1 resin, where ^{134}Ce is eluted with 0.05 M HNO$_3$. ^{134}Ce can then be used to label DTPA in its 3+ oxidation state, allowing ^{134}Ce to act as a ^{225}Ac imaging surrogate, while ^{134}Ce can label 3,4,3-LI(1,2-HOPO) in its 4+ oxidation state and act as a ^{227}Th imaging surrogate [53,54]. A PET imaging phantom study investigating the spatial resolution and recovery coefficient of ^{134}La was found to be inferior and similar to ^{18}F, respectively [52].

Strengths of ^{134}Ce/^{134}La include the 3.2 d half-life of ^{134}Ce, which permits PET imaging at extended time points after injection to track ^{225}Ac and ^{227}Th radiopharmaceuticals; the significant 63.6% positron branching ratio of ^{134}La [9]; the stable ^{134}Ba decay daughter of ^{134}La; and the ability for ^{134}Ce to act as a surrogate for both ^{225}Ac and ^{227}Th. Limitations include a scarcity of production facilities capable of achieving a ~100 MeV proton beam energy; the high positron emission energy of ^{134}La, which would result in lower PET spatial resolution; unavoidable co-produced radionuclidic impurities (^{139}Ce, t$_{1/2}$ = 137.6); and the potential for in vivo ^{134}La daughter redistribution following decay from ^{134}Ce that could blur PET imaging [9,39].

3.4. Actinium-226 (SPECT)

Actinium-226 (t$_{1/2}$ = 29.4 h) can be produced via high-energy proton spallation of a uranium carbide target or lower-energy proton bombardment of ^{226}Ra (t$_{1/2}$ = 1600 y) target material. This involved bombarding a uranium carbide target with 480 MeV protons, with ^{226}Ac separated using isotope separation online. This approach yielded 33.8 ± 2.7 MBq ^{226}Ac for imaging purposes with high radionuclidic purity [55].

An alternative production route could employ ^{226}Ra target material and the ^{226}Ra(p,n)^{226}Ac nuclear reaction on a lower energy proton cyclotron [9,55–57].

A phantom assembly with rods between 0.85 and 1.7 mm in diameter and a microSPECT/CT system was used to assess resolution using a high-energy ultra-high resolution (HEUHR) collimator and an extra ultra-high sensitivity (UHS) collimator. The primary 158 keV and 230 keV gamma photopeaks were reconstructed, with the 158 keV photopeak images demonstrating slightly better contrast recovery. For resolution, as depicted in Figure 3, the HEUHR collimator resolved all rods, while the UHS collimator could only resolve rods >1.3 mm and >1.5 mm for the 158 keV and 230 keV photopeaks, respectively [55]. This demonstrated the feasibility of using ^{226}Ac as a SPECT imaging surrogate for ^{225}Ac.

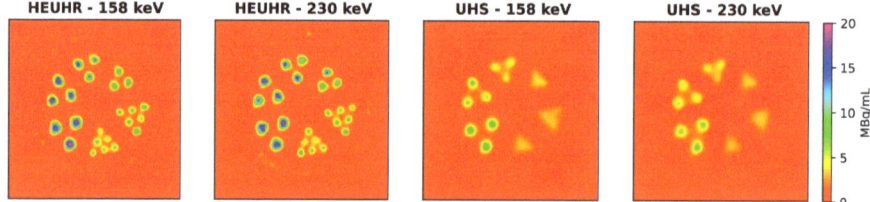

Figure 3. Inter-rod contrast measurements were used to assess image resolution from ^{226}Ac SPECT images acquired using two collimators. Figure from Koniar et al. [55].

Advantages of ^{226}Ac include its relatively long 29.4 h half-life compared to ^{132}La and ^{133}La, permitting imaging at extended time points, and its identical chemical properties to ^{225}Ac. Limitations include challenges associated with routine irradiation of hazardous ^{226}Ra target material, significant β$^-$ co-emissions that would increase patient dose, and its decay to β$^-$ emitting ^{226}Th (t$_{1/2}$ = 30 min), which further decays via multiple alpha and β$^-$ emitting progeny before stabilizing at ^{206}Pb [9].

4. Theranostic Imaging Surrogates Proposed for Lead-212

Lead-212 (t$_{1/2}$ = 10.6 h) has cultivated a significant interest for TAT due to its payload of one alpha and two β$^-$ particles in its decay chain and the rapid decay of its progeny to stable ^{208}Pb. A recent study using a ^{212}Pb somatostatin analogue demonstrated a significant antitumor effect in patients with metastatic neuroendocrine tumors, and additional radiopharmaceuticals are under development to treat other cancers [1,58–62]. Production of ^{212}Pb involves synthesizing its parent radionuclide, ^{228}Th ($t_{1/2}$ = 1.9 y), via ^{226}Ra irradiation in a nuclear reactor or high-energy proton spallation of ^{232}Th target material. ^{212}Pb can then be extracted in a convenient generator setup from ^{228}Th or one of its intermediate progeny, ^{224}Ra ($t_{1/2}$ = 3.6 d) [12,63–67].

Previous clinical trials have employed imaging techniques with conventional radiometals such as ^{68}Ga [58]. While direct SPECT imaging of ^{212}Pb can be performed using its 239 keV (44%) gamma emissions [9], it is desirable to have an imaging surrogate that can be used for research owing to the limited supply of ^{212}Pb and to provide the most accurate pre-therapy scans to assess patient eligibility for ^{212}Pb TAT radiopharmaceuticals. While no positron-emitting Pb isotopes are suitable for use as ^{212}Pb imaging surrogates, multiple gamma-ray emitters exist, with ^{203}Pb being a prime candidate for SPECT imaging.

Lead-203 (SPECT)

Lead-203 ($t_{1/2}$ = 51.9 h) emits X-rays and a primary 279 keV (81%) gamma photon that can be used for SPECT imaging. ^{203}Pb has been synthesized via ^{203}Tl(p,n)^{203}Pb, ^{203}Tl(d,2n)^{203}Pb, and ^{205}Tl(p,3n)^{203}Pb nuclear reactions on cyclotrons [21,45,63,64,68–71]. Natural thallium metal can be used as a target material; however, significant precautions must be taken owing to the high toxicity of Tl, and its low thermal conductivity and melting point (304 °C) that makes it prone to melt or sublime under intense heat of a cyclotron beam. Natural Tl metal has been used as a target material, with one technique bombarding ^{nat}Tl at 25–26 MeV, producing up to 21 GBq ^{203}Pb five days after end of bombardment [61]. However, irradiating ^{nat}Tl produces significant activities of ^{201}Pb ($t_{1/2}$ = 9.3 h), which must be permitted to decay significantly to achieve a ^{203}Pb product with high radionuclidic impurity. ^{203}Pb can be produced at lower proton energies using natural or isotopically enriched ^{203}Tl and the ^{203}Tl(p,n)^{203}Pb nuclear reaction ^{63,71}, with one process yielding up to 138.7 ± 5.1 MBq ^{203}Pb [64]. However, yields are limited due to the low nuclear reaction cross-section in this energy window [45]. Alternatively, isotopically enriched ^{205}Tl can be irradiated at 23–24 MeV proton energies to produce ^{203}Pb via the ^{205}Tl(p,3n)^{203}Pb reaction. This produces significant activities of ^{203}Pb (>12 GBq at the end of purification) with a high radionuclidic purity (>99.9%) made possible by the near absence of ^{203}Tl and its resulting ^{201}Pb co-production ^{21,63}. Enriched ^{203}Tl can also be bombarded with deuterons to produce ^{203}Pb via the ^{203}Tl(d,2n)^{203}Pb reaction; however, this production route has a lower maximum cross-section compared to the ^{205}Tl(p,3n)^{203}Pb reaction, and ^{203}Tl (29.5% natural isotopic abundance) is more expensive to enrich than ^{205}Tl (70.5% natural isotopic abundance).

^{203}Pb can be separated using ion exchange resins such as Pb resin, carboxymethyl resin, and Dowex-1X8 anion exchange resin. This can yield a concentrated ^{203}Pb product in [^{203}Pb]PbCl$_2$ or [^{203}Pb]Pb(OAc)$_2$, with direct and rapid room temperature radiolabeling of [^{203}Pb]Pb(OAc)$_2$ using chelators such as DOTA, PSC, and TCMC. Radiolabeling achieves very high molar activities, and ^{203}Pb chelate complexes have been shown to be highly stable in human serum up to 120 h [21,63,64,69,70].

Phantom imaging of ^{203}Pb has been performed, with imaging spatial-resolution results comparable to ^{99m}Tc for 1.6–4.8 mm diameter fillable rod regions [72]. In vivo preclinical and clinical SPECT imaging of uncomplexed and chelated ^{203}Pb has been performed [71,73]. Studies have included $^{203/212}$Pb-labeled PSMA and gastrin-releasing peptide receptor-targeting agents for imaging and radiotherapy of prostate-cancer-bearing mice [60,61,74,75], and $^{203/212}$Pb-labeled anti-melanin antibodies and melanocortin subtype 1 receptor targeting ligands for imaging and therapy of melanoma-bearing mice [59,72,73,76–79]. As shown in Figure 4, a PSMA-targeting ^{203}Pb agent, [^{203}Pb]Pb-CA012, exhibited a comparable biodistribution to [^{177}Lu]Lu-PSMA 617 with high tumor uptake relative to other tissues [74].

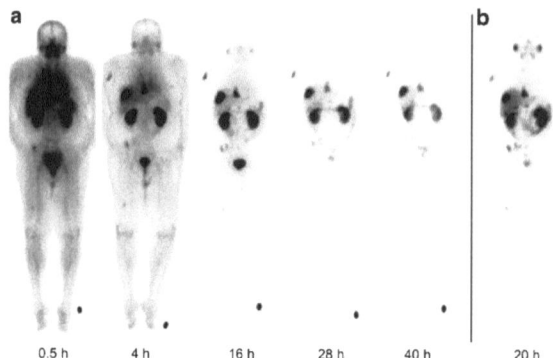

Figure 4. Planar scans of a PSMA targeting ligand [^{203}Pb]Pb-CA012 (**a**), versus a [^{177}Lu]Lu-PSMA 617 treatment scan (**b**). Figure from dos Santos et al. [74].

Strengths of ^{203}Pb include its relatively long 51.9 h half-life, which permits imaging at extended time points to inform ^{212}Pb TAT dosimetry; its relatively clean X-ray and gamma photon emission spectrum that enables SPECT imaging using a low or high-energy collimator; its ability to rapidly and stably radiolabel targeting vectors under mild chemical conditions at room temperature (similar to ^{212}Pb); and established production processes that provide ^{203}Pb with high radionuclidic purity in yields suitable for multiple patients per production run. Limitations include risks associated with preparing and irradiating highly toxic thallium targets and potential uncertainties with using ^{203}Pb pharmacokinetic data for ^{212}Pb therapy planning due to the release of ^{212}Bi progeny during ^{212}Pb decay [80].

5. Theranostic Imaging Surrogates Proposed for Radium-223/224

Radium-223 ($t_{1/2}$ = 11.4 d) is used as an alpha therapy for men with bone-metastatic castration-resistant prostate cancer. It works as a calcium-mimetic by accumulating in and irradiating osteoblastic lesions, while sparing most surrounding healthy tissue [81]. It is the only FDA-proved alpha-particle-emitting radiopharmaceutical (Xofigo®) and has been used to treat over 18,000 patients since 2013 [82]. However, unlike targeted alpha therapy, ^{223}Ra is currently administered as a [^{223}Ra]RaCl$_2$ salt in an aqueous buffer without a chelator or biological-targeting agent. Therefore, the established clinical efficacy and safety of ^{223}Ra makes it an attractive TAT candidate [82]. Similarly, ^{224}Ra ($t_{1/2}$ = 3.6 d) has been employed in a dual targeting strategy with ^{212}Pb, where ^{224}Ra accumulates at primary bone cancer sites or bone metastases, while extra-skeletal metastases can be targeted with a ^{212}Pb-labeled cancer-specific vector [83,84]. [^{224}Ra]RaCl$_2$ (marketed as ^{224}SpondylAT® (Eckert & Ziegler, Berlin, Germany) has also been used to treat bone and joint disease, ankylosing spondylitis [85], while ^{224}Ra is also under investigation for a novel brachytherapy called diffusing alpha-emitter radiation therapy (DaRT). In DaRT, ^{224}Ra-infused seeds are inserted into solid tumors, which are then irradiated with alpha emissions released during the diffusion and subsequent decay cascade of its ^{220}Rn progeny [86–95]. Both ^{223}Ra and ^{224}Ra are currently produced in significant activities as by-products and decay daughters of neutron irradiation of ^{226}Ra in a nuclear reactor. With proven purification techniques, this positions these radionuclides well for TAT [67,96,97].

^{223}Ra has recently been stably complexed with the chelator macropa, where a [^{223}Ra]Ra–macropa complex exhibited rapid clearance and low ^{223}Ra bone absorption, suggesting in vivo stability. This has opened the possibility of using ^{223}Ra complexed using functionalized chelators to target metastases beyond the bone, similar to other radionuclides used in targeted alpha therapy [82,98].

While ^{223}Ra possesses several gamma emissions within an energy window suitable for SPECT imaging (^{223}Ra: 269 keV, (13%); 154 keV (6%); ^{224}Ra: 241 keV (4.1%)), the low intensity of these gamma photons would likely be insufficient to generate a high-quality

SPECT image when considering the relatively low injected therapeutic activity (~50 kBq/kg) injected [9,81]. Similarly, a relatively low injection activity of ^{224}Ra due to its 3.6 d half-life could complicate direct SPECT imaging. Therefore, an imaging surrogate is desirable to assess the viability of $^{223/224}$Ra radiopharmaceuticals, with ^{131}Ba emerging as a candidate.

Barium-131 (SPECT)

Barium-131 ($t_{1/2}$ = 11.5 d) decays via electron capture to ^{131}Cs ($t_{1/2}$ = 9.7 d) and subsequently to stable ^{131}Xe, emitting gamma rays suitable for SPECT imaging (496 keV (48%); 216 keV (20%); 124 keV (30%); 371 keV (14%)) [9]. Additionally, approaches designed to sequester Ra (nanoparticles, chelation via macropa or ligands based on the arene scaffold) [99,100] should be transferrable owing to the proven use of Ba as a non-radioactive surrogate for Ra [101]. Therefore, the favorable imaging emissions of ^{131}Ba compared to other Ba radionuclides (^{135m}Ba, ^{133m}Ba), and the similar half-life and chemistry of ^{131}Ba to $^{223/224}$Ra positions ^{131}Ba as a promising surrogate to track in vivo $^{223/224}$Ra biodistribution.

^{131}Ba can be produced via neutron irradiation of isotopically enriched ^{130}Ba (natural abundance = 0.1%) in a nuclear reactor, which would co-produce significant activities of ^{133}Ba [45,102]. Alternatively, ^{131}Ba can be produced via proton irradiation of natural cesium target material in a cyclotron via the ^{133}Cs(p,3n)^{133}Ba nuclear reaction with a small ^{133}Ba contamination (0.01%) at beam energies of 27.5 MeV [45,101]. A 4 h irradiation yielded 190 ± 26 MBq ^{131}Ba, and an SR resin was used to separate ^{131}Ba from the Cs target material. ^{131}Ba was subsequently successfully radiolabeled to macropa, and exhibited stability in human serum [101].

SPECT imaging was performed in a cylindrical syringe, which enabled visualization of the radionuclide distribution. However, image quality was limited due to artifacts caused by the higher energy gamma photon emissions. As highlighted in Figure 5, small animal SPECT/CT was performed with [^{131}Ba]Ba(NO$_3$)$_2$, showing ^{131}Ba accumulation within the entire skeleton 1 h post-injection, which was still present 24 h after injection. Additional SPECT imaging was performed with [^{131}Ba]Ba-macropa, with rapid clearance observed through the intestines and gallbladder [101]. This demonstrated the feasibility of using ^{131}Ba as a SPECT imaging surrogate for $^{223/224}$Ra.

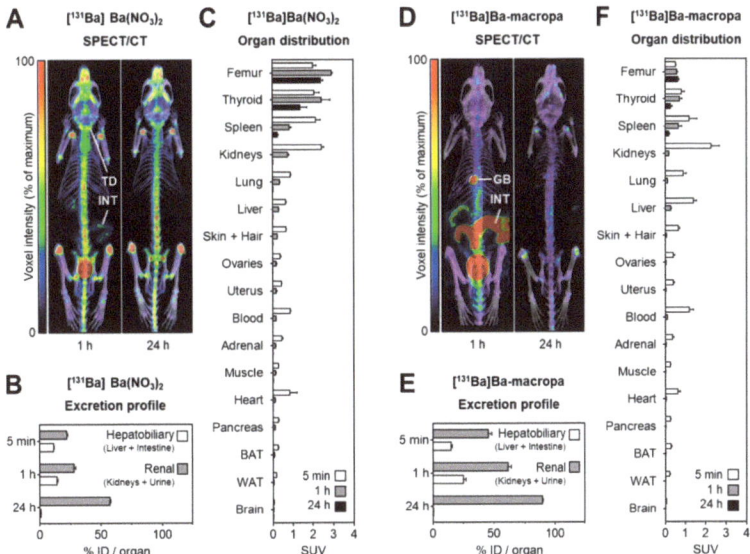

Figure 5. (**A**) SPECT/CT images of [^{131}Ba]Ba(NO$_3$)$_2$; (**B**,**C**) excretion profile and organ distribution of [^{131}Ba]Ba(NO$_3$)$_2$; (**D**) SPECT/CT images of [^{131}Ba]Ba-macropa; and (**E**,**F**) excretion profile and organ distribution of [^{131}Ba]Ba-macropa [101].

Advantages of ^{131}Ba include its relatively long half-life, which is similar to ^{223}Ra, permitting imaging at extended time points; the ability to sequester ^{131}Ba in the macropa chelator similar to ^{223}Ra; and established ^{131}Ba production routes. Limitations include higher energy gamma photon emissions, which increase unintended patient dose and can cause image artifacts. The presence of co-produced ^{133}Ba may also require additional dosimetric analysis. Additionally, the decay of ^{131}Ba to ^{131}Cs with X-ray emissions adds a suboptimal patient radioactive dose compared to an imaging radionuclide with direct decay to stable progeny. Finally, further improvements in the cyclotron production route would be required to synthesize enough activity for multiple patients in a single batch.

6. Theranostic Imaging Surrogates Proposed for Astatine-211

Astatine-211 ($t_{1/2}$ = 7.2 h) has garnered interest for TAT owing to its decay to either ^{207}Bi ($t_{1/2}$ = 31.6 y) via alpha emission or to ^{211}Pb via electron capture followed by alpha decay to stable ^{207}Pb [9]. Therefore, each ^{211}At decay yields one alpha particle. The ^{211}At decay chain also emits few high-energy gamma photons, which avoids excess radiation dose [8]. ^{211}At can be produced in medium-energy alpha cyclotrons using bismuth target material and the ^{209}Bi(α,2n)^{211}At nuclear reaction or via heavy ion irradiation and the ^{209}Bi(^{7}Li,5n)^{211}Rn reaction, where ^{211}At is obtained via decay of its longer-lived parent ^{211}Rn ($t_{1/2}$ = 14.6 h) in a generator configuration [8,103,104]. Production yields of up to 6.6 GBq have been reported, which would be sufficient for clinical radiopharmaceutical production for several patients and distribution several hours from the production site [8,105].

^{211}At was initially investigated for treating thyroid disorders and is currently being evaluated in clinical trials for multiple myeloma, leukemia, myelodysplastic syndromes, thyroid cancer, and malignant pheochromocytoma [106]. While direct SPECT imaging of ^{211}At is possible using the X-rays emitted during ^{211}At decay to ^{211}Po, it is desirable to have an imaging surrogate to perform pre-therapy assessment scans and research, owing to the limited supply and short half-life of ^{211}At that generally precludes its use at facilities located more than several hours from a production site. Several candidates exist for use as ^{211}At diagnostic imaging surrogates: chemically identical ^{209}At, or chemically similar ^{123}I, ^{124}I and ^{131}I.

6.1. Iodine-123 (SPECT)

Iodine-123 ($t_{1/2}$ = 13.2 h) decays via electron capture to near-stable ^{123}Te, and is commonly used in nuclear medicine and research of various malignancies and biological processes, including thyroid diseases and tumor imaging [107]. Its X-ray emissions and primary gamma photopeak of 159 keV (83.6%) are well suited for SPECT imaging [9].

^{123}I is primarily produced via the ^{124}Xe(p,2n)^{123}I nuclear reaction using a highly enriched ^{124}Xe gas target, which enables ^{123}I production with a high yield and radionuclidic purity. The subsequent ^{123}I product is commercially available in dilute NaOH solutions [108,109].

Strengths of ^{123}I include its favorable emission spectrum for SPECT imaging, similar half-life relative to ^{211}At, and commercial availability. Limitations include hazards associated with volatile radioactive products, the lower image quality of SPECT images to PET imaging, and the low natural abundance (0.095%) of ^{124}Xe target material.

6.2. Iodine-124 (PET)

Iodine-124 ($t_{1/2}$ = 4.2 d) undergoes positron decay to stable ^{124}Te and is employed for PET imaging studies. Its relatively long half-life allows extended radiosynthesis, quantitative imaging over several days, and distribution to sites far from production facilities [9]. ^{124}I is typically produced using isotopically enriched ^{124}Te and the ^{124}Te(d,2n)^{124}I or ^{124}Te(p,n)^{124}I nuclear reactions [110,111]. Applications in nuclear medicine and research have been extensive, including thyroid and parathyroid imaging, studies of neurotransmitter receptors, and monoclonal antibody imaging in cancer [110].

Strengths of ^{124}I include its long half-life that eases logistics and allows imaging at extended time points. Limitations include hazards associated with volatile radioactive products; a relatively low positron branching ratio (22.7%); relatively high average positron emission energy (E_{mean} = 820 keV) that results in a lower spatial resolution compared to other PET radionuclides; and co-emitted gamma rays (603 keV (63%), 1691 keV (11%)) that increase dose and shielding requirements [9].

6.3. Iodine-131 (SPECT)

Iodine-131 ($t_{1/2}$ = 8.0 d) undergoes β^- decay to stable ^{131}Xe, and similar to ^{123}I and ^{124}I, it is primarily used for treating thyroid malignancies [107]. ^{131}I can be produced in a nuclear reactor by irradiating either ^{130}Te or uranium targets [112].

Strengths of ^{131}I include its 8 d half-life that permits imaging at extended time points, commercial availability, and primary 364 keV (81.5%) gamma emission that is well suited for SPECT imaging. However, limitations include hazards associated with volatile radioactive products and significant β^- emissions that would increase patient dose [9].

6.4. Astatine-209 (SPECT)

Astatine-209 ($t_{1/2}$ = 5.4 h) decays via alpha emissions (4%) to ^{205}Bi ($t_{1/2}$ = 14.9 d) followed by decay to stable ^{205}Pb, or via electron capture (96%) to ^{209}Po ($t_{1/2}$ = 124 y). During decay to ^{209}Po, X-rays and gamma emissions (545 keV (91.0%), 195 keV (22.6%), and 239 keV (12.4%)) enable SPECT imaging. ^{209}At can be produced via high-energy proton spallation of a uranium carbide target, followed by online surface ionization and A = 213 isobars separation. This can yield ^{209}At in activities on the order of 10^2 MBq [113]. Subsequent chemical purification employs a Te column to obtain purified ^{209}At [113,114]. As shown in Figure 6, subsequent studies using ^{209}At for phantom imaging demonstrated that image reconstruction with ^{209}At X-ray emissions was superior to using its gamma emissions [114]. Additionally, in vivo imaging measurements of ^{209}At uptake in mice matched ex vivo measurements within 10%. This demonstrated the potential of using ^{209}At to accurately determine astatine biodistributions [114].

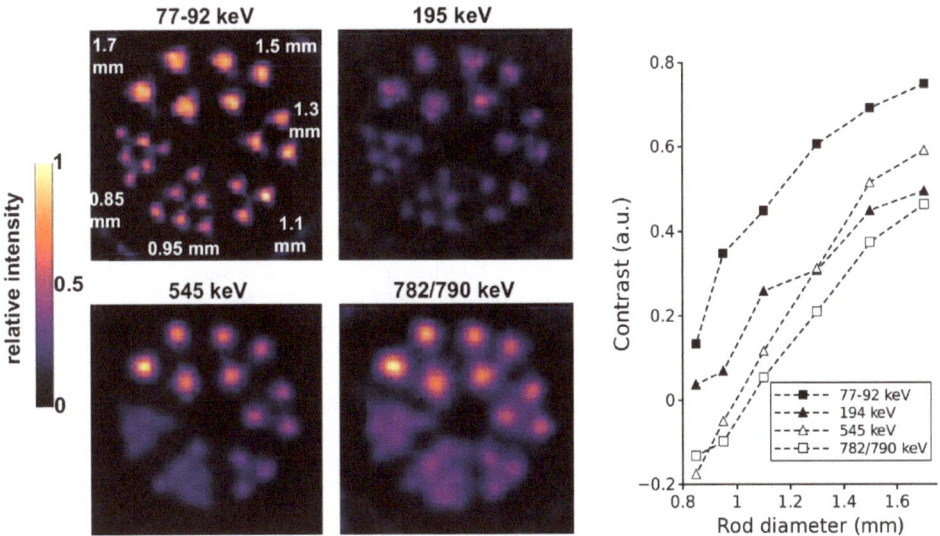

Figure 6. SPECT images and inter-rod contrast data for a phantom containing ^{209}At [114].

Strengths include identical chemistry to ^{211}At, which would give more certainty to ^{209}At pharmacokinetic data. Limitations include alpha emissions in ^{209}At decay that would require dosimetric evaluation; numerous high-energy gamma rays that complicate shielding and increase patient dose; the need to consider longer-lived ^{205}Bi in dosimetry evaluations; and production/logistical challenges associated with distributing relatively short-lived ^{209}At from a limited number of facilities capable of high-energy proton spallation and separation of ^{211}At from actinide targets [8].

7. Theranostic Imaging Surrogates Proposed for Thorium-227

Thorium-227 ($t_{1/2}$ = 18.7 d) decays via alpha emission to ^{223}Ra and can be harvested from a generator containing ^{227}Ac ($t_{1/2}$ = 21.8 y) that is produced via nuclear reactor irradiation of ^{226}Ra [115]. Thorium can be complexed with octadentate 3,2-hydroxypyridinone (3,2-HOPO) chelators attached to biological-targeting vectors [115]. Ongoing clinical studies involving ^{227}Th TAT include targeting tumors expressing human epidermal growth factor receptor 2 (HER2), PSMA, mesothelin (MSLN), and CD22 [116]. ^{227}Th does emit a 236 keV (12.9%) gamma photon that would be suitable for SPECT imaging. However, the long half-life of ^{227}Th relative to other TAT radionuclides would likely result in a low injected therapeutic activity, which could be insufficient for direct imaging [9]. Therefore, an imaging surrogate to assess ^{227}Th radiopharmaceutical pharmacokinetics is desirable, with the ^{134}Ce/^{134}La PET imaging pair showing promise (see Section 3.3). A significant uncertainty of using any theranostic imaging pair with ^{227}Th involves its long-lived ^{223}Ra progeny, which has the potential for substantial redistribution and alpha irradiation of healthy tissue after decay from ^{227}Th. This would significantly complicate direct comparisons between imaging and inferred therapeutic dosimetry and require further study.

8. Theranostic Imaging Surrogates Proposed for Terbium-149

Terbium-149 ($t_{1/2}$ = 4.1 h) is a unique radionuclide for TAT. It emits low-energy alpha particles with a short tissue range and decays via several daughter radionuclides to stable ^{145}Nd and ^{141}Pr, without any subsequent alpha emissions [9]. This absence of alpha-emitting progeny is regarded as a potential strength for ^{149}Tb TAT. ^{149}Tb is produced via high-energy proton spallation of a tantalum target followed by online isotope separation or ^{3}He bombardment of a ^{151}Eu target [19,20,117,118]. 100 MBq of ^{149}Tb was obtained in a solution suitable for preclinical applications and successfully labeled to a DOTANOC targeting vector [118]. While PET images were successfully obtained using [^{149}Tb]Tb-DOTANOC in a mouse model, ^{149}Tb possesses a relatively low positron branching ratio (21%) and relatively high positron emission energy (E_{mean} = 805 keV). These physical factors could present challenges to obtaining high-quality clinical PET images. Additionally, due to limited production and the resulting extreme scarcity of ^{149}Tb, imaging surrogates would be helpful research tools to evaluate its potential for TAT. Two surrogate candidates are ^{155}Tb and ^{152}Tb.

8.1. Terbium-155 (SPECT)

Terbium-155 ($t_{1/2}$ = 5.3 d) decays via electron capture to stable ^{155}Gd, with X-ray and gamma-ray emissions including 87 keV (32%), 105 keV (25%), 180 keV (7.5%), and 262 keV (5%) [9]. ^{155}Tb can be produced via the ^{156}Gd(p,2n)^{155}Tb reaction at 23 MeV, or the ^{155}Gd(p,n)^{155}Tb reaction at 10 MeV [119]. The ^{156}Gd(p,2n)^{155}Tb has higher demonstrated production yields (up to 1.7 GBq); however, it has a lower radionuclidic purity compared to the final product of the ^{155}Gd(p,n)^{155}Tb reaction (200 MBq yield). Subsequently, phantom and in vivo SPECT/CT studies were successfully performed with [^{155}Tb]Tb-DOTATOC, demonstrating a similar image quality to ^{111}In [119,120].

Advantages of ^{155}Tb include its accessible production routes that can synthesize multi-patient activities per run, decay to stable ^{155}Gd, and its long half-life that enables long-duration imaging. Limitations include relatively low imaging performance compared to other diagnostic radionuclides, such as PET emitters.

8.2. Terbium-152 (PET)

Terbium-152 ($t_{1/2}$ = 17.5 h) decays via positron emission to near-stable ^{152}Gd with a positron branching ratio of 20.3% and an average positron energy of 1140 keV [121]. Several primary co-emitted gamma rays include 344 keV (63.5%), 271 keV (9.5%), 586 keV (9.2%), and 779 keV (5.5%). ^{152}Tb synthesis is extremely limited, with the existing production route involving high-energy proton spallation of a tantalum target at 1.4 GeV and online isotope separation [122]. Following chemical separation, phantom studies revealed increased image noise due to the smaller positron branching ratio of ^{152}Tb, and subsequently [^{152}Tb]Tb-DOTANOC was administered to a patient and used to acquire PET scans [121].

Advantages of ^{152}Tb include a relatively long half-life permitting imaging at extended time points and its decay to near-stable ^{152}Gd. Limitations include the scarcity of facilities capable of achieving proton energies for production, the higher average positron emission energy, and significant co-emitted gamma rays that increase the radioactive dose.

9. Summary and Outlook for Alpha-Emitter Imaging Surrogates

As highlighted in this article, multiple SPECT and PET imaging surrogates have demonstrated the potential to enhance clinical TAT applications and research. Table 1 presents a summary of proposed theranostic imaging surrogates for alpha emitters, along with their properties and production status.

Table 1. Summary of prominent TAT radionuclides and their proposed theranostic SPECT and PET imaging surrogates.

Alpha Emitter	Proposed Imaging Surrogate	Half-Life	Key Decay Progeny	Key Imaging Emissions	Primary Production Routes	Production Status and References
^{225}Ac		9.9 d	^{211}Fr, ^{217}At, ^{213}Bi, ^{213}Po, ^{209}Tl, ^{209}Pb, ^{209}Bi (stable)	γ: 100 keV (1%), 218 keV (11.4%)	^{229}Th generator, ^{226}Ra proton/photonuclear reactions, ^{232}Th spallation	Routine production [31–34]
	^{133}La	3.9 h	^{133}Ba	β$^+$: 460 keV (mean), 7.2%	^{135}Ba or ^{134}Ba proton irradiation	Research [40–42]
	^{132}La	4.8 h	^{132}Ba (stable)	β$^+$: 1290 keV (mean), 42.1%	^{132}Ba proton irradiation	Research [48–50]
	^{134}Ce/^{134}La	3.2 d/ 6.5 min	^{134}Ba (stable)	β$^+$: 1217 keV (mean), 63.6%	High-energy ^{139}La proton irradiation	Research [52–54]
	^{226}Ac	29.4 h	^{226}Ra, ^{226}Th, ^{222}Ra, ^{218}Rn, ^{214}Po, ^{210}Pb, ^{210}Bi, ^{210}Po, ^{206}Pb (stable)	γ: 230 keV (26.9%), 158 keV (17.5%)	^{226}Ra proton irradiation	Research [55]
^{212}Pb		10.6 h	^{212}Bi, ^{212}Po, ^{208}Tl, ^{208}Pb (stable)	γ: 239 keV (44%)	^{228}Th generator	Routine production [12,63–67]
	^{203}Pb	51.9 h	^{203}Tl (stable)	γ: 279 keV (81%) X-ray: 73 keV (37%), 71 keV (22%)	^{205}Tl proton irradiation, ^{203}Tl proton or deuteron irradiation	Routine production [21,63,64,68–71]
^{223}Ra		11.4 d	^{219}Rn, ^{215}Po, ^{215}At, ^{211}Pb, ^{211}Bi, ^{211}Po, ^{207}Tl, ^{207}Pb (stable)	γ: 269 keV (13%), 154 keV (6%)	^{226}Ra nuclear reactor irradiation	Routine production [67,96,97]

Table 1. Cont.

Alpha Emitter	Proposed Imaging Surrogate	Half-Life	Key Decay Progeny	Key Imaging Emissions	Primary Production Routes	Production Status and References
^{224}Ra		3.6 d	^{220}Rn, ^{216}Po, ^{212}Pb, ^{212}Bi, ^{212}Po, ^{208}Tl, ^{208}Pb (stable)	γ: 241 keV (4%)	^{228}Th generator	Routine production [67,96,97]
	^{131}Ba	11.5 d	^{131}Cs	γ: 496 keV (48%), 124 keV (30%), 216 keV (20%), 371 keV (14%)	^{133}Cs proton irradiation	Research [101,102]
^{211}At		7.2 h	^{207}Bi, ^{211}Po, ^{207}Pb (stable)	X-ray: 79 keV (21%)	^{209}Bi alpha particle irradiation	Routine production [8,103–105]
	^{123}I	13.2 h	^{123}Te (near stable)	γ: 159 keV (83.6%)	^{124}Xe proton irradiation	Routine production [108,109]
	^{124}I	4.2 d	^{123}Te (stable)	β+: 820 keV (mean), 22.7%	^{124}Te proton or deuteron irradiation	Routine production [110,111]
	^{131}I	8.0 d	^{131}Xe (stable)	γ: 364 keV (89.6%)	^{130}Te or uranium nuclear reactor irradiation	Routine production [112]
	^{209}At	5.4 h	^{209}Po, ^{209}Bi, ^{205}Bi, ^{205}Pb, ^{205}Tl	γ: 545 keV (91%), 239 keV (12.4%), 195 keV (22.6%)	Proton spallation of uranium carbide	Research [113,114]
^{227}Th		18.7 d	^{223}Ra, ^{219}Rn, ^{215}Po, ^{215}At, ^{211}Pb, ^{211}Bi, ^{211}Po, ^{207}Tl, ^{207}Pb (stable)	γ: 235 keV (12.9%)	^{226}Ra nuclear reactor irradiation	Routine production [115]
	^{134}Ce/^{134}La	3.2 d/6.5 min	^{134}Ba (stable)	β+: 1217 keV (mean), 63.6%	High-energy ^{139}La proton irradiation	Research [52–54]
^{149}Tb		4.1 h	^{149}Gd, ^{149}Eu, ^{149}Sm (stable), ^{145}Eu, ^{145}Sm, ^{145}Pm, ^{145}Nd (stable)	β+: 720 keV (mean), 7.1% γ: 165 keV (26.4%)	^{151}Eu helium-3 bombardment, proton spallation of Ta	Research [19,20,117,118]
	^{155}Tb	5.3 d	^{155}Gd (stable)	γ: 87 keV (32%), 105 keV (25%), 180 keV (7.5%), and 262 keV (5%).	^{155}Gd proton irradiation	Research [119]
	^{152}Tb	17.5 h	^{152}Gd (near stable)	β+: 1140 keV (mean), 20.3%	Proton spallation of Ta	Research [122]

Production capabilities must be augmented to enable more patients and research efforts to benefit from TAT imaging surrogates. Existing medium-energy cyclotron facilities are well positioned to improve the supply chain of imaging surrogates such as ^{133}La, ^{203}Pb, and ^{155}Tb by adapting and optimizing established production techniques to the unique capabilities of each facility. A stable supply of isotopically enriched accelerator target material will be required to support growing production efforts for many of these radionuclides. Other imaging surrogates such as ^{226}Ra, ^{152}Tb, ^{209}At, and ^{134}Ce/^{134}La require high-energy accelerators, bombarding hazardous target material, and techniques such as mass separation to enable their production. While these surrogates have demonstrated research potential, their widespread deployment for radiopharmaceutical development and clinical application may be limited owing to the scarcity of facilities capable of their production.

Except for ^{149}Tb, which possesses a single alpha emission in its decay chain, most TAT radionuclides, including ^{225}Ac, ^{212}Pb, ^{223}Ra, ^{224}Ra, ^{227}Th, and ^{211}At, possess a cascade of decay progeny that are released from the original target site due to recoil energy and deposit additional alpha radiation in surrounding healthy tissues. While the highlighted imaging surrogates are well positioned to provide more accurate dosimetry data for the TAT parent radionuclide decay, there will be a degree of uncertainty regarding the dose from alpha-emitting decay progeny. This uncertainty will depend on the type of malignancy, internalization within targeted cells, and other factors within the disease microenvironment that influence the radiopharmaceutical pharmacokinetics. However, this limitation does not negate the improved accuracy of biodistribution dosimetry data conferred by using imaging surrogates matched to the TAT parent radionuclide, particularly when radionuclides are stably bound to their targeting vector. Therefore, TAT imaging surrogates have the potential to assist the preclinical development and clinical deployment of TAT radiopharmaceuticals and represent a significant improvement over conventional PET and SPECT imaging radionuclides currently paired with TAT.

10. Conclusions

Recent preclinical and clinical advances in targeted alpha therapy have spurred significant interest in utilizing alpha-emitting radiopharmaceuticals to treat metastatic cancers and other malignancies. Despite their strong potential, TAT radiopharmaceuticals suffer from an acute supply shortage of alpha-emitting radionuclides due to production constraints. This severely restricts the availability for patient therapy and slows the development of new TAT radiopharmaceuticals. Additionally, many alpha-emitting radionuclides do not possess radioactive emissions suitable for diagnostic imaging. This often leads to diagnostic radiopharmaceuticals being employed with suboptimally paired imaging radionuclides that possess different chemistries from their therapeutic counterpart, which can potentially result in different radiopharmaceutical biodistributions. Therefore, increasing the availability of SPECT and PET imaging TAT surrogates has strong potential to improve the accuracy of dosimetry and treatment tracking, and enhance TAT research output by using more economical and less potent diagnostic radionuclides for preclinical radiopharmaceutical development. Therefore, TAT imaging surrogates hold potential to improve the accuracy of diagnostic scans, equipping clinicians and researchers with more accurate biodistribution and dosimetry data that they can use to expedite the development and deployment of novel TAT radiopharmaceuticals.

Author Contributions: B.J.B.N. prepared the manuscript draft; B.J.B.N., J.W., J.D.A. and F.W. performed review and editing; and J.D.A. and F.W. provided supervision. All authors have read and agreed to the published version of the manuscript.

Funding: The authors would like to thank the Dianne and Irving Kipnes Foundation for supporting this work.

Data Availability Statement: Data sharing is not applicable.

Conflicts of Interest: The authors declare no conflict of interest.

References

1. Schultz, M.K.; Pouget, J.P.; Wuest, F.; Nelson, B.; Andersson, J.; Cheal, S.; Li, M.; Ianzini, F.; Sangeeta, R.; Graves, S.; et al. Radiobiology of Targeted Alpha Therapy. In *Nuclear Medicine and Molecular Imaging*; Signore, A., Ed.; Elsevier: Amsterdam, The Netherlands, 2022; pp. 380–403. [CrossRef]
2. Nelson, B.J.B.; Andersson, J.D.; Wuest, F. Targeted alpha therapy: Progress in radionuclide production, radiochemistry and applications. *Pharmaceutics* 2021, 13, 49. [CrossRef] [PubMed]
3. Sartor, O.; de Bono, J.; Chi, K.N.; Fizazi, K.; Herrmann, K.; Rahbar, K.; Tagawa, S.T.; Nordquist, L.T.; Vaishampayan, N.; El-Haddad, G.; et al. Lutetium-177–PSMA-617 for Metastatic Castration-Resistant Prostate Cancer. *NEJM* 2021, 385, 1091–1103. [CrossRef]

4. Strosberg, J.; El-Haddad, G.; Wolin, E.; Hendifar, A.; Yao, J.; Chasen, B.; Mittra, E.; Kunz, P.L.; Kulke, M.H.; Jacene, H.; et al. Phase 3 Trial of ^{177}Lu-Dotatate for Midgut Neuroendocrine Tumors. *NEJM* **2017**, *376*, 125–135. [CrossRef] [PubMed]
5. Garg, R.; Mills, K.; Allen, K.J.H.; Causey, P.; Perron, R.W.; Gendron, D.; Sanche, S.; Berman, J.W.; Gorny, M.K.; Dadachova, E. Comparison of various radioactive payloads for a human monoclonal antibody to glycoprotein 41 for elimination of HIV-infected cells. *Nucl. Med. Biol.* **2020**, *82–83*, 80–88. [CrossRef]
6. Elgqvist, J.; Frost, S.; Pouget, J.P.; Albertsson, P. The Potential and Hurdles of Targeted Alpha Therapy–Clinical Trials and Beyond. *Front. Oncol.* **2014**, *3*, 324. Available online: https://www.frontiersin.org/articles/10.3389/fonc.2013.00324 (accessed on 29 September 2023). [CrossRef] [PubMed]
7. Sollini, M.; Marzo, K.; Chiti, A.; Kirienko, M. The five "W"s and "How" of Targeted Alpha Therapy: Why? Who? What? Where? When? and How? *Rend. Lincei* **2020**, *31*, 231–247. [CrossRef]
8. Lindegren, S.; Albertsson, P.; Bäck, T.; Jensen, H.; Palm, S.; Aneheim, E. Realizing Clinical Trials with Astatine-211: The Chemistry Infrastructure. *Cancer Biother. Radiopharm.* **2020**, *35*, 425–436. [CrossRef]
9. Sonzogni, A.; Shu, B. Nudat 2.8 (Nuclear Structure and Decay Data). 2020. Available online: https://www.nndc.bnl.gov/nudat2/reCenter.jsp?z=56&n=77\T1\textgreater{} (accessed on 20 September 2023).
10. Bannik, K.; Madas, B.; Jarzombek, M.; Sutter, A.; Siemeister, G.; Mumberg, D.; Zitzmann-Kolbe, S. Radiobiological effects of the alpha emitter Ra-223 on tumor cells. *Sci. Rep.* **2019**, *9*, 18489. [CrossRef]
11. Morgenstern, A.; Apostolidis, C.; Kratochwil, C.; Sathekge, M.; Krolicki, L.; Bruchertseifer, F. An Overview of Targeted Alpha Therapy with [225]Actinium and [213]Bismuth. *Curr. Radiopharm.* **2018**, *11*, 200–208. [CrossRef]
12. Kokov, K.V.; Egorova, B.V.; German, M.N.; Klabukov, I.D.; Krasheninnikov, M.E.; Larkin-Kondrov, A.A.; Makoveeva, K.A.; Ovchinnikov, M.V.; Sidorova, M.V.; Chuvilin, D.Y. [212]Pb: Production Approaches and Targeted Therapy Applications. *Pharmaceutics* **2022**, *14*, 189. [CrossRef]
13. Abou, D.S.; Fears, A.; Summer, L.; Longtine, M.; Benabdallah, N.; Riddle, R.C.; Ulmert, D.; Michalski, J.; Wahl, R.L.; Chesner, D.; et al. Improved Radium-223 Therapy with Combination Epithelial Sodium Channel Blockade. *J. Nucl. Med.* **2021**, *62*, 1751–1758. [CrossRef] [PubMed]
14. Hosono, M.; Ikebuchi, H.; Nakamura, Y.; Yanagida, S.; Kinuya, S. Introduction of the targeted alpha therapy (with Radium-223) into clinical practice in Japan: Learnings and implementation. *Ann. Nucl. Med.* **2019**, *33*, 211–221. [CrossRef] [PubMed]
15. Mikalsen, L.T.G.; Kvassheim, M.; Stokke, C. Optimized SPECT Imaging of [224]Ra α-Particle Therapy by [212]Pb Photon Emissions. *J. Nucl. Med.* **2023**, *64*, 1131–1137. [CrossRef] [PubMed]
16. Watabe, T.; Kaneda-Nakashima, K.; Shirakami, Y.; Kadonaga, Y.; Ooe, K.; Wang, Y.; Haba, H.; Toyoshima, A.; Cardinale, J.; Giesel, F.L.; et al. Targeted α-therapy using astatine ([211]At)-labeled PSMA1, 5, and 6: A preclinical evaluation as a novel compound. *Eur. J. Nucl. Med. Mol. Imaging* **2023**, *50*, 849–858. [CrossRef] [PubMed]
17. Jang, A.; Kendi, A.T.; Johnson, G.B.; Halfdanarson, T.R.; Sartor, O. Targeted Alpha-Particle Therapy: A Review of Current Trials. *Int. J. Mol. Sci.* **2023**, *24*, 11626. [CrossRef] [PubMed]
18. Beyer, G.J.; Miederer, M.; Vranjes-Durić, S.; Comor, J.J.; Künzi, G.; Hartley, O.; Senekowitsch-Schmidtke, R.; Soloviev, D.; Buchegger, F. Targeted alpha therapy in vivo: Direct evidence for single cancer cell kill using [149]Tb-rituximab. *Eur. J. Nucl. Med. Mol. Imaging* **2004**, *31*, 547–554. [CrossRef]
19. Umbricht, C.A.; Köster, U.; Bernhardt, P.; Gracheva, N.; Johnston, K.; Schibli, R.; van der Meulen, N.P.; Müller, C. Alpha-PET for Prostate Cancer: Preclinical investigation using [149]Tb-PSMA-617. *Sci. Rep.* **2019**, *9*, 17800. [CrossRef]
20. Aliev, R.A.; Zagryadskiy, V.A.; Latushkin, S.T.; Moiseeva, A.N.; Novikov, A.N.; Unezhev, V.N.; Kazakov, A.G. Production of a Short-Lived Therapeutic α-Emitter [149]Tb by Irradiation of Europium by 63 MeV α-Particles. *At. Energy* **2021**, *129*, 337–340. [CrossRef]
21. Saini, S.; Bartels, J.L.; Appiah, J.K.; Rider, J.H.; Baumhover, N.; Schultz, M.K.; Lapi, S.E. Optimized Methods for the Production of High-Purity [203]Pb Using Electroplated Thallium Targets. *J. Nucl. Med.* **2023**, *64*, 1791–1797. [CrossRef]
22. Fani, M.; Del Pozzo, L.; Abiraj, K.; Mansi, R.; Tamma, M.L.; Cescato, R.; Waser, B.; Weber, W.A.; Reubi, J.C.; Maecke, H.R. PET of Somatostatin Receptor–Positive Tumors Using 64Cu- and 68Ga-Somatostatin Antagonists: The Chelate Makes the Difference. *J. Nucl. Med.* **2011**, *52*, 1110. [CrossRef]
23. Fani, M.; Braun, F.; Waser, B.; Beetschen, K.; Cescato, R.; Erchegyi, J.; Rivier, J.E.; Weber, W.A.; Maecke, H.R.; Reubi, J.C. Unexpected sensitivity of sst2 antagonists to N-Terminal radiometal modifications. *J. Nucl. Med.* **2012**, *53*, 1481. [CrossRef] [PubMed]
24. Busslinger, S.D.; Tschan, V.J.; Richard, O.K.; Talip, Z.; Schibli, R.; Müller, C. [225Ac]Ac-SibuDAB for Targeted Alpha Therapy of Prostate Cancer: Preclinical Evaluation and Comparison with [225Ac]Ac-PSMA-617. *Cancers* **2022**, *14*, 5651. [CrossRef] [PubMed]
25. King, A.P.; Gutsche, N.T.; Raju, N.; Fayn, S.; Baidoo, K.E.; Bell, M.M.; Olkowski, C.S.; Swenson, R.E.; Lin, F.I.; Sadowski, S.M. [225]Ac-Macropatate: A Novel α-Particle Peptide Receptor Radionuclide Therapy for Neuroendocrine Tumors. *J. Nucl. Med.* **2023**, *64*, 549. [CrossRef]
26. Yadav, M.P.; Ballal, S.; Sahoo, R.K.; Bal, C. Efficacy and safety of [225]Ac-DOTATATE targeted alpha therapy in metastatic paragangliomas: A pilot study. *Eur. J. Nucl. Med. Mol. Imaging* **2022**, *49*, 1595–1606. [CrossRef] [PubMed]
27. Kratochwil, C.; Bruchertseifer, F.; Giesel, F.L.; Weis, M.; Verburg, F.A.; Mottaghy, F.; Kopka, K.; Apostolidis, C.; Haberkorn, U.; Morgenstern, A. 225Ac-PSMA-617 for PSMA-targeted a-radiation therapy of metastatic castration-resistant prostate cancer. *J. Nucl. Med.* **2016**, *57*, 1941–1944. [CrossRef]

28. Rathke, H.; Bruchertseifer, F.; Kratochwil, C.; Keller, H.; Giesel, F.L.; Apostolidis, C.; Haberkorn, U.; Morgenstern, A. First patient exceeding 5-year complete remission after ^{225}Ac-PSMA-TAT. *Eur. J. Nucl. Med. Mol. Imaging* **2021**, *48*, 311–312. [CrossRef]
29. Zacherl, M.J.; Gildehaus, F.J.; Mittlmeier, L.; Böning, G.; Gosewisch, A.; Wenter, V.; Unterrainer, M.; Schmidt-Hegemann, N.; Belka, C.; Kretschmer, A.; et al. First Clinical Results for PSMA-Targeted α-Therapy Using ^{225}Ac-PSMA-I&T in Advanced-mCRPC Patients. *J. Nucl. Med.* **2021**, *62*, 669–674. [CrossRef] [PubMed]
30. Sathekge, M.; Bruchertseifer, F.; Vorster, M.; Lawal, I.O.; Knoesen, O.; Mahapane, J.; Davis, C.; Reyneke, F.; Maes, A.; Kratochwil, C. Predictors of overall and disease-free survival in metastatic castration-resistant prostate cancer patients receiving ^{225}Ac-PSMA-617 radioligand therapy. *J. Nucl. Med.* **2020**, *61*, 62–69. [CrossRef]
31. Zimmermann, R. Is Actinium Really Happening? *J. Nucl. Med.* **2023**, *64*, 1516–1518. [CrossRef]
32. Robertson, A.K.H.; Ramogida, C.F.; Schaffer, P.; Radchenko, V. Development of ^{225}Ac Radiopharmaceuticals: TRIUMF Perspectives and Experiences. *Curr. Radiopharm.* **2018**, *11*, 156–172. [CrossRef]
33. Engle, J. The Production of Ac-225. *Curr. Radiopharm.* **2018**, *11*, 173–179. [CrossRef] [PubMed]
34. Grimm, T.; Grimm, A.; Peters, W.; Zamiara, M. High-Purity Actinium-225 Production from Radium-226 using a Superconducting Electron Linac. *J. Med. Imaging Radiat. Sci.* **2019**, *50*, S12–S13. [CrossRef]
35. Augusto, R.S.; Smith, J.; Varah, S.; Paley, W.; Egoriti, L.; McEwen, S.; Day Goodacre, T.; Mildenberger, J.; Gottberg, A.; Trudel, A.; et al. Design and radiological study of the ^{225}Ac medical target at the TRIUMF-ARIEL proton-target station. *Radiat. Phys. Chem.* **2022**, *201*, 110491. [CrossRef]
36. Robertson, A.K.H.; Lobbezoo, A.; Moskven, L.; Schaffer, P.; Hoehr, C. Design of a thorium metal target for ^{225}Ac production at TRIUMF. *Instruments* **2019**, *3*, 18. [CrossRef]
37. Deblonde, G.J.P.; Zavarin, M.; Kersting, A.B. The coordination properties and ionic radius of actinium: A 120-year-old enigma. *Coord. Chem. Rev.* **2021**, *446*, 214130. [CrossRef]
38. Shannon, R.D. Revised effective ionic radii and systematic studies of interatomic distances in halides and chalcogenides. *Acta Crystallogr.* **1976**, *32*, 751–767. [CrossRef]
39. Nelson, B.J.B.; Andersson, J.D.; Wuest, F. Radiolanthanum: Promising theranostic radionuclides for PET, alpha, and Auger-Meitner therapy. *Nucl. Med. Biol.* **2022**, *110–111*, 59–66. [CrossRef]
40. Nelson, B.J.B.; Wilson, J.; Andersson, J.D.; Wuest, F. High yield cyclotron production of a novel $^{133/135}$La theranostic pair for nuclear medicine. *Sci. Rep.* **2020**, *10*, 22203. [CrossRef]
41. Nelson, B.J.B.; Ferguson, S.; Wuest, M.; Wilson, J.; Duke, M.J.M.; Richter, S.; Soenke-Jans, H.; Andersson, J.D.; Juengling, F.; Wuest, F. First in vivo and phantom imaging of cyclotron produced ^{133}La as a theranostic radionuclide for ^{225}Ac and ^{135}La. *J. Nucl. Med.* **2022**, *63*, 584–590. [CrossRef]
42. Brühlmann, S.A.; Kreller, M.; Pietzsch, H.J.; Kopka, K.; Mamat, C.; Walther, M.; Reissig, F. Efficient Production of the PET Radionuclide ^{133}La for Theranostic Purposes in Targeted Alpha Therapy Using the ^{134}Ba(p,2n)^{133}La Reaction. *Pharmaceuticals* **2022**, *15*, 1167. [CrossRef]
43. Yang, H.; Zhang, C.; Yuan, Z.; Rodriguez-Rodriguez, C.; Robertson, A.; Radchenko, V.; Perron, R.; Gendron, D.; Causey, P.; Gao, F.; et al. Synthesis and Evaluation of a Macrocyclic Actinium-225 Chelator, Quality Control and In Vivo Evaluation of ^{225}Ac-crown-αMSH Peptide. *Chem. Eur. J.* **2020**, *26*, 11435–11440. [CrossRef]
44. Thiele, N.A.; Brown, V.; Kelly, J.M.; Amor-Coarasa, A.; Jermilova, U.; MacMillan, S.N.; Nikolopoulou, A.; Ponnala, S.; Ramogida, C.F.; Robertson, A.K.H.; et al. An Eighteen-Membered Macrocyclic Ligand for Actinium-225 Targeted Alpha Therapy. *Angew. Chem. Int. Ed. Engl.* **2017**, *129*, 14904–14909. [CrossRef]
45. Rochman, D.; Koning, A.J.; Sublet, J.C.; Fleming, M.; Bauge, E.; Hilaire, S.; Romain, P.; Morillon, B.; Duarte, H.; Goriely, S.; et al. The TENDL Library: Hope, Reality, and Future. In Proceedings of the International Conference on Nuclear Data for Science and Technology, Bruges, Belgium, 11–16 September 2016; EDP Sciences: Les Ulis, France, 2017.
46. Ferguson, S.; Jans, H.S.; Wuest, M.; Riauka, T.; Wuest, F. Comparison of scandium-44 g with other PET radionuclides in preclinical PET phantom imaging. *EJNMMI Phys.* **2019**, *6*, 23. [CrossRef] [PubMed]
47. Levin, C.S.; Hoffman, E.J. Calculation of positron range and its effect on the fundamental limit of positron emission tomography system spatial resolution. *Phys. Med. Biol.* **1999**, *44*, 781–799. [CrossRef] [PubMed]
48. Aluicio-Sarduy, E.; Barnhart, T.E.; Weichert, J.; Hernandez, R.; Engle, J.W. Cyclotron-Produced ^{132}La as a PET Imaging Surrogate for Therapeutic ^{225}Ac. *J. Nucl. Med.* **2021**, *62*, 1012–1015. [CrossRef] [PubMed]
49. Aluicio-Sarduy, E.; Hernandez, R.; Olson, A.P.; Barnhart, T.E.; Cai, W.; Ellison, P.A.; Engle, J.W. Production and in vivo PET/CT imaging of the theranostic pair $^{132/135}$La. *Sci. Rep.* **2019**, *9*, 10658. [CrossRef] [PubMed]
50. Aluicio-Sarduy, E.; Thiele, N.A.; Martin, K.E.; Vaughn, B.A.; Devaraj, J.; Olson, A.P.; Barnhart, T.E.; Wilson, J.J.; Boros, E.; Engle, J.W. Establishing Radiolanthanum Chemistry for Targeted Nuclear Medicine Applications. *Chem. Eur. J.* **2020**, *26*, 1238–1242. [CrossRef] [PubMed]
51. Abel, E.P.; Clause, H.K.; Fonslet, J.; Nickles, R.J.; Severin, G.W. Half-lives of ^{132}La and ^{135}La. *Phys. Rev. C* **2018**, *97*, 034312. [CrossRef]
52. Lubberink, M.; Lundqvist, H.; Tolmachev, V. Production, PET performance and dosimetric considerations of ^{134}Ce/^{134}La, an Auger electron and positron-emitting generator for radionuclide therapy. *Phys. Med. Biol.* **2002**, *47*, 615–629. [CrossRef]

53. Bailey, T.A.; Mocko, V.; Shield, K.M.; An, D.D.; Akin, A.C.; Birnbaum, E.R.; Brugh, M.; Cooley, J.C.; Engle, J.W.; Fassbender, M.E.; et al. Developing the ^{134}Ce and ^{134}La pair as companion positron emission tomography diagnostic isotopes for ^{225}Ac and ^{227}Th radiotherapeutics. *Nat. Chem.* **2021**, *13*, 284–289. [CrossRef]
54. Bailey, T.A.; Lakes, A.; An, D.; Gauny, S.; Abergel, R.J. Biodistribution Studies of Chelated Ce-134/La-134 as Positron-Emitting Analogues of Alpha-Emitting Therapy Radionuclides. *J. Nucl. Med.* **2019**, *60* (Suppl. S1), 130. Available online: https://jnm.snmjournals.org/content/60/supplement_1/130 (accessed on 29 September 2023).
55. Koniar, H.; Rodríguez-Rodríguez, C.; Radchenko, V.; Yang, H.; Kunz, P.; Rahmim, A.; Uribe, C.; Schaffer, P. SPECT imaging of Ac-226 for radiopharmaceutical development: Performance evaluation as a theranostic isotope pair for Ac-225. *J. Nucl. Med.* **2022**, *63* (Suppl. S2), 2341. Available online: http://jnm.snmjournals.org/content/63/supplement_2/2341.abstract (accessed on 29 September 2023).
56. Nagatsu, K.; Suzuki, H.; Fukada, M.; Ito, T.; Ichinose, J.; Honda, Y.; Minegishi, K.; Higashi, T.; Zhang, M.R. Cyclotron production of ^{225}Ac from an electroplated ^{226}Ra target. *Eur. J. Nucl. Med. Mol. Imaging* **2021**, *49*, 279–289. [CrossRef] [PubMed]
57. Apostolidis, C.; Molinet, R.; McGinley, J.; Abbas, K.; Möllenbeck, J.; Morgenstern, A. Cyclotron production of Ac-225 for targeted alpha therapy. *Appl. Radiat. Isot.* **2005**, *62*, 383–387. [CrossRef] [PubMed]
58. Delpassand, E.S.; Tworowska, I.; Esfandiari, R.; Torgue, J.; Hurt, J.; Shafie, A.; Núñez, R. Targeted α-Emitter Therapy with ^{212}Pb-DOTAMTATE for the Treatment of Metastatic SSTR-Expressing Neuroendocrine Tumors: First-in-Humans Dose-Escalation Clinical Trial. *J. Nucl. Med.* **2022**, *63*, 1326. [CrossRef] [PubMed]
59. Li, M.; Zhang, X.; Quinn, T.P.; Lee, D.; Liu, D.; Kunkel, F.; Zimmerman, B.E.; McAlister, D.; Olewein, K.; Menda, Y.; et al. Automated cassette-based production of high specific activity [$^{203/212}$Pb]peptide-based theranostic radiopharmaceuticals for image-guided radionuclide therapy for cancer. *Appl. Radiat. Isot.* **2017**, *127*, 52–60. [CrossRef]
60. Banerjee, S.R.; Minn, I.; Kumar, V.; Josefsson, A.; Lisok, A.; Brummet, M.; Chen, J.; Kiess, A.P.; Baidoo, K.; Brayton, C.; et al. Preclinical evaluation of $^{203/212}$Pb-labeled low-molecular-weight compounds for targeted radiopharmaceutical therapy of prostate cancer. *J. Nucl. Med.* **2020**, *61*, 80–88. [CrossRef] [PubMed]
61. Li, M.; Sagastume, E.A.; Lee, D.; McAlister, D.; DeGraffenreid, A.J.; Olewine, K.R.; Graves, S.; Copping, R.; Mirzadeh, S.; Zimmerman, B.E.; et al. $^{203/212}$Pb Theranostic Radiopharmaceuticals for Image-guided Radionuclide Therapy for Cancer. *Curr. Med. Chem.* **2020**, *27*, 7003–7031. [CrossRef]
62. Yong, K.; Brechbiel, M. Application of ^{212}Pb for Targeted α-particle Therapy (TAT): Preclinical and Mechanistic Understanding through to Clinical Translation. *AIMS Med. Sci.* **2015**, *2*, 228–245. [CrossRef]
63. McNeil, B.L.; Robertson, A.K.H.; Fu, W.; Yang, H.; Hoehr, C.; Ramogida, C.F.; Schaffer, P. Production, purification, and radiolabeling of the ^{203}Pb/^{212}Pb theranostic pair. *EJNMMI Radiopharm. Chem.* **2021**, *6*, 6. [CrossRef]
64. McNeil, B.L.; Mastroianni, S.A.; McNeil, S.W.; Zeisler, S.; Kumlin, J.; Borjian, S.; McDonagh, A.W.; Cross, M.; Schaffer, P.; Ramogida, C.F. Optimized production, purification, and radiolabeling of the ^{203}Pb/^{212}Pb theranostic pair for nuclear medicine. *Sci. Rep.* **2023**, *13*, 10623. [CrossRef]
65. Li, R.G.; Stenberg, V.Y.; Larsen, R.H. An Experimental Generator for Production of High-Purity ^{212}Pb for Use in Radiopharmaceuticals. *J. Nucl. Med.* **2023**, *64*, 173–176. [CrossRef] [PubMed]
66. Artun, O. The investigation of the production of Ac-227, Ra-228, Th-228, and U-232 in thorium by particle accelerators for use in radioisotope power systems and nuclear batteries. *Nucl. Instrum. Methods Phys. Res. B* **2022**, *512*, 12–20. [CrossRef]
67. Radchenko, V.; Morgenstern, A.; Jalilian, A.R.; Ramogida, C.F.; Cutler, C.; Duchemin, C.; Hoehr, C.; Haddad, F.; Bruchertseifer, F.; Gausemel, H.; et al. Production and supply of α-particle-emitting radionuclides for targeted α-therapy. *J. Nucl. Med.* **2021**, *62*, 1495–1503. [CrossRef] [PubMed]
68. Horlock, P.L.; Thakur, M.L.; Watson, I.A. Cyclotron produced lead-203. *Postgrad. Med. J.* **1975**, *51*, 751–754. [CrossRef] [PubMed]
69. Nelson, B.J.B.; Wilson, J.; Schultz, M.K.; Andersson, J.D.; Wuest, F. High-yield cyclotron production of ^{203}Pb using a sealed ^{205}Tl solid target. *Nucl. Med. Biol.* **2023**, *116–117*, 108314. [CrossRef]
70. Nelson, B.; Wilson, J.; Andersson, J.; Wuest, F. O-18-High yield lead-203 cyclotron production using a thallium-205 sealed solid target for diagnostic SPECT imaging. *Nucl. Med. Biol.* **2022**, *114–115*, S12. [CrossRef]
71. Máthé, D.; Szigeti, K.; Hegedűs, N.; Horváth, I.; Veres, D.S.; Kovács, B.; Szűcs, Z. Production and in vivo imaging of ^{203}Pb as a surrogate isotope for in vivo ^{212}Pb internal absorbed dose studies. *Appl. Radiat. Isot.* **2016**, *114*, 1–6. [CrossRef]
72. Miao, Y.; Figueroa, S.D.; Fisher, D.R.; Moore, H.A.; Testa, R.F.; Hoffman, T.J.; Quinn, T.P. 203Pb-labeled α-melanocyte-stimulating hormone peptide as an imaging probe for melanoma detection. *J. Nucl. Med.* **2008**, *49*, 823–829. [CrossRef]
73. Jiao, R.; Allen, K.J.H.; Malo, M.E.; Yilmaz, O.; Wilson, J.; Nelson, B.J.B.; Wuest, F.; Dadachova, E. A Theranostic Approach to Imaging and Treating Melanoma with ^{203}Pb/^{212}Pb-Labeled Antibody Targeting Melanin. *Cancers* **2023**, *15*, 3856. [CrossRef]
74. Dos Santos, J.C.; Schäfer, M.; Bauder-Wüst, U.; Lehnert, W.; Leotta, K.; Morgenstern, A.; Kopka, K.; Haberkorn, U.; Mier, W.; Kratochwil, C. Development and dosimetry of ^{203}Pb/^{212}Pb-labelled PSMA ligands: Bringing "the lead" into PSMA-targeted alpha therapy? *Eur. J. Nucl. Med. Mol. Imaging* **2019**, *46*, 1081–1091. [CrossRef]
75. Okoye, N.; Rold, T.; Berendzen, A.; Zhang, X.; White, R.; Schultz, M.; Li, M.; Dresser, T.; Jurisson, S.; Quinn, T.; et al. Targeting the BB2 receptor in prostate cancer using a Pb-203 labeled peptide. *J. Nucl. Med.* **2017**, *58* (Suppl. S1), 321. Available online: http://jnm.snmjournals.org/content/58/supplement_1/321.abstract (accessed on 29 September 2023).
76. Miao, Y.; Hylarides, M.; Fisher, D.R.; Shelton, T.; Moore, H.; Wester, D.W.; Fritzberg, A.R.; Winkelmann, C.T.; Hoffman, T.; Quinn, T.P. Melanoma therapy via peptide-targeted {alpha}-radiation. *Clin. Cancer Res.* **2005**, *11*, 5616–5621. [CrossRef]

77. Yang, J.; Xu, J.; Cheuy, L.; Gonzalez, R.; Fisher, D.R.; Miao, Y. Evaluation of a Novel Pb-203-Labeled Lactam-Cyclized Alpha-Melanocyte-Stimulating Hormone Peptide for Melanoma Targeting. *Mol. Pharm.* **2019**, *16*, 1694–1702. [CrossRef] [PubMed]
78. Li, M.; Liu, D.; Lee, D.; Kapoor, S.; Gibson-Corley, K.N.; Quinn, T.P.; Sagastume, E.A.; Mott, S.L.; Walsh, S.A.; Acevedo, M.R.; et al. Enhancing the Efficacy of Melanocortin 1 Receptor-Targeted Radiotherapy by Pharmacologically Upregulating the Receptor in Metastatic Melanoma. *Mol. Pharm.* **2019**, *16*, 3904–3915. [CrossRef] [PubMed]
79. Allen, K.J.H.; Malo, M.E.; Jiao, R.; Dadachova, E. Targeting Melanin in Melanoma with Radionuclide Therapy. *Int. J. Mol. Sci.* **2022**, *23*, 9520. [CrossRef] [PubMed]
80. Li, M.; Baumhover, N.J.; Liu, D.; Cagle, B.S.; Boschetti, F.; Paulin, G.; Lee, D.; Dai, Z.; Obot, E.R.; Marks, B.M.; et al. Preclinical Evaluation of a Lead Specific Chelator (PSC) Conjugated to Radiopeptides for ^{203}Pb and ^{212}Pb-Based Theranostics. *Pharmaceutics* **2023**, *15*, 414. [CrossRef] [PubMed]
81. Parker, C.; Nilsson, S.; Heinrich, D.; Helle, S.I.; O'Sullivan, J.M.; Fosså, S.D.; Chodacki, A.; Wiechno, P.; Logue, J.; Seke, M.; et al. Alpha Emitter Radium-223 and Survival in Metastatic Prostate Cancer. *NEJM* **2013**, *369*, 213–223. [CrossRef] [PubMed]
82. Abou, D.S.; Thiele, N.A.; Gutsche, N.T.; Villmer, A.; Zhang, H.; Woods, J.J.; Baidoo, K.E.; Escorcia, F.E.; Wilson, J.J.; Thorek, D.L.J. Towards the stable chelation of radium for biomedical applications with an 18-membered macrocyclic ligand. *Chem. Sci.* **2021**, *12*, 3733–3742. [CrossRef]
83. Tornes, A.J.K.; Stenberg, V.Y.; Larsen, R.H.; Bruland, Ø.S.; Revheim, M.E.; Juzeniene, A. Targeted alpha therapy with the ^{224}Ra/^{212}Pb-TCMC-TP-3 dual alpha solution in a multicellular tumor spheroid model of osteosarcoma. *Front. Med.* **2022**, *9*, 1058863. [CrossRef]
84. Juzeniene, A.; Stenberg, V.Y.; Bruland, Ø.S.; Revheim, M.E.; Larsen, R.H. Dual targeting with ^{224}Ra/^{212}Pb-conjugates for targeted alpha therapy of disseminated cancers: A conceptual approach. *Front. Med* **2023**, *9*, 1051825. [CrossRef]
85. Braun, J.; Lemmel, E.M.; Manger, B.; Rau, R.; Sörensen, H.; Sieper, J. Therapie der ankylosierenden Spondylitis (AS) mit Radiumchlorid (224SpondylAT®). *Z. Rheumatol.* **2001**, *60*, 74–83. [CrossRef] [PubMed]
86. Alpha Tau. AlphaDaRT Revolutionary Alpha-Emitters Radiotherapy. Alpha DaRT Technology Brochure. 2022. Available online: https://www.alphatau.com/_files/ugd/74925d_d8c28da928ba46bdab3f0272d356a8d9.pdf (accessed on 20 September 2023).
87. Yang, G.Q.; Harrison, L.B. A Hard Target Needs a Sharper DaRT. *Int. J. Radiat. Oncol. Biol. Phys.* **2020**, *107*, 152–153. [CrossRef] [PubMed]
88. Cooks, T.; Tal, M.; Raab, S.; Efrati, M.; Reitkopf, S.; Lazarov, E.; Etzyoni, R.; Schmidt, M.; Arazi, L.; Kelson, I.; et al. Intratumoral 224Ra-Loaded Wires Spread Alpha-Emitters Inside Solid Human Tumors in Athymic Mice Achieving Tumor Control. *Anticancer Res.* **2012**, *32*, 5315–5321. [PubMed]
89. Reitkopf-Brodutch, S.; Confino, H.; Schmidt, M.; Cooks, T.; Efrati, M.; Arazi, L.; Rath-Wolfson, L.; Marshak, G.; Kelson, I.; Keisari, Y.; et al. Ablation of experimental colon cancer by intratumoral 224Radium-loaded wires is mediated by alpha particles released from atoms which spread in the tumor and can be augmented by chemotherapy. *Int. J. Radiat. Biol.* **2015**, *91*, 179–186. [CrossRef]
90. Keisari, Y.; Popovtzer, A.; Kelson, I. Effective treatment of metastatic cancer by an innovative intratumoral alpha particle-mediated radiotherapy in combination with immunotherapy: A short review. *J. Phys. Conf. Ser.* **2020**, *1662*, 012016. [CrossRef]
91. Confino, H.; Schmidt, M.; Efrati, M.; Hochman, I.; Umansky, V.; Kelson, I.; Keisari, Y. Inhibition of mouse breast adenocarcinoma growth by ablation with intratumoral alpha-irradiation combined with inhibitors of immunosuppression and CpG. *Cancer Immunol. Immunother.* **2016**, *65*, 1149–1158. [CrossRef]
92. Confino, H.; Hochman, I.; Efrati, M.; Schmidt, M.; Umansky, V.; Kelson, I.; Keisari, Y. Tumor ablation by intratumoral Ra-224-loaded wires induces anti-tumor immunity against experimental metastatic tumors. *Cancer Immunol. Immunother.* **2015**, *64*, 191–199. [CrossRef]
93. Feliciani, G.; Bellia, S.R.; Del Duca, M.; Mazzotti, G.; Monti, M.; Stanganelli, I.; Keisari, Y.; Kelson, I.; Popovtzer, A.; Romeo, A.; et al. A New Approach for a Safe and Reproducible Seeds Positioning for Diffusing Alpha-Emitters Radiation Therapy of Squamous Cell Skin Cancer: A Feasibility Study. *Cancers* **2022**, *14*, 240. [CrossRef]
94. Domankevich, V.; Efrati, M.; Schmidt, M.; Glikson, E.; Mansour, F.; Shai, A.; Cohen, A.; Zilberstein, Y.; Flaisher, E.; Galalae, R.; et al. RIG-1-Like Receptor Activation Synergizes with Intratumoral Alpha Radiation to Induce Pancreatic Tumor Rejection, Triple-Negative Breast Metastases Clearance, and Antitumor Immune Memory in Mice. *Front. Oncol.* **2020**, *10*, 990. [CrossRef]
95. Nishri, Y.; Vatarescu, M.; Luz, I.; Epstein, L.; Dumančić, M.; Del Mare, S.; Shai, A.; Schmidt, M.; Deutsch, L.; Den, R.B.; et al. Diffusing alpha-emitters radiation therapy in combination with temozolomide or bevacizumab in human glioblastoma multiforme xenografts. *Front. Oncol.* **2022**, *12*, 888100. [CrossRef]
96. Bagheri, R.; Afarideh, H.; Ghannadi-Maragheh, M.; Bahrami-Samani, A.; Shirvani-Arani, S. Production of ^{223}Ra from ^{226}Ra in Tehran Research Reactor for treatment of bone metastases. *J. Radioanal. Nucl. Chem.* **2015**, *304*, 1185–1191. [CrossRef]
97. Pruszyński, M.; Walczak, R.; Rodak, M.; Bruchertseifer, F.; Morgenstern, A.; Bilewicz, A. Radiochemical separation of ^{224}Ra from ^{232}U and ^{228}Th sources for ^{224}Ra/^{212}Pb/^{212}Bi generator. *Appl. Radiat. Isot.* **2021**, *172*, 109655. [CrossRef]
98. Abou, D.; Thiele, N.; Villmer, A.; Gustche, N.; Escorcia, F.; Wilson, J.; Thorek, D. MACROPA highly stable chelator of Radium-223 and functionalization attempts for targeted treatment of cancer. *J. Nucl. Med.* **2020**, *61* (Suppl. S1), 587. Available online: http://jnm.snmjournals.org/content/61/supplement_1/587.abstract (accessed on 29 September 2023).
99. Bauer, D.; Blumberg, M.; Köckerling, M.; Mamat, C. A comparative evaluation of calix[4]arene-1,3-crown-6 as a ligand for selected divalent cations of radiopharmaceutical interest. *RSC Adv.* **2019**, *9*, 32357–32366. [CrossRef]

100. Steinberg, J.; Bauer, D.; Reissig, F.; Köckerling, M.; Pietzsch, H.J.; Mamat, C. Modified Calix[4]crowns as Molecular Receptors for Barium. *ChemistryOpen* **2018**, *7*, 432–438. [CrossRef]
101. Reissig, F.; Bauer, D.; Ullrich, M.; Kreller, M.; Pietzsch, J.; Mamat, C.; Kopka, K.; Pietzsch, H.J.; Walther, M. Recent insights in barium-131 as a diagnostic match for radium-223: Cyclotron production, separation, radiolabeling, and imaging. *Pharmaceuticals* **2020**, *13*, 272. [CrossRef]
102. Kulage, Z.; Cantrell, T.; Griswold, J.; Denton, D.; Garland, M.; Copping, R.; Mirzadeh, S. Nuclear data for reactor production of ^{131}Ba and ^{133}Ba. *Appl. Radiat. Isot.* **2021**, *172*, 109645. [CrossRef]
103. Feng, Y.; Zalutsky, M.R. Production, purification and availability of ^{211}At: Near term steps towards global access. *Nucl. Med. Biol.* **2021**, *100–101*, 12–23. [CrossRef]
104. Nolen, J.; Mustapha, B.; Gott, M.; Washiyama, K.; Sampathkumaran, U.; Winter, R. Development of ^{211}At Production via Continuous Extraction of ^{211}Rn. *J. Med. Imaging Radiat. Sci.* **2019**, *50*, S35–S36. [CrossRef]
105. Zalutsky, M.R.; Zhao, X.G.; Alston, K.L.; Bigner, D. High-level production of alpha-particle-emitting (211)At and preparation of (211)At-labeled antibodies for clinical use. *J. Nucl. Med.* **2001**, *42*, 1508–1515.
106. Albertsson, P.; Bäck, T.; Bergmark, K.; Hallqvist, A.; Johansson, M.; Aneheim, E.; Lindegren, S.; Timperanza, C.; Smerud, K.; Palm, S. Astatine-211 based radionuclide therapy: Current clinical trial landscape. *Front. Med.* **2023**, *9*, 1076210. [CrossRef] [PubMed]
107. Urhan, M.; Dadparvar, S.; Mavi, A.; Houseni, M.; Chamroonrat, W.; Alavi, A.; Mandel, S.J. Iodine-123 as a diagnostic imaging agent in differentiated thyroid carcinoma: A comparison with iodine-131 post-treatment scanning and serum thyroglobulin measurement. *Eur. J. Nucl. Med. Mol. Imaging* **2007**, *34*, 1012–1017. [CrossRef] [PubMed]
108. Ardisson, V.; Lepareur, N. Chapter 76-Labeling Techniques with 123I: Application to Clinical Settings. In *Comprehensive Handbook of Iodine*; Preedy, V.R., Burrow, G.N., Watson, R., Eds.; Academic Press: Cambridge, MA, USA, 2009; pp. 741–756. [CrossRef]
109. Costa, O.D.; Barcellos, H.; Matsuda, H.; Sumiya, L.D.; Junqueira, F.C.; Matsuda, M.M.N.; Lapolli, A.L. A new ^{124}Xe irradiation system for ^{123}I production. *Appl. Radiat. Isot.* **2023**, *200*, 110926. [CrossRef]
110. Lamparter, D.; Hallmann, B.; Hänscheid, H.; Boschi, F.; Malinconico, M.; Samnick, S. Improved small scale production of iodine-124 for radiolabeling and clinical applications. *Appl. Radiat. Isot.* **2018**, *140*, 24–28. [CrossRef] [PubMed]
111. Cascini, G.L.; Niccoli Asabella, A.; Notaristefano, A.; Restuccia, A.; Ferrari, C.; Rubini, D.; Altini, C.; Rubini, G. 124 iodine: A longer-life positron emitter isotope-new opportunities in molecular imaging. *Biomed. Res. Int.* **2014**, *2014*, 672094. [CrossRef]
112. Khalafi, H.; Nazari, K.; Ghannadi-Maragheh, M. Investigation of efficient ^{131}I production from natural uranium at Tehran research reactor. *Ann. Nucl. Energy* **2005**, *32*, 729–740. [CrossRef]
113. Crawford, J.R.; Kunz, P.; Yang, H.; Schaffer, P.; Ruth, T.J. ^{211}Rn/^{211}At and ^{209}At production with intense mass separated Fr ion beams for preclinical 211At-based α-therapy research. *Appl. Radiat. Isot.* **2017**, *122*, 222–228. [CrossRef]
114. Crawford, J.R.; Robertson, A.K.H.; Yang, H.; Rodríguez-Rodríguez, C.; Esquinas, P.L.; Kunz, P.; Blinder, S.; Sossi, V.; Schaffer, P.; Ruth, T.J. Evaluation of ^{209}At as a theranostic isotope for ^{209}At-radiopharmaceutical development using high-energy SPECT. *Phys. Med. Biol.* **2018**, *63*, 045025. [CrossRef]
115. Hagemann, U.B.; Wickstroem, K.; Hammer, S.; Bjerke, R.M.; Zitzmann-Kolbe, S.; Ryan, O.B.; Karlsson, J.; Scholz, A.; Hennekes, H.; Mumberg, D.; et al. Advances in Precision Oncology: Targeted Thorium-227 Conjugates as a New Modality in Targeted Alpha Therapy. *Cancer Biother. Radiopharm.* **2020**, *35*, 497–510. [CrossRef]
116. Karlsson, J.; Schatz, C.A.; Wengner, A.M.; Hammer, S.; Scholz, A.; Cuthbertson, A.; Wagner, V.; Hennekes, H.; Jardine, V.; Hagemann, U.B. Targeted thorium-227 conjugates as treatment options in oncology. *Front. Med.* **2023**, *9*, 1071086. [CrossRef]
117. Moiseeva, A.N.; Aliev, R.A.; Unezhev, V.N.; Zagryadskiy, V.A.; Latushkin, S.T.; Aksenov, N.V.; Gustova, N.S.; Voronuk, M.G.; Starodub, G.Y.; Ogloblin, A.A. Cross section measurements of ^{151}Eu(^{3}He,5n) reaction: New opportunities for medical alpha emitter ^{149}Tb production. *Sci. Rep.* **2020**, *10*, 508. [CrossRef]
118. Müller, C.; Vermeulen, C.; Köster, U.; Johnston, K.; Türler, A.; Schibli, R.; van der Meulen, N.P. Alpha-PET with terbium-149: Evidence and perspectives for radiotheragnostics. *EJNMMI Radiopharm. Chem.* **2016**, *1*, 5. [CrossRef] [PubMed]
119. Müller, C.; Fischer, E.; Behe, M.; Köster, U.; Dorrer, H.; Reber, J.; Haller, S.; Cohrs, S.; Blanc, A.; Grünberg, J.; et al. Future prospects for SPECT imaging using the radiolanthanide terbium-155—Production and preclinical evaluation in tumor-bearing mice. *Nucl. Med. Biol.* **2014**, *41*, e58–e65. [CrossRef]
120. Favaretto, C.; Talip, Z.; Borgna, F.; Grundler, P.V.; Dellepiane, G.; Sommerhalder, A.; Zhang, H.; Schibli, R.; Braccini, S.; Müller, C.; et al. Cyclotron production and radiochemical purification of terbium-155 for SPECT imaging. *EJNMMI Radiopharm. Chem.* **2021**, *6*, 37. [CrossRef]
121. Baum, R.P.; Singh, A.; Benešová, M.; Vermeulen, C.; Gnesin, S.; Köster, U.; Johnston, K.; Müller, D.; Senftleben, S.; Kulkarni, H.R.; et al. Clinical evaluation of the radiolanthanide terbium-152: First-in-human PET/CT with ^{152}Tb-DOTATOC. *Dalton Trans.* **2017**, *46*, 14638–14646. [CrossRef] [PubMed]
122. Naskar, N.; Lahiri, S. Theranostic Terbium Radioisotopes: Challenges in Production for Clinical Application. *Front. Med.* **2021**, *8*, 675014. [CrossRef]

Disclaimer/Publisher's Note: The statements, opinions and data contained in all publications are solely those of the individual author(s) and contributor(s) and not of MDPI and/or the editor(s). MDPI and/or the editor(s) disclaim responsibility for any injury to people or property resulting from any ideas, methods, instructions or products referred to in the content.

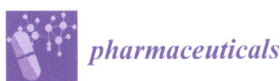

Article

Influence of the Molar Activity of $^{203/212}$Pb-PSC-PEG$_2$-TOC on Somatostatin Receptor Type 2-Binding and Cell Uptake

Marc Pretze [1,*,†], Enrico Michler [1,†], Roswitha Runge [1], Kerstin Wetzig [1], Katja Tietze [1], Florian Brandt [1], Michael K. Schultz [2,3,4,5] and Jörg Kotzerke [1]

1. Department of Nuclear Medicine, University Hospital Carl Gustav Carus, Technical University Dresden, Fetscherstr. 74, 01307 Dresden, Germany; enrico.michler@ukdd.de (E.M.); roswitha.runge@ukdd.de (R.R.); kerstin.wetzig@ukdd.de (K.W.); katja.tietze@ukdd.de (K.T.); florian.brandt@ukdd.de (F.B.); joerg.kotzerke@ukdd.de (J.K.)
2. Department of Radiology, University of Iowa, Iowa City, IA 52240, USA; mschultz@perspectivetherapeutics.com
3. Viewpoint Molecular Targeting, Inc. (DBA Perspective Therapeutics), Coralville, IA 52241, USA
4. Department of Chemistry, University of Iowa, Iowa City, IA 52241, USA
5. Department of Radiation Oncology, University of Iowa, Iowa City, IA 52242, USA
* Correspondence: marc.pretze@ukdd.de; Tel.: +49-351-458-5417
† These authors contributed equally to this work.

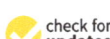

Citation: Pretze, M.; Michler, E.; Runge, R.; Wetzig, K.; Tietze, K.; Brandt, F.; Schultz, M.K.; Kotzerke, J. Influence of the Molar Activity of $^{203/212}$Pb-PSC-PEG$_2$-TOC on Somatostatin Receptor Type 2-Binding and Cell Uptake. *Pharmaceuticals* 2023, *16*, 1605. https://doi.org/10.3390/ph16111605

Academic Editor: Martina Benešová-Schäfer

Received: 10 October 2023
Revised: 6 November 2023
Accepted: 10 November 2023
Published: 14 November 2023

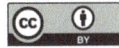

Copyright: © 2023 by the authors. Licensee MDPI, Basel, Switzerland. This article is an open access article distributed under the terms and conditions of the Creative Commons Attribution (CC BY) license (https:// creativecommons.org/licenses/by/ 4.0/).

Abstract: (1) Background: In neuroendocrine tumors (NETs), somatostatin receptor subtype 2 is highly expressed, which can be targeted by a radioactive ligand such as [^{177}Lu]Lu-1,4,7,10-tetraazacyclododecane-*N*,*N'*,*N''*,*N'''*-tetraacetic acid-[Tyr^3,Thr^8]-octreotide (^{177}Lu-DOTA-TOC) and, more recently, by a lead specific chelator (PSC) containing $^{203/212}$Pb-PSC-PEG$_2$-TOC (PSC-TOC). The molar activity (A_M) can play a crucial role in tumor uptake, especially in receptor-mediated uptake, such as in NETs. Therefore, an investigation of the influence of different molar activities of $^{203/212}$Pb-PSC-TOC on cell uptake was investigated. (2) Methods: Optimized radiolabeling of $^{203/212}$Pb-PSC-TOC was performed with 50 µg of precursor in a NaAc/AcOH buffer at pH 5.3–5.5 within 15–45 min at 95° C. Cell uptake was studied in AR42 J, HEK293 sst2, and ZR75-1 cells. (3) Results: $^{203/212}$Pb-PSC-TOC was radiolabeled with high radiochemical purity >95% and high radiochemical yield >95%, with A_M ranging from 0.2 to 61.6 MBq/nmol. The cell uptake of ^{203}Pb-PSC-TOC (A_M = 38 MBq/nmol) was highest in AR42 J (17.9%), moderate in HEK293 sstr (9.1%) and lowest in ZR75-1 (0.6%). Cell uptake increased with the level of A_M. (4) Conclusions: A moderate A_M of 15–40 MBq/nmol showed the highest cell uptake. No uptake limitation was found in the first 24–48 h. Further escalation experiments with even higher A_M should be performed in the future. It was shown that A_M plays an important role because of its direct dependence on the cellular uptake levels, possibly due to less receptor saturation with non-radioactive ligands at higher A_M.

Keywords: ^{203}Pb; ^{212}Pb; TOC; cell uptake; AR42 J; molar activity (A_M); neuroendocrine tumor (NET); somatostatin receptor (SST2); targeted alpha-therapy (TAT)

1. Introduction

Recently, receptor-targeted α-therapy (TAT) has gained importance in nuclear medicine clinical routine, especially for tumor patients who develop resistance to β$^-$-therapy [1,2]. Typically, patients receive multiple doses of ^{90}Y or ^{177}Lu (dose of 5–8 GBq per patient) at periodic intervals of administration (e.g., 8-week intervals) [3]. Unfortunately, a significant proportion of these patients will eventually experience progressive disease and discontinue therapy. On the other hand, it has been observed that further responses and prolonged survival can be achieved by initiating α-therapy after disease progression. For example, the use of ^{225}Ac (dose: 100 kBq/kg, four α-particles per decay) can dramatically reduce the required level of administered radioactivity (by a factor of about 1000 compared to

^{177}Lu). However, the behavior of α-particles in tumor cells is complicated by α-emitting radionuclide progeny in the ^{225}Ac series. Of particular interest are ^{221}Fr, ^{217}At, ^{213}Bi, and ^{213}Po. A key issue is the biological fate of ^{213}Bi ($t_{1/2}$ 46 min), which is transported out of the tumor cells (by its own escape or by the escape of ^{221}Fr or ^{217}At) and accumulates mainly in the kidneys, delivering an α-emitting dose of ^{213}Po, which, in turn, could have a higher negative impact on renal function [4]. Therefore, it is often suggested that only patients with an efficient renal function can be considered eligible for ^{225}Ac therapy, while patients with impaired renal function may not be eligible for these therapies.

^{212}Pb is a promising radionuclide for targeted alpha particle therapy that emits only one α-particle per β$^-$-decay of ^{212}Pb to ^{212}Bi and then either 64% to ^{212}Po or 36% to ^{208}Tl [5,6]. Therefore, a ^{212}Pb-labeled radiopharmaceutical, once accumulated in the tumor tissue, will deposit its highest dose in the form of the α-particle specifically in the tumor cells, with a lower probability of further α-decay occurring in healthy organs. Thus, ^{212}Pb represents a more favorable choice for cancer α-therapy patients who are naïve to (or who have progressed on) β$^-$-therapy, including patients with reduced renal function. Ongoing preclinical and clinical studies are investigating the potential of ^{212}Pb-labeled peptides and antibodies (at a dose of approximately 2 MBq/kg) [4] or approximately between ^{177}Lu and ^{225}Ac administered doses of radioactivity. Lead specific chelator-PEG$_2$-[Tyr^3,Thr^8]-octreotide (PSC-PEG-TOC) (VMT-α-NET) is a somatostatin subtype 2 (SST2) receptor targeting peptide for the treatment of neuroendocrine tumors (NETs) that exhibits rapid tumor accumulation, high tumor retention, and rapid renal excretion [7]. It carries the chelator PSC [7], which forms highly stable complexes with $^{203/212}$Pb and, in contrast to less stable 1,4,7,10-tetraazacyclododecane-N,N',N'',N'''-tetraacetic acid (DOTA) complexes, remains intact even after β$^-$ conversion to ^{212}Bi [8]. Recently, the true matched pair $^{203/212}$Pb has come into focus through several first in-human theranostic applications [9–11]. While ^{203}Pb ($t_{1/2}$ = 52 h; 279 keV gamma ray; 81% intensity) represents an ideal elementally matched imaging surrogate, ^{212}Pb itself can be used for SPECT imaging [12]. A true matched pair could finally overcome the differential pharmacokinetic/pharmacological properties observed between diagnostic and therapeutic radiotracers with unmatched radionuclides pairs [13].

In addition to somatostatin analogs, such as PSC-TOC, other radiopharmaceuticals targeting other receptors (e.g., PSMA derivatives) for radiolabeling with $^{203/212}$Pb are under preclinical investigation and may soon be translated into clinical use [4,14–16]. Emerging evidence suggests that α-particles have the potential to overcome resistance to β$^-$-therapy and could lead to further therapeutic options for patients with palliative effects and, in some cases, even complete remission [17]. Furthermore, the appearance of Cherenkov light due to the decay of ^{212}Pb may be useful not only for diagnostics but also for further treatment options [18]. The optimal mass of the precursor peptide for radiopharmaceuticals is an important parameter in radiopharmaceutical development to ensure that the highest degree of tumor targeting with the lowest accumulation and retention in normal organs and healthy tissues is achieved. This parameter is also important in achieving a formulation that results in smooth radiometallation and a high radiochemical yield and purity. In general, this parameter is known as the molar activity (A_M), which plays a crucial role for all PET radiotracers targeting saturable binding sites (e.g., receptors) but is secondary or negligible for many metabolic PET radiotracers, where the endogenous levels of the compound are in great excess of the radiotracer itself due to saturation of the receptors at the tumor site [19].

In this work, the influence of the A_M-to-cell uptake of $^{203/212}$Pb-PSC-TOC was investigated in different cell lines (AR42 J, HEK293 sst2, and ZR75-1) to develop a more detailed understanding of the tracer in preparation for clinical use.

2. Results

2.1. Radiochemistry

The radiochemical yield (RCY) was 74–97% for ^{203}Pb-PSC-TOC (Table 1) and 22–99% for ^{212}Pb-PSC-TOC, depending on the reaction conditions (Tables 2 and 4). The radiochemical purity (RCP) was always >95%. Stabilities greater than 95% of the formulated $^{203/212}$Pb-PSC-TOC were found up to 16 h at r.t. and for ^{203}Pb-PSC-TOC up to 11 d at 4 °C by RP-HPLC. For ^{212}Pb-PSC-TOC, HPLC is very useful for determining the identity of the product but not for the direct determination of RCY, according to the approach used here. A free ^{208}Tl daughter nuclide was observed up to 20% in the chromatogram 4 h after radiosynthesis. Isothermal titration calorimetry (ITC) experiments confirmed the stability of the ^{212}Bi daughter radionuclide in the PSC chelator to >95% at 2 h after radiolabeling. Importantly, the contribution of free ^{208}Tl to the total body dose was shown to be negligible [20].

Table 1. ^{203}Pb-PSC-TOC reactions.

Reactions [1]	Starting Activity (MBq)	Product Activity (MBq)	RCY (%)	A_M (MBq/nmol)
1	74	72	97	2.3
2	174	128	74	5.4
3	40	36	90	1.3
4	302	249	82	7.9
5	536	488	91	15.3
6	455	438	96	13.7
7	2105	1972	94	61.6
8 [2]	125	109	87	1.1
9	1301	1226	94	38.3

[1] Reactions were always performed with 50 µg (31.7 nmol) VTM-α-NET for 15 min at 95 °C. [2] Exception: here, it is 156 µg (98.8 nmol) PSC-TOC.

Table 2. ^{212}Pb-PSC-TOC reactions.

Reactions [1]	Starting Activity (MBq)	Product Activity (MBq)	RCY (%)	A_M (MBq/nmol)
1	24	10	40	0.8
2	4	2	53	0.2
3	490 *	176 *	36	13.9
4	214 *	48 *	22	3.8
5 [2]	24	11	48	0.8

[1] Reactions were always performed with 20 µg (12.7 nmol) VTM-α-NET for 15 min at 95 °C. [2] Exception: here, it is 20 µg (13.7 nmol) DOTA-TATE. * Normalization was performed (see Table 3).

Table 3. Normalization factors for the activity measurements of ^{212}Pb after separation from the daughter nuclides by Pb resin for the ISOMED 2010 dose calibrator.

Time after Separation (min)	Normalization Factor
0	1.86
5	1.80
30	1.58
60	1.37
90	1.26
120	1.18

Table 4. Optimized ^{212}Pb-PSC-TOC reactions.

Reactions [1]	Starting Activity (MBq)	Product Activity (MBq)	RCY (%)	A_M (MBq/nmol)
1	522 *	490 *	98	15.5
2	328	315	97	9.9
3	274	260	99	8.2
4	177	165 *	93	5.2
5	146	104 *	71	3.3
6	95	78 *	82	2.5
7	32	31	99	1.0

[1] Reactions were always performed with 50 µg (31.7 nmol) VTM-α-NET for 45 min at 95 °C. * Normalization was performed (see Table 3).

The optimization of the radiochemical labeling procedure included steps to overcome the loss of activity due to several purification steps: The freshly eluted activity from the ^{224}Ra/^{212}Pb generator is partitioned into Pb resin 10–12%, waste ~2%, and product 84–86%.

The purification of ^{212}Pb by Pb resin removes potential traces of the parent nuclide ^{224}Ra, as well as the daughter nuclides ^{212}Bi and ^{208}Tl [21]. Therefore, activity measurements with a dose calibrator (ISOMED 2010, Nuvia Instruments GmbH, Dresden, Germany) in equilibrium of the mother and daughter nuclides show different values before and after Pb resin purification. Therefore, a normalization factor for the dose calibrator is required immediately after purification (Table 3). Further purification with C18 or Maxi-Clean (MC) SPE cartridges results in a further loss of product activity. The C18 contained 6–10% of the product activity, and the MC cartridge contained up to 40% of the product activity. It appears that the chelated ^{212}Pb-PSC complex has strong binding competition with the sorbent material of the MC cartridges. Therefore, these cartridges are not suitable for purification. However, the cartridge purifications were later found to be obsolete due to further development of optimized radiolabeling conditions.

2.2. Cell Uptake Studies with Different Molar Activities

During the studies with ^{203}Pb-PSC-TOC, it was found that SST2-transfected HEK293 cells showed a moderate cell uptake compared to endogenously SST2-positive AR42J cells, which showed a higher cell uptake. Compared to the routinely used ^{68}Ga-DOTA-[Tyr^3,Thr^8]-octreotate (TATE) with a cell uptake in AR42J of about 8.7 ± 0.4% after 1 h, the uptake of $^{203/212}$Pb-PSC-TOC reached a comparable level 24 h after incubation only at the highest $A_M > 7.9$ MBq/nmol (^{203}Pb-PSC-TOC) and $A_M > 3.3$ MBq/nmol (^{212}Pb-PSC-TOC). ZR75-1 cells were used as a negative control and showed no significant uptake for all radiotracers used in this work.

It was found that cell uptake was strongly influenced by the number of cells seeded 1–2 days prior to the uptake experiments. With 100,000 cells seeded, very low cell uptake was observed, and the cell uptake increased with the number of cells seeded. The optimal number of cells for uptake was 1.0 million cells per well. Seeding cells three days prior to uptake had no further effect on cell uptake.

The optimum activity of ^{203}Pb-PSC-TOC for incubation was found to be 100 kBq per well on a six-well plate, and cell viability was good for over 72 h. For ^{212}Pb-PSC-TOC, activities greater than 50 kBq per well lead to a decrease in cell uptake and even lower cell viability (11% viability after 72 h), which affected the credibility of the cell uptake values. Therefore, activities of 25 kBq per well were used for ^{212}Pb-PSC-TOC.

Figure 1 shows the cell uptake for ^{203}Pb-PSC-TOC, and Figure 2 shows the cell uptake for ^{212}Pb-PSC-TOC. It was found that the uptake increased with the A_M for both radioligands. In most of the experiments, only timeframes between 1 and 24 h were considered, because, for diagnostic purposes, patients are measured only within a timeframe of 24 h, and, for therapeutic purposes, most of the dose is already deposited (two half-lives = 75% of the dose, $t_{1/2} = 10.64$ h). In the case of the highest produced A_M of $^{203/212}$Pb-PSC-TOC, the timeframe was extended to 72 h in order to find a possible plateau or decrease in cell uptake. ^{203}Pb-PSC-TOC showed an increase of relative cell uptake per 1 million cells up to 24.0 ± 0.8% even 149 h after incubation ($2.9 \times t_{1/2}$ of ^{203}Pb). For ^{212}Pb-PSC-TOC, the cell uptake still increased up to 25.0 ± 0.5% 72 h after incubation. Increased uptake values were found at the lowest excess of cold peptide (25%). These results could support the hypothesis that free binding sites of SST2 receptors are still available (Figure 2).

Tables 5 and 6 show the statistical evaluation of the cell accumulation of $^{203/212}$Pb-PSC-TOC. Each cell line was incubated with the respective A_M in triplicate. The standard deviation of the mean accumulation was less than 10%, confirming that the data were consistent with the conclusions. The standard deviation for ZR75-1 uptake was not shown, because it was less than 0.04% in each experiment.

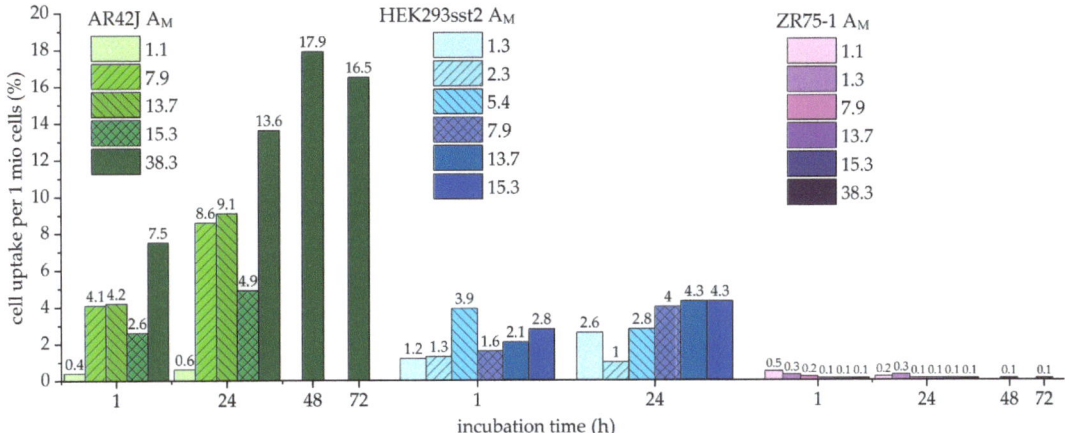

Figure 1. The cell uptake of ^{203}Pb-PSC-TOC in different cell lines is shown. The values above the columns represent the relative mean cell uptake in percent. A_M is given in MBq/nmol. Each column represents the mean value of a triplicate. Shades of green: AR42J; shades of blue: HEK293 sst2; shades of purple: ZR75-1.

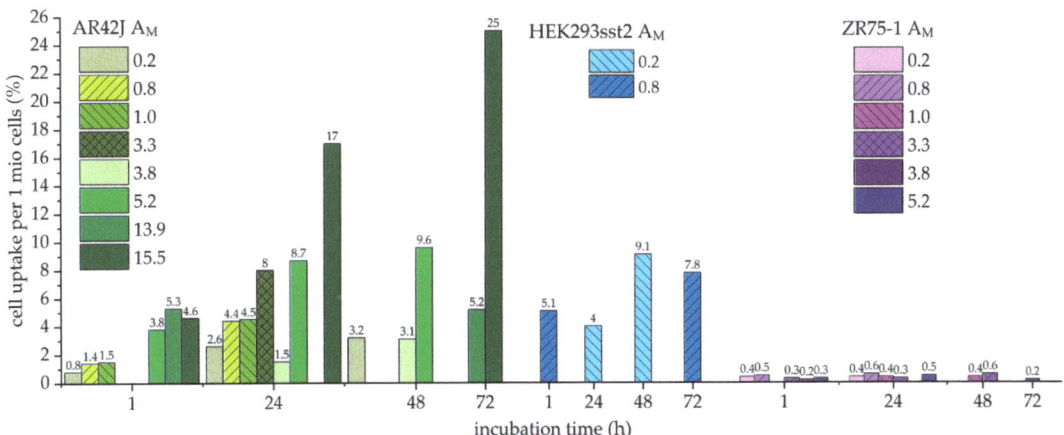

Figure 2. Cell uptake of ^{212}Pb-PSC-TOC in different cell lines is shown. The values above the columns represent the relative mean cell uptake in percent. A_M is given in MBq/nmol. Each column represents the mean value of a triplicate. Shades of green: AR42J; shades of blue: HEK293 sst2; shades of purple: ZR75-1.

Table 5. Cell uptake statistics for ^{203}Pb-PSC-TOC.

Cells	Incubation Time (h)	Molar Activity (MBq/nmol)							
		1.1	1.3	2.3	5.4	7.9	13.7	15.3	38.3
AR42J uptake (%)	1	0.4 ± 0.1				4.1 ± 0.2	4.2 ± 0.0	2.6 ± 0.2	7.5 ± 0.4
	24	0.6 ± 0.0				8.6 ± 0.5	9.1 ± 0.4	4.9 ± 0.6	13.6 ± 0.2
	48								17.9 ± 0.7
	72								16.5 ± 1.3
HEK293 sst2 uptake (%)	1		1.2 ± 0.3	1.3 ± 0.1	3.9 ± 0.2	1.6 ± 0.3	2.1 ± 0.1	2.8 ± 0.1	1.2 ± 0.3
	24		2.6 ± 0.6	1.0 ± 0.0	2.8 ± 0.2	4.0 ± 0.3	4.3 ± 0.2	4.3 ± 0.9	2.6 ± 0.6

Table 6. Cell uptake statistics for ^{212}Pb-PSC-TOC.

Cells	Incubation Time (h)	Molar Activity (MBq/nmol)							
		0.2	0.8	1.0	3.3	3.8	5.2	13.9	15.5
AR42J uptake (%)	1	0.8 ± 0.1	1.4 ± 0.1	1.5 ± 0.1		n.d.	3.8 ± 0.2	5.3 ± 0.3	4.6 ± 0.3
	24	2.6 ± 0.2	4.4 ± 0.4	4.5 ± 0.0	8.0 ± 1.0	1.5 ± 0.1	8.7 ± 0.7		17.0 ± 0.7
	48	3.2 ± 0.4				3.1 ± 0.1	9.6 ± 0.7		
	72							5.2 ± 0.4	25.0 ± 0.5
HEK293 sst2 uptake (%)	1							5.1 ± 0.5	
	24					4.0 ± 0.5			
	48					9.1 ± 0.5			
	72							7.8 ± 0.0	

3. Discussion

3.1. Radiochemistry

Radiolabeling of PSC-TOC with ^{203}Pb proceeded smoothly under standard labeling conditions. Challenges were observed with ^{212}Pb when using the same conditions as for ^{203}Pb that needed to be overcome. However, the addition of a higher mass of peptide precursor and slightly longer reaction times solved this problem [21]. The quality control showed an RCY >95% in most cases for $^{203/212}$Pb-PSC-TOC. It is noteworthy that, when the RCP for ^{212}Pb-PSC-TOC was only >90%, this was due to ejected daughter nuclides that transferred to a solvent form [22]. When the developed TLC was remeasured after 2 h, the RCP increased to >95% (24 h later, the RCP was even >99%), as the free daughter nuclides decayed on the TLC within this time, confirming the radiochemical purity of ^{212}Pb-PSC-TOC.

3.2. Influence of Molar Activity on Cell Uptake

For the cell uptake experiments performed in this work, it was observed that, the higher the A_M, the higher the cell uptake. An uptake limit was not found in these experiments, but there may be one, as can be found in the literature [19]. Furthermore, neither PSMA nor TATE peptides reached tumor saturation in the patients [23]. AR42J cells always showed the highest cell uptake for each A_M compared to HEK293 sst2 cells, which showed lower cell uptake. ZR75-1 cells as a negative control did not show significant cell uptake due to the lack of SST2 receptor. Therefore, AR42J cells may have the highest SST2 receptor expression of the cells used in this study. For further studies in this direction, transfected cells with even higher SST2 receptor expression than in AR42J cells could be used [24].

The high uptake of SST2-specific radioligands has been well examined for agonists and antagonists. It is known that agonists like TOC effectuate the internalization of SST2 receptors after stimulation in vivo and that this is the reason for the high and long-lasting uptake of SST2 radioligands [25]. However, this high accumulation seems to reduce after several treatments with β$^-$-radioligands, due to differentiation of the SST2 expressing tumor cells. With only low SST2 expression at the tumor site, this could be one reason for the "β$^-$ resistance" when only low amounts of radioligands reach the tumor site. The lower expression of SST2 receptor may merely be overcome by TAT, which seem to have a similar impact in tumor therapy at much lower doses compared to β$^-$-therapy [26]. Therefore, antagonists like JR11, which have a similar accumulation to the agonistic radioligands, even after several treatments, may be a solution for this issue, since the SST2 expressing tumors do not differentiate when blocked by antagonists [27]. Another instrument to overcome the lowering SST2-specific tumor accumulation may be epigenetic stimulation before treatment or during a series of treatments. Experimental data have shown higher uptake rates in HEK293 sst2 cells up to 28 times versus untreated cells [28].

In radioligand therapy, a medium A_M tracer could reduce radiation exposure to dose-limiting organs with only a limited effect on radionuclide accumulation in the tumor. In this case, high A_M is considered to be 200 MBq/nmol, and low A_M is considered to be 2 MBq/nmol. Therefore, it can be assumed that the moderate A_M level of 15–40 MBq/nmol (Tables 1 and 4) achieved in this work may be the optimal amount for application. Nevertheless, further cell studies with even higher A_M should be performed to confirm this. One way to achieve higher A_M is HPLC purification, which has been shown to increase the A_M of a ^{68}Ga ligand by a factor of 10,000 [29]. In addition, a pilot therapy study with the optimal A_M can be performed against low A_M and high A_M to validate the observations from the cell studies. This experimental comparison may provide evidence to support the idea that moderate molar activities may indeed provide superior tumor uptake while minimizing radiation exposure to dose-limiting organs.

The amount of somatostatin analog administered varies with the analog used and the intended purpose of the administered drug. The TATE analog is administered at a high tracer level (100 nmol) in α- and β⁻-therapy, which is in the range of physiologically applied concentrations. This could lead to a lower tumor uptake if tumor receptors are blocked with an unlabeled peptide. Conversely, a higher A_M could negatively affect the tumor-to-organ ratio by saturating the physiologically expressing organs. For ^{212}Pb therapy, this would mean that A_M = 1 MBq/nmol is closer to the amount of, e.g., Luthathera (50 MBq/nmol, 148 nmol for 7.4 GBq [30]) than A_M = 10 MBq/nmol.

A comparable study on the influence of the A_M applied with ^{68}Ga or ^{177}Lu was not found in the scientific literature. The results of an Al^{18}F-labeled PSMA-11 study were presented [31], where it was found that the administration of a high A_M tracer increased the detection of low expression tumors while also increasing uptake in PSMA-expressing tissues, potentially leading to false-positive findings.

Taken together, variations in A_M may have different implications for diagnostic and therapeutic use. However, the moderate A_M of 15–40 MBq/nmol investigated in this work showed the highest cell uptake and should be used when administered to patients. For patients, a lower amount of peptide could increase tumor uptake while decreasing side effects.

4. Materials and Methods

All reagents and solvents were purchased from commercial suppliers at the highest purity and used without further purification. PSC-PEG$_2$-TOC (VMT-α-NET) and ^{224}Ra/^{212}Pb generator (VMT-α-GEN) were obtained from Perspective Therapeutics Inc., Coralville, IA, USA. ^{203}Pb solution in 8 M HCl was obtained from Cross Cancer Institute, Edmonton, AB, Canada. RCP was monitored by thin-layer chromatography (TLC) on iTLC-SG plates (Agilent, Santa Clara, CA, USA). Measurement of the radionuclide purity (RNP) and evaluation of the radio-TLC was performed with a thin-layer scanner (MiniScanPRO+, Eckert&Ziegler Eurotope GmbH, Berlin, Germany) equipped with a Model 43-2 alpha detector ZnS(Ag) scintillator (Ludlum Measurements, Sweetwater, TX, USA) and a build-in multi-channel analyzer (MCA) for gamma spectroscopy. Radio-HPLC was performed on a Shimadzu HPLC system (Thermo Scientific, Dreieich, Germany), equipped with a reverse-phase column (Merck Chromolith RP-18e; 100 × 4.6 mm plus a 5 × 4.6 mm guard column, Darmstadt, Germany) and a UV diode array detector (220 nm). The solvent system used was a gradient of acetonitrile:water (containing 0.05% TFA) (0–13 min: 0–60% MeCN) at a flow rate of 1.6 mL/min, unless otherwise stated. The pH was measured using a reflectance photometer (QUANTOFIX Relax, Macherey-Nagel GmbH & Co. KG, Düren, Germany).

4.1. Radiochemistry

Radiolabeling of the DOTA and PSC conjugates was performed according to standard protocols for these chelators [7]. Briefly, 50 µg precursor (DOTA-TATE (M = 1435.6 g/mol) or PSC-PEG$_2$-TOC (PSC-PEG$_2$-TOC, M = 1578.7 g/mol)) in H$_2$O$_{suprapure}$ was added to a 10 mL reaction vial together with 100 µL EtOH$_{absolute}$, 290 µL 1 M NaAc/AcOH buffer (pH 4, 99.99% trace metal), and 2 mg sodium ascorbate (Ph.Eur.).

$^{203/212}$Pb in 5–10 mL 1.6 M HCl$_{suprapure}$ was trapped on a custom-made Pb resin cartridge (100 mg PB-B10-F, Triskem, Bruz, France) preconditioned with 1 mL 2 M HCl$_{suprapure}$. The captured activity was rinsed with 1 mL 2 M HCl$_{suprapure}$. The activity was eluted with 2 mL NaAc/AcOH buffer (pH 6, 99.99% trace metal) directly into the reaction vial. The solution was heated at 95 °C for 15 min for ^{203}Pb and 15 or 45 min for ^{212}Pb. The reaction solution was then diluted with 4 mL of 0.9% NaCl solution and cooled.

Finally, the product was purified by using a C18 Plus light cartridge (WAT023501, Waters, Eschborn, Germany) preconditioned with 1 mL EtOH and 3 mL H_2O (wet condition). The cooled and diluted product solution (4 mL 0.9% NaCl) was slowly passed through the C18 cartridge. The C18 cartridge containing the product was rinsed with 2 mL of 0.9% NaCl solution and was directly eluted with 1 mL of 50% EtOH for injection directly through a vented sterile filter (0.22 µm, SLGVV255F, Millex-GV, Merck-Millipore, Darmstadt, Germany) into a product vial. Finally, the product was diluted with 7 mL of 0.9% NaCl solution.

Another purification method was performed using a Maxi-Clean (MC) SPE 0.5 mL IC-Chelate cartridge (5122565, S*Pure, Mainz, Germany) preconditioned with 5 mL $H_2O_{suprapure}$ (wet condition). The cooled and diluted product solution (4 mL 0.9% NaCl) was slowly transferred through a vented sterile filter into the product vial via the MC cartridge and washed with an additional 2 mL 0.9% NaCl into the product vial.

4.2. Quality Control of Radiotracer

Quality control included several standard tests established in the clinical manufacturing:
- TLC with eluent 0.1 M Na-citrate pH 5 (Start: $^{203/212}$Pb-PSC-TOC and particles ($R_f < 0.4$), end: $^{203/212}$Pb-chloride) (Figure 3).
- TLC with eluent 1M NH$_4$ Ac: MeOH 1:1 (Start: $^{203/212}$Pb-particles, end: $^{203/212}$Pb-PSC-TOC and $^{203/212}$Pb-chloride) (Figure 4).
- HPLC $^{203/212}$Pb-PSC-TOC t_R = 7.4 min. $^{203/212}$Pb-DOTA-TATE t_R = 7.1 min.
- pH value: 5.3 ± 0.5.
- RNP: ^{212}Pb: 75 and 238 keV; ^{212}Bi: 727 keV (6.7%); and ^{208}Tl: 510 (22.6%), 583 (85.0%), and 860 (12.5%) keV (Figure 5).

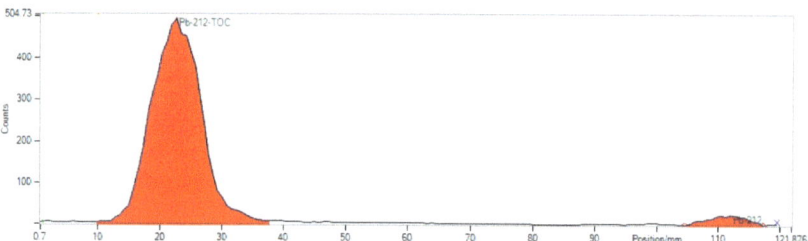

Figure 3. Corresponding TLC with Na-citrate as the eluent for the detection of unlabeled $^{203/212}$Pb at the front (position 115 mm, 3.9%) of the TLC. ^{212}Pb-TOC runs at the origin (position 25 mm, 96.1%).

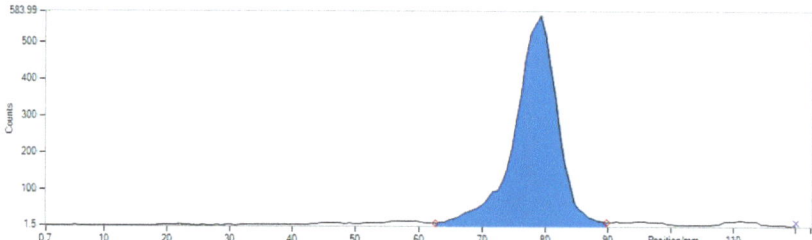

Figure 4. Corresponding TLC with NH$_4$ Az:MeOH as the eluent for the detection of $^{203/212}$Pb-particles at the origin (position 20 mm, 0.6%) of the TLC. ^{212}Pb-TOC runs at the front (position 80 mm, 99.4%.)

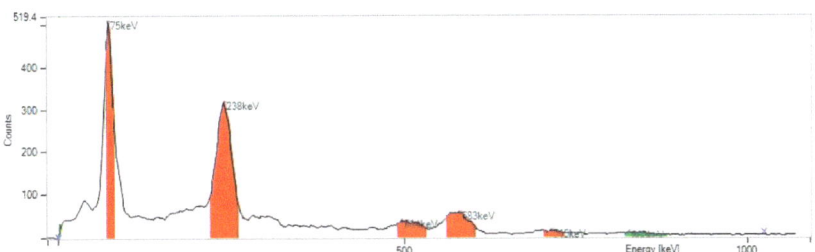

Figure 5. Corresponding gamma spectrum via MCA for verification of the RNP. Gamma lines found: ^{212}Pb: 75, 238 keV; ^{208}Tl: 510, 583, 860 keV; ^{212}Bi: 727 keV.

4.3. Cell Uptake Experiments

Cell uptake of $^{203/212}$Pb-PSC-TOC was tested against our gold standard ^{68}Ga-DOTATATE. AR42J (CRL-1492, ATCC®, Manassas, VA, USA), HEK293 sst2 (stably SST2 receptor transfected cells derived from Andrea Kliewer, University Hospital, Jena, Germany), and ZR75-1 (CRL-1500, ATCC®, Manassas, VA, USA); cells were seeded 1–2 days prior to the assay in 6-well plates to reach 0.5×10^6 cells per well in a humidified atmosphere containing 5% CO_2.

Each cell line was grown in its own medium:

- AR42J: Gibco RPMI 1640 medium (ATCC-Modification) supplemented with 10% fetal calf serum (FCS)
- HEK293 sst2 (stably transfected HEK293 cells): Dulbecco's modified Eagle's medium supplemented with 10% fetal calf serum (FCS), L-glutamine (2 mM = 1%), G-418 (50 mg/mL)
- ZR75-1: Gibco RPMI 1640 medium (w/o glutamine) supplemented with 10% fetal calf serum (FCS), 1% NEAA, 1 mM sodium pyruvate (1%), and 2 mM *N*-acetyl-alanyl-L-glutamine (1%)

After incubation with the respective radiotracer for 1 h, 24 h, 48 h, and 72 h, the medium, wash fraction (2×1 mL cold PBS 4 °C), and cell fraction (lysed with 1 mL 0.1 M NaOH and cell scraper) were collected, and the remaining activity in the fractions was measured with a gamma counter (HIDEX). The relative cell uptake in percent per 1 million cells was calculated between the medium, wash fraction, and lysate. Each cell incubation was performed in triplicate.

5. Conclusions

It was shown that the A_M of $^{203/212}$Pb-PSC-TOC has an effect on the cell uptake. No saturation was found in this work, but it is known from the literature that higher A_M > 100 MBq/nmol could have a negative effect on tumor uptake due to non-specific binding of the radioligand. It is noteworthy that higher A_M leads to higher cell uptake due to receptor-specific binding, and the values found in this work can be used as a reference for clinical application.

Another interesting radiochemical observation of this investigation is that the ^{212}Pb labeling benefited from a longer reaction time and a larger amount of precursor to achieve a high RCY. Since ^{203}Pb and ^{212}Pb are elementally identical, the apparent differences must necessarily be due to the differences in stable Pb found in the solutions provided (generator eluant versus ^{203}Pb solution), and thus, further investigation of the relative specific activity of the solutions is required.

In conclusion, for high tumor uptake, radiolabeling of 50 µg of PSC-TOC precursor should be performed with >1000 MBq ^{203}Pb and with >500 MBq ^{212}Pb.

Author Contributions: Conceptualization, M.P., E.M., R.R. and J.K.; methodology, M.P., R.R., K.W. and K.T.; software, R.R.; validation, M.P. and R.R.; formal analysis, R.R.; investigation, M.P. and R.R.; resources, M.K.S. and J.K.; data curation, M.P., K.W. and R.R.; writing—original draft preparation, M.P. and F.B.; writing—review and editing, M.P., E.M., R.R., K.W., K.T., M.K.S. and J.K.; visualization, M.P.; supervision, M.P. and R.R.; project administration, E.M. and J.K.; funding acquisition, M.K.S. and J.K. All authors have read and agreed to the published version of the manuscript.

Funding: This research received no external funding.

Data Availability Statement: All data can be referred to on request to the corresponding author.

Acknowledgments: The authors would like to thank Andrea Kliewer from University Hospital Jena for providing the transfected HEKsst2 cells. Moreover, we thank Fiorenza Ianzini and Lisa Hübinger for the extensive proofreading of the manuscript.

Conflicts of Interest: The MiniScanPRO+ was provided by Eckert&Ziegler especially for the evaluation of α-particles on TLC. M.K.S. is employed by Perspective Therapeutics, which has financial interest in the VMT-α-NET radiopharmaceutical. The authors declare no further conflict of interest.

References

1. Kratochwil, C.; Bruchertseifer, F.; Giesel, F.L.; Weis, M.; Verburg, F.A.; Mottaghy, F.; Kopka, K.; Apostolidis, C.; Haberkorn, U.; Morgenstern, A. ^{225}Ac-PSMA-617 for PSMA-targeted α-radiation therapy of metastatic castration-resistant prostate cancer. *J. Nucl. Med.* **2016**, *57*, 1941–1944. [CrossRef] [PubMed]
2. Guerra Liberal, F.D.C.; O'Sullivan, J.M.; McMahon, S.J.; Prise, K.M. Targeted alpha therapy: Current clinical applications. *Cancer Biother. Radiopharm.* **2020**, *35*, 404–417. [CrossRef] [PubMed]
3. Brogsitter, C.; Hartmann, H.; Wunderlich, G.; Schottelius, M.; Wester, H.J.; Kotzerke, J. Twins in spirit part IV—[^{177}Lu] high affinity DOTATATE. A promising new tracer for peptide receptor radiotherapy? *Nuklearmedizin* **2017**, *56*, 1–8. [CrossRef] [PubMed]
4. Dos Santos, J.C.; Schäfer, M.; Bauder-Wüst, U.; Lehnert, W.; Leotta, K.; Morgenstern, A.; Kopka, K.; Haberkorn, U.; Mier, W.; Kratochwil, C. Development and dosimetry of ^{203}Pb/^{212}Pb-labelled PSMA ligands: Bringing "the lead" into PSMA-targeted alpha therapy? *Eur. J. Nucl. Med. Mol. Imaging* **2019**, *46*, 1081–1091. [CrossRef]
5. Li, M.; Sagastume, E.A.; Lee, D.; McAlister, D.; DeGraffenreid, A.J.; Olewine, K.R.; Graves, S.; Copping, R.; Mirzadeh, S.; Zimmerman, B.E.; et al. $^{203/212}$Pb theranostic radiopharmaceuticals for image-guided radionuclide therapy for cancer. *Curr. Med. Chem.* **2020**, *27*, 7003–7031. [CrossRef]
6. McNeil, B.L.; Mastroianni, S.A.; McNeil, S.W.; Zeisler, S.; Kumlin, J.; Borjian, S.; McDonagh, A.W.; Cross, M.; Schaffer, P.; Ramogida, C.F. Optimized production, purification, and radiolabeling of the ^{203}Pb/^{212}Pb theranostic pair for nuclear medicine. *Sci. Rep.* **2023**, *13*, 10623. [CrossRef]
7. Li, M.; Baumhover, N.J.; Liu, D.; Cagle, B.S.; Boschetti, F.; Paulin, G.; Lee, D.; Dai, Z.; Obot, E.R.; Marks, B.M.; et al. Preclinical evaluation of a lead specific chelator (PSC) conjugated to radiopeptides for ^{203}Pb and ^{212}Pb-Based theranostics. *Pharmaceutics* **2023**, *15*, 414. [CrossRef]
8. Mirzadeh, S.; Kumar, K.; Gansow, O.A. The chemical fate of ^{212}Bi-DOTA formed by β$^-$ decay of ^{212}Pb(DOTA)$^{2-}$. *Radiochim. Acta* **1993**, *60*, 1–10. [CrossRef]
9. Meredith, R.; Torgue, J.; Shen, S.; Fisher, D.R.; Banaga, E.; Bunch, P.; Morgan, D.; Fan, J.; Straughn, J.M., Jr. Dose escalation and dosimetry of first-in-human alpha radioimmunotherapy with ^{212}Pb-TCMC-trastuzumab. *J. Nucl. Med.* **2014**, *55*, 1636–1642. [CrossRef]
10. Delpassand, E.S.; Tworowska, I.; Esfandiari, R.; Torgue, J.; Hurt, J.; Shafie, A.; Núñez, R. Targeted α-emitter therapy with ^{212}Pb-DOTAMTATE for the treatment of metastatic SSTR-expressing neuroendocrine tumors: First-in-humans dose-escalation clinical trial. *J. Nucl. Med.* **2022**, *63*, 1326–1333. [CrossRef]
11. Müller, D.; Herrmann, H.; Schultz, M.K.; Solbach, C.; Ettrich, T.; Prasad, V. ^{203}Pb-VMT-α-NET scintigraphy of a patient with neuroendocrine tumor. *Clin. Nucl. Med.* **2023**, *48*, 54–55. [CrossRef] [PubMed]
12. Mikalsen, L.T.G.; Kvassheim, M.; Stokke, C. Optimized SPECT Imaging of ^{224}Ra α-particle therapy by ^{212}Pb photon emissions. *J. Nucl. Med.* **2023**, *64*, 1131–1137. [CrossRef]
13. Kotzerke, J.; Runge, R.; Braune, A.; Wunderlich, G. Different Radionuclides in DOTA-EB-TATE Effect Different Uptake in Somatostatin Receptor-Positive HEK293 Cells. *J. Nucl. Med.* **2019**, *60*, 436. [CrossRef] [PubMed]
14. Stenberg, V.Y.; Juzeniene, A.; Chen, Q.; Yang, X.; Bruland, Ø.S.; Larsen, R.H. Preparation of the alpha-emitting prostate-specific membrane antigen targeted radioligand [^{212}Pb]Pb-NG001 for prostate cancer. *J. Label. Comp. Radiopharm.* **2020**, *63*, 129–143. [CrossRef]
15. Durand-Panteix, S.; Monteil, J.; Sage, M.; Garot, A.; Clavel, M.; Saidi, A.; Torgue, J.; Cogne, M.; Quelven, I. Preclinical study of ^{212}Pb alpha-radioimmunotherapy targeting CD20 in non-Hodgkin lymphoma. *Br. J. Cancer* **2021**, *125*, 1657–1665. [CrossRef]
16. Li, J.; Huang, T.; Hua, J.; Wang, Q.; Su, Y.; Chen, P.; Bidlingmaier, S.; Li, A.; Xie, Z.; Bidkar, A.P.; et al. CD46 targeted ^{212}Pb alpha particle radioimmunotherapy for prostate cancer treatment. *J. Exp. Clin. Cancer Res.* **2023**, *42*, 61. [CrossRef] [PubMed]

17. Rathke, H.; Bruchertseifer, F.; Kratochwil, C.; Keller, H.; Giesel, F.L.; Apostolidis, C.; Haberkorn, U.; Morgenstern, A. First patient exceeding 5-year complete remission after ^{225}Ac-PSMA-TAT. *Eur. J. Nucl. Med. Mol. Imaging* **2021**, *48*, 311–312. [CrossRef]
18. Wood, V.; Ackerman, N.L. Cherenkov light production from the alpha-emitting decay chains of ^{223}Ra, ^{212}Pb, and ^{149}Tb for Cherenkov luminescence imaging. *Appl. Radiat. Isot.* **2016**, *118*, 354–360. [CrossRef] [PubMed]
19. Luurtsema, G.; Pichler, V.; Bongarzone, S.; Seimbille, Y.; Elsinga, P.; Gee, A.; Vercouillie, J. EANM guideline for harmonisation on molar activity or specific activity of radiopharmaceuticals: Impact on safety and imaging quality. *EJNMMI Radiopharm. Chem.* **2021**, *6*, 34. [CrossRef]
20. Orcutt, K.D.; Henry, K.E.; Habjan, C.; Palmer, K.; Heimann, J.; Cupido, J.M.; Gottumukkala, V.; Cissell, D.D.; Lyon, M.C.; Hussein, A.I.; et al. Dosimetry of [^{212}Pb]VMT01, a MC1R-targeted alpha therapeutic compound, and effect of free ^{208}Tl on tissue absorbed doses. *Molecules* **2022**, *27*, 5831. [CrossRef]
21. Li, M.; Zhang, X.; Quinn, T.P.; Lee, D.; Liu, D.; Kunkel, F.; Zimmerman, B.E.; McAlister, D.; Olewein, K.R.; Menda, Y.; et al. Automated cassette-based production of high specific activity [$^{203/212}$Pb] peptide-based theranostic radiopharmaceuticals for image-guided radionuclide therapy for cancer. *Appl. Radiat. Isot.* **2017**, *127*, 52–60. [CrossRef] [PubMed]
22. Bobba, K.N.; Bidkar, A.P.; Meher, N.; Fong, C.; Wadhwa, A.; Dhrona, S.; Sorlin, A.; Bidlingmaier, S.; Shuere, B.; He, J.; et al. Evaluation of ^{134}Ce/^{134}La as a PET imaging theranostic pair for ^{225}Ac α-radiotherapeutics. *J. Nucl. Med.* **2023**, *64*, 1076–1082. [CrossRef] [PubMed]
23. Sabet, A.; Nagarajah, J.; Dogan, A.S.; Biersack, H.-J.; Sabet, A.; Guhlke, S.; Ezziddin, S. Does PRRT with standard activities of ^{177}Lu-octreotate really achieve relevant somatostatin receptor saturation in target tumor lesions?: Insights from intra-therapeutic receptor imaging in patients with metastatic gastroenteropancreatic neuroendocrine tumors. *EJNMMI Res.* **2013**, *3*, 82. [PubMed]
24. Tian, R.; Jacobson, O.; Niu, G.; Kiesewetter, D.O.; Wang, Z.; Zhu, G.; Ma, Y.; Liu, G.; Chen, X. Evans Blue attachment enhances somatostatin receptor subtype-2 imaging and radiotherapy. *Theranostics* **2018**, *8*, 735–745. [CrossRef]
25. Waser, B.; Tamma, M.L.; Cescato, R.; Maecke, H.R.; Reubi, J.C. Highly efficient in vivo agonist-induced internalization of sst$_2$ receptors in somatostatin target tissues. *J. Nucl. Med.* **2009**, *50*, 936–941. [CrossRef]
26. Kratochwil, C.; Apostolidis, L.; Rathke, H.; Apostolidis, C.; Bicu, F.; Bruchertseifer, F.; Choyke, P.L.; Haberkorn, U.; Giesel, F.L.; Morgenstern, A. Dosing ^{225}Ac-DOTATOC in patients with somatostatin-receptor-positive solid tumors: 5-year follow-up of hematological and renal toxicity. *Eur. J. Nucl. Med. Mol. Imaging* **2021**, *49*, 54–63. [CrossRef]
27. Nicolas, G.P.; Schreiter, N.; Kaul, F.; Uiters, H.; Bouterfa, H.; Kaufmann, J.; Erlanger, T.E.; Cathomas, R.; Christ, E.; Fani, M.; et al. Sensitivity Comparison of ^{68}Ga-OPS202 and ^{68}Ga-DOTATOC PET/CT in patients with gastroenteropancreatic neuroendocrine tumors: A prospective phase II imaging study. *J. Nucl. Med.* **2018**, *59*, 915–921. [CrossRef]
28. Kotzerke, J.; Buesser, D.; Naumann, A.; Runge, R.; Huebinger, L.; Kliewer, A.; Freudenberg, R.; Brogsitter, C. Epigenetic-like stimulation of receptor expression in SSTR2 transfected HEK293 cells as a new therapeutic strategy. *Cancers* **2022**, *14*, 2513. [CrossRef]
29. von Hacht, J.L.; Erdmann, S.; Niederstadt, L.; Prasad, S.; Wagener, A.; Exner, S.; Beindorff, N.; Brenner, W.; Grötzinger, C. Increasing molar activity by HPLC purification improves ^{68}Ga-DOTA-NAPamide tumor accumulation in a B16/F1 melanoma xenograft model. *PLoS ONE* **2019**, *14*, e0217883. [CrossRef]
30. Hennrich, U.; Kopka, K. Lutathera®: The First FDA- and EMA-approved radiopharmaceutical for peptide receptor radionuclide therapy. *Pharmaceuticals* **2019**, *12*, 114. [CrossRef]
31. Piron, S.; Verhoeven, J.; De Coster, E.; Descamps, B.; Kersemans, K.; Pieters, L.; Vral, A.; Vanhove, C.; De Vos, F. Impact of the molar activity and PSMA expression level on [^{18}F]AlF-PSMA-11 uptake in prostate cancer. *Sci. Rep.* **2021**, *11*, 22623. [CrossRef] [PubMed]

Disclaimer/Publisher's Note: The statements, opinions and data contained in all publications are solely those of the individual author(s) and contributor(s) and not of MDPI and/or the editor(s). MDPI and/or the editor(s) disclaim responsibility for any injury to people or property resulting from any ideas, methods, instructions or products referred to in the content.

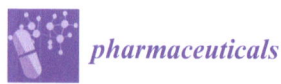 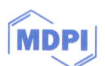

Review

Towards Effective Targeted Alpha Therapy for Neuroendocrine Tumours: A Review

Paul M. D. Gape [1,*], Michael K. Schultz [2,3], Graeme J. Stasiuk [1] and Samantha Y. A. Terry [1]

1. School of Biomedical Engineering & Imaging Sciences, King's College London, London SE1 7EP, UK; graeme.stasiuk@kcl.ac.uk (G.J.S.); samantha.terry@kcl.ac.uk (S.Y.A.T.)
2. Departments of Radiology, Radiation Oncology, Free Radical and Radiation Biology Program, University of Iowa, Iowa City, IA 52242, USA; mschultz@perspectivetherapeutics.com
3. Perspective Therapeutics, Coralville, IA 52241, USA
* Correspondence: paul.m.gape@kcl.ac.uk

Abstract: This review article explores the evolving landscape of Molecular Radiotherapy (MRT), emphasizing Peptide Receptor Radionuclide Therapy (PRRT) for neuroendocrine tumours (NETs). The primary focus is on the transition from β-emitting radiopharmaceuticals to α-emitting agents in PRRT, offering a critical analysis of the radiobiological basis, clinical applications, and ongoing developments in Targeted Alpha Therapy (TAT). Through an extensive literature review, the article delves into the mechanisms and effectiveness of PRRT in targeting somatostatin subtype 2 receptors, highlighting both its successes and limitations. The discussion extends to the emerging paradigm of TAT, underlining its higher potency and specificity with α-particle emissions, which promise enhanced therapeutic efficacy and reduced toxicity. The review critically evaluates preclinical and clinical data, emphasizing the need for standardised dosimetry and a deeper understanding of the dose-response relationship in TAT. The review concludes by underscoring the significant potential of TAT in treating SSTR2-overexpressing cancers, especially in patients refractory to β-PRRT, while also acknowledging the current challenges and the necessity for further research to optimize treatment protocols.

Keywords: molecular radiotherapy; targeted radionuclide therapy; targeted alpha therapy; peptide receptor radionuclide therapy; neuroendocrine tumours

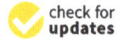

Citation: Gape, P.M.D.; Schultz, M.K.; Stasiuk, G.J.; Terry, S.Y.A. Towards Effective Targeted Alpha Therapy for Neuroendocrine Tumours: A Review. *Pharmaceuticals* 2024, 17, 334. https://doi.org/10.3390/ph17030334

Academic Editor: Hirofumi Hanaoka

Received: 8 February 2024
Revised: 22 February 2024
Accepted: 26 February 2024
Published: 4 March 2024

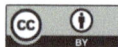

Copyright: © 2024 by the authors. Licensee MDPI, Basel, Switzerland. This article is an open access article distributed under the terms and conditions of the Creative Commons Attribution (CC BY) license (https://creativecommons.org/licenses/by/4.0/).

1. Introduction

1.1. Molecular Radiotherapy

MRT consists of the administration of a radiopharmaceutical, composed of an unstable radionuclide attached to a targeting ligand via a chelator. The ligand binds cellular sites that are overexpressed in tumour cells, but have low expression in healthy cells, therefore delivering cytotoxic radiation specifically to tumour cells and the associated tumour microenvironment, while sparing healthy tissue. As such, MRT has the potential to simultaneously irradiate all cancer cells within the patient, in contrast to local external beam radiation therapies targeting a single site of disease. The use of MRT for the treatment of neuroendocrine tumours has been employed as an effective therapy for several decades. Until recently, MRT targeted to neuroendocrine tumours has primarily employed beta(β)-particle emitters (e.g., ^{177}Lu). However, over the last several years, the use of alpha(α)-particle emitters for this application has emerged as potentially transformative. In this review, the transition from β-emitting radiopharmaceuticals to α-emitting agents in PRRT is presented. A critical analysis of the radiobiological basis, clinical applications, and ongoing developments in Targeted Alpha Therapy (TAT) is presented through an extensive literature review that explores this emerging paradigm of TAT and the promise of enhanced therapeutic efficacy and reduced toxicity. The review critically evaluates preclinical and clinical data, emphasizing the need for standardised dosimetry and a deeper understanding of the dose-response relationship in TAT. The review concludes by underscoring the significant potential of TAT in treating SSTR2-overexpressing cancers, especially in patients refractory to β-PRRT, while also acknowledging the current challenges and the necessity for further research to optimize treatment protocols. A complete review of the biology and pathophysiology of neuroendocrine tumours is beyond the scope of this review, which focuses on the use of MRT for the treatment of this disease. Nonetheless, a brief review of this family of malignancies is included here to provide context for the ensuing discussion.

1.2. Neuroendocrine Tumours

Neuroendocrine neoplasms are sub-classified by site of origin and pathology. Well-differentiated neoplasms are often referred to as NETs, and poorly differentiated neoplasms as neuroendocrine carcinomas [1]. NETs are further sub-classified according to their Ki-67 proliferation rate as G1, G2 or G3. G1 represents low-proliferative NETs, associated with good prognosis, and G3 represents high grade NETs, associated with poor prognosis [2]. The most common sites of origin are gastroenteropancreatic (GEP) structures and the lung. Tumours can also vary according to their functional status, with some NETs secreting excess hormones. NETs are considered rare cancers, accounting for roughly 0.5% of cancers, but their prevalence has increased in recent years, although it is generally accepted that the increase in prevalence can be attributed to some degree to improved imaging agents [3]. It is common to see NETs referred to as heterogeneous or diverse. This means they arise from a range of tissues and that patients present with a diverse range of symptoms, requiring a multidisciplinary approach to treatment [4]. In patients with localised disease, the first therapeutic option is surgery with curative intent. However, in the case of non-localised (metastasised disease), surgery is generally not considered feasible. In this patient cohort, systemic treatment is necessary and typically starts with a somatostatin analogue (SSA), for example, octreotide or lanreotide. This treatment is not curative in intent but aims to control symptoms. Further treatment options include systemic chemotherapy, though it has been shown that chemotherapy is of limited benefit [5]. This is the point in a patient's journey at which peptide receptor radionuclide therapy (PRRT) is typically offered [6].

1.3. PRRT for NETs—Targeting the Somatostatin Subtype 2 Receptor

PRRT targeting the somatostatin receptor (SSTR) is a specific example of MRT. SSTRs of various subtypes are overexpressed on the cell surface of a range of cancers. Most notably, over 80% of NETs overexpress SSTRs, particularly SSTR subtype 2 ($SSTR_2$), making this a suitable target for PRRT [7]. However, as well as being expressed on the surface of neuroendocrine tumour cells, $SSTR_2$ is widely expressed in normal tissues, particularly of the endocrine system [8]. Expression of $SSTR_2$ in normal tissue is shown anatomically in Figure 1 [9]. Imaging agents targeting $SSTR_2$ have shown physiological uptake in the spleen, kidneys, adrenal glands, liver, stomach, and small intestine [10]. While the present discussion is focused on NETs, SSTRs are also expressed in a range of other malignancies, such as lymphoma, several brain tumours, and in breast tumours, which are areas for a future investigation and review [11].

1.4. Evolving Standard of Care in PRRT

The most logical choice of targeting ligand may appear to be somatostatin, the native peptide hormone consisting of 14 amino acids. However, the somatostatin peptide-hormone is subject to rapid enzymatic degradation in vivo [12], motivating attempts to develop synthetic somatostatin analogues (SSAs) in order to provide tumour targeting with sufficient stability and affinity.

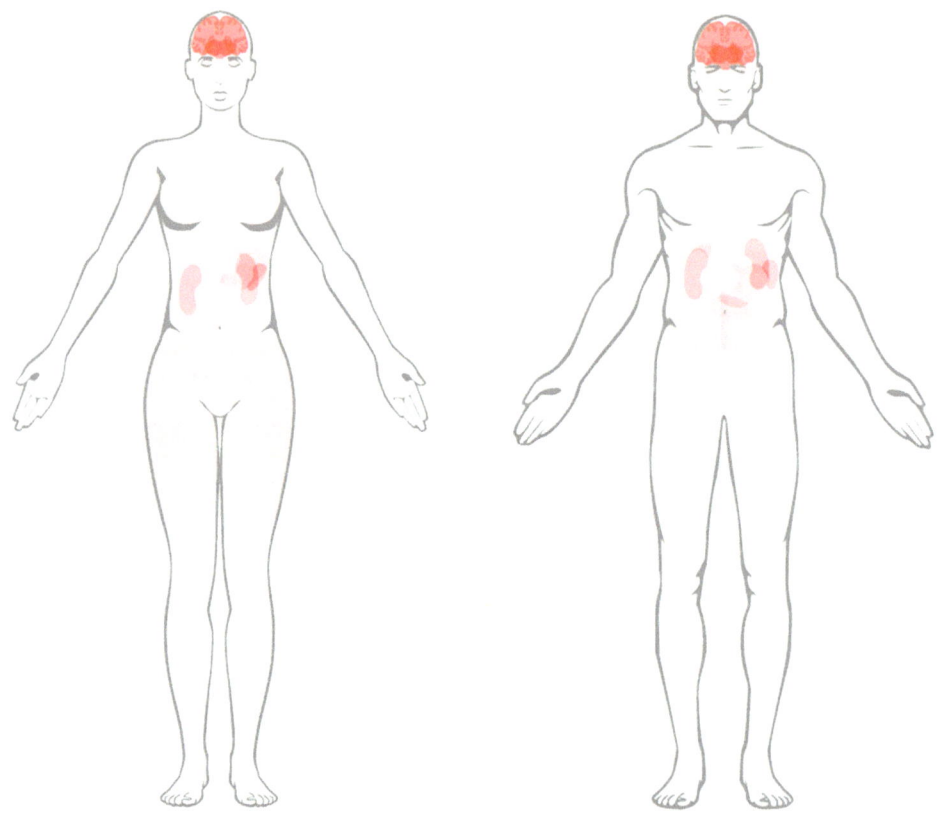

Figure 1. Anatomical depiction of SSTR 2 expression in human tissue in female (**left**) and male (**right**). Image credit: Human Protein Atlas version 23.0 (www.proteinatlas.org/ENSG00000180616-SSTR2 /tissue, accessed on 22 February 2024) [9].

These earliest iterations of PRRT focused on the development of [^{111}In-DTPA-$_D$-Phe1]-octreotide ([^{111}In]In-pentetreotide), initially for imaging. The utility of the newly developed radiopharmaceutical was initially demonstrated in 1050 patients [13,14]. The uptake demonstrated on imaging subsequently motivated the use of [^{111}In]In-pentetreotide for therapy [15]. This demonstrates an early application of the so-called "theragnostic principle", by which radiolabelled somatostatin analogues can target the same receptor for use in imaging and therapy.

Although the decay of ^{111}In results in the release of potentially therapeutic Auger and conversion electrons, the observed efficacy of the ^{111}In-labelled agent was modest and several patients developed leukaemia or myelodysplastic syndrome at high activities (>100 GBq) [16]. Given these shortcomings, β-emitters were later favoured due to their higher energy and longer range emissions. Higher energy β-emitters, such as ^{90}Y, were considered more promising for the treatment of bulky disease [7], whereas lower energy (thus shorter range) β-emitters, for instance ^{177}Lu, result in a lower radiation-absorbed dose to the kidney. ^{177}Lu also has the advantage of being directly imageable via the gamma photons in its decay scheme [17].

A novel targeting ligand with higher affinity for SSTR$_2$, [Tyr^3]-octreotide, was developed and combined with the chelator 1,4,7,10-tetra-azacyclododecane-tetra-acetic acid (DOTA), allowing for reliable and stable radiolabelling of ^{111}In and ^{90}Y ([^{90}Y]Y-DOTATOC; as well as ^{177}Lu- and ^{68}Ga-labelled agents introduced later). The [^{90}Y]Y-DOTATOC radiopharmaceutical was shown to be effective in stabilizing disease and slowing the rate of tumour progression, hence becoming the predominant choice of treatment in the early years of PRRT [18,19].

Later iterations of PRRT have utilised a newer somatostatin analogue, DOTA-[Tyr^3]-octreotate (DOTATATE), due to its higher binding affinity and in vivo uptake in target tissues compared to competitor SSAs [20]. A number of clinical trials have investigated the safety and efficacy of [^{177}Lu]Lu-DOTATATE, leading to the international phase three trial, NETTER-1 [21]. This trial established PRRT as standard of care for patients with metastatic SSTR$_2$-positive GEP-NETs, demonstrating a significantly higher response rate and extending progression-free survival (PFS) when compared with the control arm (high-dose of long-acting repeatable octreotide administrations). This positive result led to the approval of [^{177}Lu]Lu-DOTATATE, under the name Lutathera, in Europe by the European Medicines Agency in late 2017 and in America by the Food and Drug Administration in early 2018 [22]. Notably, while considered safe and effective by these agencies, the objective tumour response rate observed was 18% in the NETTER-1 trial (subsequently revised to 13% in post-trial analysis [1,23]), providing a basis for improvement that is being explored using α-emitting radionuclides. Current clinical practice, as recommended by the joint IAEA, EANM and SNMMI guidance on PRRT, consists of the systemic administration of the radiopharmaceutical over multiple cycles with 6–12 week intervals [7]. Administered activities are generally fixed at 3.7 GBq for [^{90}Y]Y-DOTA-TATE/TOC and 5.5–7.4 GBq for [^{177}Lu]Lu-DOTATATE and not varied between patients.

Based on the fundamental principle of maximizing the absorbed dose of radiation to tumour tissue, while minimizing radiation exposure to all other normal healthy organs and tissues, the next generation of PRRT may be realised through improvements in targeting ligand, chelator, and/or radionuclide. In the following, the argument for transitioning from β-emitters to α-emitters is considered, and the available literature reviewed critically.

2. Targeted Alpha Therapy (TAT)

2.1. Radiobiological Basis for TAT

TAT is a particularly interesting and promising strategy for cancer treatment given the high potency and specificity associated with α-particle emissions. The α-particle is a helium nucleus consisting of two protons and two neutrons, creating a composite particle with a net positive charge and a mass that is much greater than that of a β$^-$-particle (approximately 7000 times greater). The mass and charge of the α-particles make them highly ionizing and limit their range in tissue to 50–100 μm, or approximately 1–3 cell diameters [24]. The energy deposition of the particle along this path, referred to as the linear energy transfer (LET), varies between roughly 60 and 200 keV/μm. For comparison, the LET of a β$^-$-particle or a photon ranges from 0.1 to 1.0 keV/μm [25], and the LET of Auger electrons is 4–25 keV/μm [26]. This pattern of energy deposition of α-particles creates a dense track of ionizations along the path of the particle through the biological material in the vicinity of the decay. Where this biological material is the DNA of a tumour cell, these ionizations lead to complex damage such as DNA double-strand breaks, which almost invariably overcome the cell's repair mechanisms [25]. Conversely, β-emitters are more likely to produce simple, repairable damage, such as well-separated DNA single-strand breaks, due to the sparse nature of their ionization track. Auger electrons produce a dense, irregular pattern of ionisations clustered within several cubic nm from the site of the initial decay. Given the high LET of these low-energy electrons, they also have the potential to produce complex damage that is less reparable than that created by low LET radiation [27]. However, the short range of the Auger electrons means there is a greater requirement for the radionuclide to be transported into the cell and ideally incorporated into the DNA to maximise effectiveness, which may prove difficult in solid tumours [28]. Few α-particles are required to produce a cytotoxic effect, with estimates ranging from 1 to 20 traversals of the nucleus [29,30], resulting in higher potency than lower LET radiations. As demonstrated in Figure 2, the short range of the α-particle and the Auger electron also reduces the irradiation of off-target tissues, potentially reducing the probability of toxicity in normal organs.

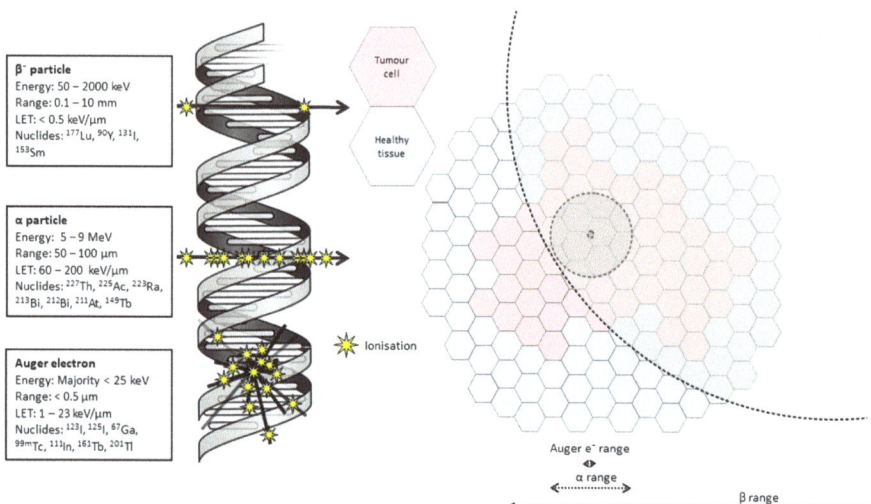

Figure 2. Radiobiological basis for TAT. High LET radiation produces a dense track of ionisations in biological target, producing complex irreparable damage to structures such as DNA. Range of Auger electron, α-particle and β-particle depicted (not to scale) to illustrate potential for sparing of healthy tissue.

Importantly, cell killing with α-emitters is less influenced by oxygen effects than β-emitters, where cytotoxicity is a product of the formation of reactive oxygen species (ROS), which subsequently damage the biological target [31]. The complex nature of the damage caused by individual α-particles also implies that cell survival should not be modulated by dose rate, whereas for low-LET radiation the biological effect of the dose is generally reduced when the dose is given over a longer period of time. This result was shown in vitro as early as 1964 [32]. In the in vivo setting, numerous other factors contribute to the effectiveness of α-emitters in potentiating tumour-specific cell death, including the tumour residence time of the agent and stability of the chelation of the parent and daughter radionuclides in the α-emitter decay chain. Thus, shorter-lived α-emitting radionuclides may provide additional benefit in ensuring a greater percentage of α-particles are localised to tumours within the expected biological residence time of the agent and daughter radionuclides.

The net effect of these differences between radiation qualities is encapsulated by the term relative biological effectiveness (RBE). This parameter is defined as the ratio of absorbed doses of two radiation types required to produce an identical, pre-defined biological effect. For RBE to be a meaningful quantity, the experimental and reference radiations must be defined, dosimetry should be performed, and the biological effect considered should be clearly stated. An RBE value for cell killing by α-particles of between three and five was recommended by a US Department of Energy Panel [33], but the accurate determination of the RBE for clinical and preclinical applications remains an important question. Broadly, the balance between response and toxicity is described by the therapeutic index, calculated as the ratio of the dose at which the treatment can be deemed effective and the dose at which the treatment results in undue toxicity. The therapeutic window may be considered as the difference between these two doses [34]. For the reasons discussed above, it is hoped that TAT will effectively widen the therapeutic window through improved tumour response and reduced off-target toxicity.

2.2. Evaluation of Candidate Radionuclides for TAT

There should not be a "one size fits all" approach for TAT. The radionuclide chosen should be matched to the requirements of the indication being treated. One example of this may be to choose an isotope with an appropriate half-life. This depends critically on the biological targeting ligand (sometimes referred to as vector) and the time taken for the radiopharmaceutical to accumulate in target tissues and to be cleared from non-target tissues. As mentioned above, for longer-lived radionuclides, the actual retention time of the agent in the tumour as well as the fate of the decay progeny in the α-emitter decay series must also be considered. The biological clearance of the agent may vary from minutes to days depending on molecular weight (antibodies for example have biological clearance rates that can be measured in days) [35]. Somatostatin analogues are relatively small biomolecules and thus clear quickly from the blood, so may be suited to a shorter half-life isotope [36]. While use of a longer-lived isotope may still be effective, their use is relatively inefficient due to potential washout of the agent from tumours and release of daughter radionuclides from the chelation moiety of the agent.

The decay schemes for a series of medically relevant α-emitters are shown in Figure 3 and their properties described in Table 1. Also included are so-called 'in vivo generators' of α-particles such as ^{212}Pb. While technically a β-emitter, the longer half-life of the parent in this case allows for the delivery of the daughter isotope, an α-emitter, to the site of interest in the body [37]. Not all α-emitters are discussed, for example ^{226}Th and ^{255}Fm. Although these isotopes may have been touted as having potential therapeutic applications, due to difficult production processes, the availability of these isotopes even for research purposes is severely limited [36].

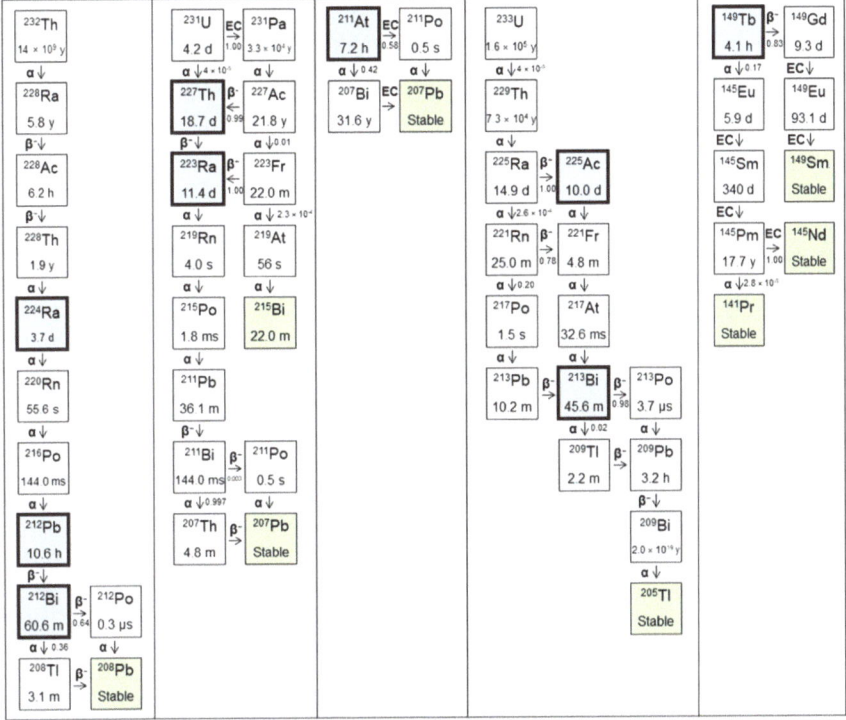

Figure 3. Decay schemes for medically relevant α-emitters. Blue indicates isotopes with potential for clinical translation, green indicates stable isotopes. Decay mode (α, β, electron capture (EC)) indicated, with associated yield where relevant.

Table 1. Relevant radionuclides for TAT, including in vivo alpha generators. Blue indicates isotopes with potential for clinical translation, green indicates stable isotopes. Emissions listed are not exhaustive but represent most of the energy in the decay scheme. ε = electron capture. Energy of β-particles refers to the mean energy. Decay data from ENSDF database as of February 2024 (http://www.nndc.bnl.gov/ensarchivals, accessed on 22 February 2024).

Parent	Daughters	$T_{1/2}$	Decay Type	Energy (MeV)	Yield	Imaging
^{227}Th		18.7 d	α	5.76, 5.98, 6.04	0.20, 0.23, 0.24	γ: 236 keV (0.13)
	^{223}Ra	11.4 d	α	5.60, 5.72	0.25, 0.51	γ: 269 keV (0.13)
	^{219}Rn	3.96 s	α	6.55, 6.82	0.13, 0.79	γ: 271 keV (0.11)
	^{215}Po	1.78 ms	α	7.39	1.00	-
	^{211}Pb	36.1 min	β-	0.16, 0.47	0.06, 0.91	γ: 405 keV (0.04)
	^{211}Bi	2.14 min	α	6.28, 6.62	0.16, 0.84	γ: 351 keV (0.13)
	^{207}Tl	4.77 min	β-	0.493	1.00	-
	^{207}Pb	Stable				
^{225}Ac		10.0 d	α	5.79, 5.83	0.18, 0.51	-
	^{221}Fr	4.80 min	α	6.13, 6.24 6.34	0.15, 0.01, 0.83	γ: 218 keV (0.13)
	^{217}At	32.6 ms	α	7.07	1.00	-
	^{213}Bi	45.6 min	α (0.02)	5.86	0.02	γ: 440 keV (0.26)
			β- (0.98)	0.32, 0.49	0.30, 0.67	
	^{213}Po	3.72 µs	α	8.38	1.00	-
	^{209}Tl	2.16 min	β-	0.660	0.97	γ: 117 keV (0.76)
	^{209}Pb	3.23 h	β-	0.198	1.00	-
	^{209}Bi	2.0 × 10^{19} y	α	2.88, 3.08	0.01, 0.99	
	^{205}Tl	Stable				
^{224}Ra		3.66 d	α	5.45, 5.69	0.05, 0.95	γ: 241 keV (0.04)
	^{220}Rn	55.6 s	α	6.29	0.99	-
	^{216}Po	144 ms	α	6.78	1.00	-
	^{212}Pb	10.6 h	β-	0.41, 0.93, 0.17	0.05, 0.81, 0.14	-
	^{212}Bi	60.6 min	α (0.36)	6.05, 6.09	0.25, 0.10	γ: 727 keV (0.07)
			β- (0.64)	0.53, 0.83	0.04, 0.55	
	^{212}Po	17.1 ns	α	10.2	0.42	-
	^{208}Tl	3.05 min	β-	0.44, 0.54, 0.65	0.24, 0.22, 0.49	γ: 277 keV (0.07)
	^{208}Pb	Stable				
^{211}At		7.21 h	α (0.42)	5.87	0.42	X: 77–92 keV
			ε (0.58)	-	-	-
	^{211}Po	0.52 s	α	7.45	0.99	-
	^{207}Bi	31.6 y	ε	-	-	γ: 570 keV (0.98)
	^{207}Pb	Stable				
^{149}Tb		4.12 h	α (0.17)	3.97	0.17	β+: 639 keV (0.04)
			ε (0.83)			γ: 165 keV (0.27)
	^{149}Gd	9.28 d	ε	-	-	γ: 150 keV (0.48)
	^{149}Eu	93.1 d	ε	-	-	-
	^{149}Sm	Stable				
	^{145}Eu	5.93 d	ε	-	-	β+: 740 keV (0.02)
	^{145}Sm	340 d	ε	-	-	-
	^{145}Pm	17.7 y	α (2.8 × 10^{-7})	2.24	2.80 × 10^{-7}	-
			ε (1.00)	-	-	-
	^{145}Nd	Stable				
	^{141}Pr	Stable				

The only α-emitting isotope currently clinically approved in the USA and Europe is ^{223}RaCl$_2$ and is indicated for castration-resistant prostate cancer and bone metastases (in males), following the results of the ALSYMPCA trial [38]. This represents a simpler scenario, in which the unconjugated radionuclide is injected. ^{223}Ra is a calcium mimic and therefore shows accumulation in sites of increased bone turnover, particularly bone metastases. However, this implies that ^{223}RaCl$_2$ is ineffective against soft tissue metastases. This demonstrates how the efficacy of ^{223}Ra could be improved by conjugation with a targeting ligand, though this has been limited due to the relative lack of chelators that demonstrate stability in vivo [39].

Much of the interest in TAT has focused on ^{225}Ac. This is principally because of the seven radionuclide daughters in its decay chain (four α and three β$^-$), meaning the total decay energy is high relative to other candidate isotopes. ^{225}Ac is also readily chelated with DOTA [40], allowing for conjugation with a range of antibodies and small molecules. However, because ^{225}Ac is itself an α-emitter, the emission of the α-particle results in the release from chelation of the entire decay series, with each decay. This is due to the recoil energy imparted to the daughter nucleus (^{221}Fr), which is more than sufficient to break all chemical bonds with each α-emission by ^{225}Ac. This is further exacerbated in that the first daughter in this decay series (i.e., ^{221}Fr) has very little affinity for chelation to DOTA-like macrocycles [41]. This leads to a redistribution of the free daughters, with potential to cause significant damage to healthy tissues. For example, ^{225}Ac decays to ^{213}Bi (through ^{221}Fr and ^{217}At), and free Bi is known to accumulate in the kidneys [42]. For most studies involving long-lived α-emitters, recoiling daughters pose a serious problem and toxic effects are likely, though the balance between anti-tumour effect and toxicity will vary and must be understood for each isotope, targeting ligand, and indication [43]. This may be less so with the use of relatively short-lived ^{212}Pb because the recoil energy of the β-particle emission of ^{212}Pb is significantly less than the binding energy of the daughter nucleus to the chelator. Although reports of Bi instability to decoupling has been reported for DOTA and TCMC [44,45], recent reports of a new chelator with improved stability of the chelator ^{212}Bi coupling represents an advance that can improve the therapeutic index for targeting ligands conjugated to this new chelator (known as Pb-Specific-Chelator or PSC) [46–49].

Given the high RBE of the α-particle, knowing the biodistribution of the radiopharmaceutical is of heightened importance to ensure targeted delivery and the minimum off-target exposure. One way to achieve this is through imaging. As shown in Table 1, all the isotopes considered have some potential to be imaged, either directly or via a daughter. However, often this potential is limited by low abundance and complicated decay schemes, as for example with ^{223}Ra, where SPECT imaging is feasible but only with long scan times [50]. In a population of patients with metastatic prostate cancer, this may not be tolerable. This limitation can be overcome through imaging with an imaging surrogate isotope. Radionuclides with elementally matched isotopes suitable for imaging offer an advantage here, because the biodistribution of the imaging agent is more likely to be representative of the therapeutic. An example of this principle is seen with ^{212}Pb and ^{203}Pb, which are suitable for SPECT imaging [47,51]. A recent development that further provides an advantage for the ^{212}Pb/^{203}Pb-matched pair of isotopes is the demonstration that ^{212}Pb SPECT imaging of NET tumours directly is feasible [52]. Quantitative imaging of a tracer amount of the therapeutic radionuclide or a theragnostic pair radionuclide enables treatment planning, as is standard in EBRT, in which target-absorbed doses to tumours and tolerance-absorbed doses to healthy organs are prescribed and the therapeutic activity is calculated to satisfy these constraints [53]. Post-therapy imaging and dosimetry then enable verification of the absorbed doses delivered in MRT.

Aside from the theoretical properties of each candidate radionuclide, translation to the clinic will be limited by availability and supply. The majority of the radionuclides in Table 1 are generator derived. Supply of ^{223}Ra via ^{227}Ac/^{227}Th generators is already established for clinical use. Generators loaded with ^{228}Th form the basis of ^{224}Ra production and can also be used to supply ^{212}Pb and ^{212}Bi. While radiolytic damage to the generator matrix material at high activities limits the level of radioactivity that can be loaded to current generators, the availability and half-life of ^{228}Th ($t_{1/2}$ = 1.9 years) inventories and the potential for continental distribution of ^{224}Ra ($t_{1/2}$ = 3.9 days) enables a system of inventory management and simple wet-chemical purifications that can be readily scaled for commercial radiopharmaceutical production facilities of ^{212}Pb radiopharmaceuticals [54]. A number of publications have demonstrated the potential for an emanation-based approach to the production of ^{212}Pb via the isolation of gaseous ^{220}Rn [55]. However, a production of ^{212}Pb using this approach at levels beyond a single clinical dose *per* day has yet to be demonstrated to our knowledge, and current emanation devices would require large inventories of ^{228}Th on site at each finished product radiopharmaceutical manufacturing facility. This is an area of intense research as the potential of next generation ^{212}Pb-based radiopharmaceuticals is increasingly recognised. To date, the vast majority of ^{225}Ac is produced from the decay of ^{229}Th, of which only three sources are currently available worldwide. This amounts to approximately 68 GBq *per* year in global production, well below the clinical demand for PRRT [40]. Accelerator and reactor-based approaches are emerging that are showing promise for alleviating this shortfall [56]. For example, the Tri-Lab effort, incorporating US National Laboratories at Oak Ridge, Los Alamos and Brookhaven, will aim to increase supply using accelerator production via ^{232}Th(p,x)^{225}Ac, with 307 mCi produced in the 2022 financial year and plans to expand production capabilities [57]. Similarly, a partnership between Canadian Nuclear Laboratories (CNL) and German radiopharmaceutical biotech company ITM has been established to increase production by a factor of 30 via irradiation of ^{226}Ra targets [58]. Production of ^{211}At requires target irradiation by an α-particle beam of energy above 28 MeV. Few accelerator facilities are able to reach this requirement [59]. Clearly, establishment of other production routes to ensure a stable supply of α-emitters for TAT is of critical importance. Continued investment in these technologies for the improved production and purity of ^{225}Ac is sought to satisfy the demand for α-emitters for radionuclide therapy.

In the following section, all experience, preclinical and clinical, with TAT of SSTR$_2$-overexpressing cancers is critically reviewed.

3. Literature Review

3.1. Overview

The published literature relating to TAT of SSTR$_2$-overexpressing cancers was reviewed via keyword database search (Pubmed, Web of Science, Ovid). Results were included up to the date of 1 December 2023. Results were screened and categorised by scope into in vitro, in vivo, clinical, in silico, case report, abstract, or review. Abstracts and reviews were excluded from further analysis. A total of 43 studies were found; the distribution of article scope and radionuclide across the studies is shown in Figure 4.

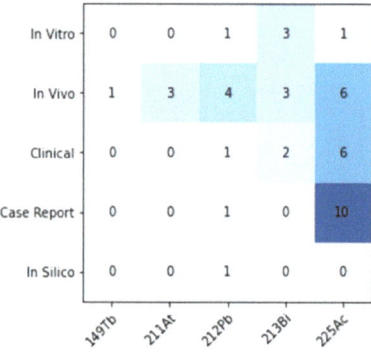

Figure 4. Literature review overview showing the scope of included studies and distribution of radionuclides reported for TAT of SSTR$_2$-overexpressing cancers.

The majority of the current clinical experience with TAT for PRRT in NETs is with ^{225}Ac. Despite theoretical feasibility and applications for other indications, no studies were found relating to ^{223}Ra, ^{224}Ra or ^{227}Th. Most studies used the DOTA chelator (29/43) and the TOC/TATE (37/43)-targeting ligand. Two SSTR antagonists (LM3, JR11) were investigated, in contrast to the conventional agonists [40,60]. Several more recent publications examined SSAs conjugated to a new chelator (via a PEG linker), developed specifically for $^{203/212}$Pb radiopharmaceuticals, and appear to improve the pharmacokinetic properties and stability of chelation [46,47,49].

3.2. Preclinical Studies

An overview of all studies containing in vitro and/or in vivo work is given in Table 2. Analysis of the specific aspects of the studies is continued in the sections below, with a focus on the relationships between activity (MBq), absorbed dose (Gy) and biological endpoint.

Table 2. Overview of in vitro and in vivo studies in α-PRRT. OS = overall survival, D_{10} = absorbed dose to reduce survival to 10%, MPC = murine pheochromocytoma cell.

Author	Radiopharmaceutical	Aim	Findings
Chan [61]	[^{213}Bi]Bi-DOTA-TATE	Determine whether TAT efficacy in vivo is related to tumour size in two SSTR$_2$ +ve cell lines.	Improved OS, increased tumour doubling time vs. control in small (50 mm^3) and large (200 mm^3) CA20948 and H69 tumours. Several cures in small tumour cohort. No toxicity.
Chan [62]	[^{213}Bi]Bi-DOTA-TATE	Investigate optimal radiolabelling conditions (peptide amount, quencher, pH) for [^{213}Bi]Bi-DOTATATE.	>3.5 nmol DOTATATE required for >99% incorporation with 100 MBq ^{213}Bi. Optimised conditions: pH = 8.3, TRIS = 0.15 mol/L in 800 µL. Ascorbic acid (0.9 mmol/L) required to avoid radiolysis.
Chan [63]	[^{213}Bi]Bi-DOTA-TATE	Evaluate the therapeutic effect of TAT with and without renal protection using L lysine in vivo.	MTA in healthy mice = 13, 21.7 MBq with/without renal protection. In tumour-bearing, median OS > 30 d at 17 MBq, severe weight loss and mortality at 33 MBq. Renal protection improved OS.
Chan [64]	[^{213}Bi]Bi-DOTA-TATE	Develop methods to determine relationship between absorbed dose and cell killing in vitro. Compare cytotoxicity across radiations in various cell lines.	In CA20948, D_{10} = 3 Gy, 18 Gy and 5 $_{Gy}$ for [^{213}Bi]Bi-DOTATATE, [^{177}Lu]Lu-DOTATATE and ^{137}Cs. In BON, [^{177}Lu]Lu-DOTATATE had no effect, D_{10} for [^{213}Bi]Bi-DOTATATE, ^{137}Cs = 2.5 Gy, 4.5 Gy.
Chapeau [65]	[^{212}Pb]Pb-eSOMA-01	Develop new octreotate derivatives with non-DOTA chelators and assess their potential for TAT of NETs with Pb.	New SSTR$_2$-targetting ligands labelled successfully with $^{212/203}$Pb, eSOMA-01 showed favourable biodistribution compared to DOTAM-TATE.
Cieslik [66]	[^{225}Ac]Ac-L1-TATE	Assess feasibility of L1 as chelator with ^{177}Lu, ^{211}At, ^{225}Ac in two SSTR$_2$ +ve cell lines, evaluate biodistribution in MPC tumour bearing mice.	L1 can bind radionuclides for imaging and therapy. Preferable fast and mild labelling compared to DOTA. [^{225}Ac]Ac-L1 produced with molar activity > 0.25 MBq/nmol.
Graf [67]	[^{225}Ac]Ac-DOTA-TOC	Assess γH2AX foci formation as biomarker of cytotoxicity and response to [^{225}Ac]Ac-DOTATOC and [^{177}Lu]Lu-DOTATOC in vitro and in vivo.	High tumour control rate with single treatment of both agents. Number of γH2AX foci correlated with apoptosis (in vitro) and tumour growth, showing potential as biomarker.
Handula [60]	[^{225}Ac]Ac-DOTA-JR11	Investigate potential of [^{225}Ac]Ac-DOTA-JR11 (antagonist) for therapy of NETs via mouse model.	Low tumour-to-kidney ratio of absorbed dose is limiting for therapeutic use of [^{225}Ac]Ac-DOTA-JR11.

Table 2. Cont.

Author	Radiopharmaceutical	Aim	Findings
King [68]	[^{225}Ac]Ac-MACROPA-TATE	Synthesise and characterise MACROPA TATE, compare performance with DOTA TATE in labelling efficiency, stability, binding, efficacy.	[^{225}Ac]Ac-MACROPATATE showed higher renal and liver uptake and toxicity at lower activities, DOTATATE deemed superior.
Lee [46]	[^{212}Pb]Pb-PSC-PEG$_2$-TOC	Improve SSTR$_2$ targeting over DOTA-based conjugates via click-chemistry-based cyclization, improved chelator design and insertion of PEG linkers.	Development of lead-specific chelator (PSC) and insertion of PEG linkers results in improved tumour uptake, retention and quicker renal clearance, and dose-dependent therapeutic effect with acceptable toxicity.
Li [47]	[^{212}Pb]Pb-PSC-PEG-TOC	Characterise Pb-specific chelator for radiolabelling yield, stability and in vivo biodistribution.	^{212}Pb and ^{212}Bi stably incorporated in PSC-PEG-TOC. Biodistribution of ^{212}Pb/^{212}Bi-PSC-PEG-TOC were comparable. $^{203/212}$Pb showed comparable biodistribution.
Miederer [69]	[^{225}Ac]Ac-DOTA-TOC	Compare biodistribution, toxicity and anti-tumour effect of [^{225}Ac]Ac-DOTATOC and [^{177}Lu]Lu-DOTATOC.	Activities > 30 kBq of ^{225}Ac-induced tubular necrosis, weight loss. ^{225}Ac (20 kBq) showed improved tumour growth delay vs. ^{177}Lu (0.45 MBq).
Müller [70]	[^{149}Tb]Tb-DOTA-NOC	Letter to the editor to highlight the potential of ^{149}Tb for 'α PET'.	High quality PET image of mouse injected with 7 MBq [^{149}Tb]Tb-DOTANOC showing high tumour uptake.
Nayak [71]	[^{213}Bi]Bi-DOTA-TOC	Compare binding, cytotoxicity, induction of apoptosis between [^{213}Bi/^{177}Lu]Lu-DOTATOC in human pancreatic adenocarcinoma cells.	RBE of [^{213}Bi]Bi-DOTATOC, [^{177}Lu]Lu-DOTATOC relative to ^{137}Cs is 3.4, 1.0. ^{213}Bi induced greater release of apoptosis markers in Capan-2 cells.
Norenberg [72]	[^{213}Bi]Bi-DOTA-TOC	Evaluate quantitative labelling methods, stability, biodistribution, safety, and efficacy in vivo.	Activity-related decrease in tumour growth rate observed (>11 MBq). Mild acute but no chronic nephrotoxicity. No haemato-toxicity.
Pretze [49]	[^{212}Pb]Pb-PSC-PEG$_2$-TOC	Investigate the influence of different molar activities of [$^{203/212}$Pb]Pb-PSC$_2$-TOC on cell uptake.	Uptake increased with molar activity, 15–40 MBq/nmol showed highest cell uptake.
Qin [73]	[^{211}At]At-SAB-Oct	Develop octreotide SAB conjugate to be labelled with ^{211}At and evaluate therapeutic efficacy against SCLC.	Anti-tumour response against SCLC model demonstrated, with acceptable toxicity profile.
Stallons [74]	[^{212}Pb]Pb-DOTAM-TATE	Determine binding and cell kill in vitro. Assess biodistribution in vivo. Establish tolerable regimen and efficacy as mono and combination therapy.	Non-toxic at <45 µCi, toxicity overcome by fractionation into 3 cycles. 79% cure rate with 3 × 10 µCi in combination with 5FU. Benefits of ascorbic acid and nephro protection demonstrated.
Tafreshi [75]	[^{225}Ac]Ac-DOTA-TATE	Assess toxicity, biodistribution, dosimetry and efficacy in lung neuroendocrine model (H727/H69) in vivo.	Chronic progressive nephropathy at >111 kBq. Single admin produced tumour growth delay and reduction in tumour volume vs. control.

Table 2. Cont.

Author	Radiopharmaceutical	Aim	Findings
Vaidyanathan [76]	[^{211}At]At-GIMBO	Synthesise octreotate analogue with guanidine-containing template for ^{211}At labelling, assess in comparison with Glu-TOCA in vitro and in vivo.	Single step process to synthesise radioiodinated and astatinated octreotide analogue with positive template reported. Affinity for SSTR$_2$ demonstrated, but high uptake in normal tissue is limiting.
Wharton [77]	[^{225}Ac]Ac-H$_4$noneupaX-TATE	Develop novel bifunctional chelator capable of complexing ^{225}Ac and ^{155}Tb for theragnostics.	H$_4$noneupaX was characterised, then labelling of ^{225}Ac and ^{155}Tb assessed. SPECT/CT imaging of ^{155}Tb demonstrates potential as theragnostic pair isotope for ^{225}Ac therapy.
Zhao [78]	[^{211}At]At-SPC-TOC	Investigate possible use of ^{211}Ac-labelled octreotide to treat NSCLC.	[^{211}At]At-SPC-octreotide showed elevated and activity-dependent apoptosis induction compared to PBS, cold peptide and unlabelled ^{211}At.

3.2.1. In Vitro RBE

Applying RBE to TAT, we may ask what absorbed dose of an α-emitter is required to produce the same biological effect as a low-LET reference radiation such as photons or electrons. Three studies report the RBE of TAT in vitro. A summary of these findings can be found in Table 3, showing the sometimes subtle differences between these studies. Averaging these estimates results in an RBE of 3.9 (SD 1.9) for cell killing with α-particles in vitro.

Table 3. Overview of in vitro RBE studies for α-emitters. $D_{10,20}$ = absorbed dose required for 10, 20% cell survival. ED_{50} = activity concentration required for 50% cell survival. ^{177}Lu is included to demonstrate reported equivalence to irradiation with ^{137}Cs.

Author	Cell Line	Radiopharmaceutical	Reference Radiation	End Point	RBE
Chan [64]	CA20948 (rat pancreatic)	[^{213}Bi]Bi-DTPA	^{137}Cs	D_{10}	2.0
		[^{213}Bi]Bi-DOTATATE	^{137}Cs	D_{10}	1.5
		[^{213}Bi]Bi-DOTATATE	[^{177}Lu]Lu-DOTATATE	D_{10}	5.4
		[^{213}Bi]Bi-DOTATATE	[^{177}Lu]Lu-DOTATATE	D_{10}	5.7
	BON (human carcinoid)	[^{213}Bi]Bi-DTPA	^{137}Cs	D_{10}	1.8
		[^{213}Bi]Bi-DOTATATE	^{137}Cs	D_{10}	1.7
Graf [67]	AR42J (rat pancreatic)	[^{225}Ac]Ac-DOTATOC	[^{177}Lu]Lu-DOTATOC	ED_{50} (kBq/mL)	5.5
Nayak [71]	Capan-2 (human pancreatic)	[^{213}Bi]Bi-DOTATOC	^{137}Cs	D_{20}	3.4
		[^{177}Lu]Lu-DOTATOC	^{137}Cs	D_{20}	1.0

The RBE can be seen to depend on several parameters, including cell line, reference radiation and biological end point. Dependence on cell line may be due to varying levels of SSTR$_2$ expression. The end points considered also differ subtly. Two studies consider the absorbed dose to produce a cell survival of 10% or 20%. Typically, cell survival curves for high-LET radiation such as α-emitters are log-linear functions of absorbed dose, meaning that RBE will vary according to the end point chosen. The parameter RBE2 has been proposed to overcome this shortcoming, and is defined as the ratio of the linear coefficients characterising the high-LET dose-response curve and the low-LET MV photon 2 Gy fraction-equivalent absorbed dose-response curve [79].

Dosimetry in this setting is not routinely carried out and lacks standardization. For example, Chan and collaborators separately consider the absorbed dose due to specific irradiation from the bound radionuclide and non-specific irradiation from the radioactive incubation medium [64]. In the specific case, the MIRD formalism is applied using the

MIRDcell software V2.0 [80], in which sub-cellular regions are considered as sources and targets, with dimensions and uptake fractions calculated and used as the basis for dosimetric estimate [81]. For the non-specific scenario, a bespoke Monte Carlo method was applied using the radiation transport code MCNPX. In this way, an estimate of the radiation dose received by the cells (grown as an adherent monolayer) from the radiation distributed throughout the total volume of liquid in the well was made. When estimating RBE, these assumptions should be communicated clearly, and it should be acknowledged that methodological differences may cause discrepancies between estimates [82].

3.2.2. In Vivo Efficacy

A total of 11 studies assessed the efficacy of TAT in vivo, with efficacy being defined according to a range of endpoints. Most commonly (5/11 studies), parameters relating to tumour growth rate were assessed, such as tumour regrowth doubling time and tumour growth delay. Also in 5/11 studies, overall survival (OS) was considered, and 4/11 studies considered tumour size. Other endpoints investigated included cure rate and various potential biomarkers of response (percentage of cells undergoing apoptosis, percentage of γH2AX positive cells, $SSTR_2$ expression).

The animal species studied were predominantly mice, apart from one study where Lewis rats were used [72]. It is noted that when assessing efficacy in athymic mice, any response attributable to the immune system cannot be studied. Increasingly, the immune response is known to play an important role in anti-tumour effects [83], leading to a potentially important discordance between the preclinical and clinical settings.

A source of heterogeneity between studies was the tumour model used. Firstly, a range of cell lines was used as a xenograft, most commonly the rat pancreatic cancer cell lines AR42J and CA20948, but also a range of non-small cell lung cancer cells showing $SSTR_2$ expression (H69, H727, A549). The fact that these cell lines are being studied preclinically is a sign that the indication for PRRT could soon expand beyond midgut NETs studied in the NETTER-1 trial. Even amongst studies considering the same tumour cell line, the number of cells inoculated and tumour size at the time of PRRT varied significantly, from non-visible to 382 mm^3 in mice and 1720 mm^3 in rats. Importantly, none of the cell lines studied represent a model of a human NET. For the best prospect of translation, the level and heterogeneity of $SSTR_2$ expression should bear similarity to the clinical scenario.

Conclusions about the efficacy of TAT, particularly in comparison to β-PRRT, are of limited use if the activities and peptide masses administered are arbitrary. The administered activity should be chosen to maximize the therapeutic index, balancing anti-tumour efficacy against the risk of toxicity. However, few studies selected a therapeutic activity based on a prior activity escalation toxicity study, King [68] and Stallons [74] being the only examples. The majority of studies (8/11) did consider some form of activity escalation when assessing therapeutic response, though a rationale for the activities chosen was rarely given. One study based administered activities on renal dose limits from the literature [46], specifically 27 Gy for β-particles (adjusted according to an RBE of 5 for α-particles), and 11 Gy and 20 Gy based on the results of Chan and collaborators [63]. The range of single cycle activity, cumulated activity and peptide amount *per* cycle are shown in Figure 5. Differences between radiopharmaceuticals are to be expected, given the differing pharmacokinetics and decay scheme energies. However, differences of several orders of magnitude were observed with the same radiopharmaceutical. The administered mass of peptide has been shown to alter biodistribution [49,84], therefore care must be taken in interpreting results if changing peptide mass and radionuclide activity simultaneously. However, Stallons and collaborators found that decreasing the specific activity by a factor of roughly 25 did not significantly alter the tumour uptake in a biodistribution study [74]. Roughly half of the studies (5/11) considered a single administration only. Of the six considering a fractionated regimen, the interval between cycles varied significantly, from a single day (42, 44 [75]) to 14–21 days [72]. Alternating the fractionation regime was shown to have a significant effect on overall survival [46,74].

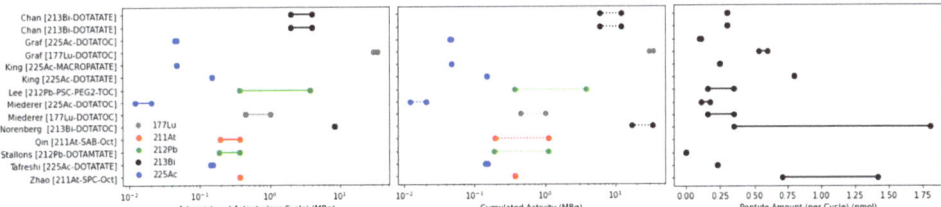

Figure 5. Range of administered activity, cumulated activity and administered peptide mass in preclinical efficacy studies.

Despite methodological differences, the results in these studies go some way to explaining the excitement around TAT. A significant anti-tumour response leading to prolonged survival is repeatedly demonstrated across a range of tumours and tumour sizes. In both studies by Chan and collaborators investigating [^{213}Bi]Bi-DOTATATE, median overall survival in a treated cohort was extended beyond the length of follow up; in the later study, complete responses were observed [61,63]. Stallons and collaborators and Lee and collaborators demonstrate complete responses to ^{212}Pb [74,82], King and collaborators reports complete response following ^{225}Ac [68]. However, this effect is not seen evenly across all treated cohorts, stressing the importance of optimising the way these novel radiopharmaceuticals are given.

3.2.3. In Vivo Healthy Tissue Toxicity

While the previous section demonstrates exciting potential efficacy, an acceptable toxicity profile is also a prerequisite for TAT. Firstly, it was observed that whether toxicity was determined in healthy or tumour-bearing animals was a source of discordance between studies. Toxicity was assessed in healthy animals in 3/10 studies, 6/10 in tumour-bearing animals and 1 study considered both scenarios. Given that tumour uptake has been shown to lead to decreased bioavailability in normal tissue [85], this introduces some uncertainty when extrapolating results from healthy animals.

Through appraising the literature, the commonly observed toxicities arising from TAT in the preclinical setting were established. The most common observation was weight loss, a non-specific marker seen in 6/10 studies that assessed toxicity. In each case, weight loss was associated with increasing administered activity.

Evidence of nephrotoxicity, a known adverse effect of PRRT, was also found in 6/10 studies. This was most commonly seen on pathological examination (5/6). Interestingly, 3/10 studies measured changes in blood urea nitrogen (BUN) and creatinine as potential biomarkers of renal injury but found no relationship between these parameters and outcome. This indicates that these commonly used biomarkers are not sensitive markers for nephrotoxicity, meaning more appropriate biomarkers are required, for example neutrophil gelatinase-associated lipocalin (NGAL), as investigated by Chan and collaborators [62] and highlighted as a potential biomarker of tubular damage and long-term nephrotoxicity evaluated by Li et al. [86]. One study did assess renal function via functional imaging with ^{99m}Tc-DMSA, but no difference in uptake between treated and control cohorts was observed [61]. Clinically, amino acids are commonly co-administered with PRRT to inhibit reabsorption of the radiopharmaceutical in proximal tubular cells, therefore significantly reducing uptake and radiation-absorbed dose [87]. Of the studies included here, 6/10 did not co-administer amino acids for renal protection. The remaining 4/10 investigated toxicity both with and without amino acids. Chan and collaborators [63] show that the renal-absorbed dose is decreased by a factor of roughly two by the co-administration of L-lysine with [^{213}Bi]Bi-DOTATATE, suggesting that the sparing remains relevant in TAT. Conclusions around renal toxicity that do not account for the sparing effect of amino acids should be considered with this potential improvement in mind.

Aside from renal toxicity, haematological toxicity was assessed in 5/10 studies. Stallons and collaborators observed decreased levels of leukocytes, erythrocytes, albumin and bone marrow depletion leading to mortality following the highest activity administration of [^{212}Pb]Pb-DOTAMTATE [74]. However, this study also showed that it was possible to manage and overcome this toxicity when using a fractionated administration regimen (3 cycles at 21-day intervals). One study reported mild hypothyroidism as a side effect, shown through low thyroid hormone level in blood sampling, but this was not considered significant. No hepatotoxicity was observed, and no toxicity associated with the administration of unlabelled peptide as a control was reported.

Maximum tolerated activity was investigated in two studies. For [^{213}Bi]Bi-DOTATATE, maximum tolerated activity with and without renal protection was determined as 21.7 and 13.0 MBq, given as three or two cycles with one day intervals, respectively. For [^{212}Pb]Pb-DOTAMTATE, the maximum tolerated activity was between 0.74 and 1.48 MBq when given as a single administration, roughly an order of magnitude lower than for ^{213}Bi. The no-observed-effect level activity was found to be 0.37 MBq, and the highest non-severely toxic dose was 0.74 MBq. Lee et al. did not observe any acute toxicity or lethal effects with activities up to 3.7 MBq using [^{212}Pb]Pb-PSC-PEG$_2$-TOC, perhaps due to the introduction of the new Pb-specific chelator and PEG$_2$ linker and improved chelation and renal clearance of this agent [46]. While not strictly defined as maximum tolerated activity within the study, Miederer and collaborators [69] showed that no histopathologic alterations were found in the kidneys after treatment with [^{225}Ac]Ac-DOTATOC at activities below 20 kBq. No studies performed dosimetry to estimate the relationship between absorbed dose and toxicity in a specific organ.

3.2.4. In Vivo Dosimetry

In attempting to understand response and toxicity quantitatively, and potentially relate this knowledge to new contexts, absorbed dose to the tumour and to organs at risk is an important parameter. Clinically, there is a growing body of evidence implying correlation between absorbed dose delivered and therapeutic response [88]. Similarly, renal-absorbed dose is considered a risk factor for long-term renal toxicity after β-PRRT [89]. Five studies estimated absorbed dose to the tumour and six studies estimated absorbed dose to the kidneys in the preclinical setting. The reported absorbed dose coefficients (ADC) are given in Table 4. The absorbed dose coefficient varied depending on the cell line used, even when the tumour size was comparable at the time of administration. The large difference in absorbed dose coefficients for [^{225}Ac]Ac-DOTATATE and for [^{213}Bi]Bi-DOTATATE reflects the net emission of four α particles *per* decay of ^{225}Ac, compared to one *per* decay of ^{213}Bi. The ratio of tumour-absorbed dose to kidney-absorbed dose is a useful metric to potentially understand the viability of a perspective therapeutic agent. The highest reported ratio is for [^{212}Pb]Pb-PSC-PEG$_2$-TOC, where structural modifications to the chelator and linker result in T:K absorbed dose >2.6. Contrastingly, Handula and collaborators conclude that [^{225}Ac]Ac-DOTA-JR11 is unsuitable for therapy based on a low T:K of 0.34 [60]. While T:K is a useful parameter, clearly more work is required to properly understand what constitutes effective tumour-absorbed doses and safe renal-absorbed doses for this class of radiopharmaceuticals.

As mentioned, RBE is an important parameter, particularly in comparison with the RBE determined in vitro. This would go some way towards answering the question of whether in vitro radiosensitivity is a relevant parameter in the more complex in vivo setting. Only two studies considered the efficacy of α and β radiation head to head, both with [^{177}Lu]Lu-DOTATOC as the β-emitting radiopharmaceutical. Graf and collaborators showed a growth delay of 20 and 15 days with ^{225}Ac and ^{177}Lu when tumour-bearing mice were treated with equitoxic activities as determined via MTT assay (44 kBq and 34 MBq, respectively). However, independent in vivo dosimetry was not carried out, meaning RBE could not be estimated [67]. Miederer and collaborators [69] found that treatment with 20 kBq of [^{225}Ac]Ac-DOTATOC showed a significantly greater reduction in tumour mass than 1 MBq of [^{177}Lu]Lu-DOTATOC, but no in vivo dosimetry was performed to quantify tumour-absorbed dose and estimate RBE directly.

Table 4. Summary of preclinical tumour- and kidney-absorbed dose coefficients for TAT. ADC = absorbed dose coefficient. Nephroprotection given as administration of L-lysine before TAT. T:K = tumour-to-kidney ratio.

Author	Radiopharmaceutical	Tumour Bearing	Cell Line	Nephro-Protection	ADC (Gy/MBq) Tumour	ADC (Gy/MBq) Kidneys	T:K
Chan [61]	[^{213}Bi]Bi-DOTATATE	+	CA20948	−	0.8	1.6	0.49
		+	H69	−	0.5	2.0	0.23
Chan [63]	[^{213}Bi]Bi-DOTATATE	+	AR42J	+	0.7	0.6	1.18
		+	AR42J	−	0.7	1.1	0.64
		−	N/A	+	N/A	0.5	N/A
		−	N/A	−	N/A	1.0	N/A
Chapeau [65]	[^{212}Pb]Pb-DOTAM-TATE	+	H69	−	26.6	140.0	0.19
	[^{212}Pb]Pb-eSOMA-01	+	H69	−	35.5	121.7	0.29
	[^{212}Pb]Pb-eSOMA-02	+	H69	−	14.7	147.4	0.10
Handula [60]	[^{225}Ac]Ac-DOTA-JR11	+	H69	−	328.5	952.6	0.34
Lee [46]	[^{212}Pb]Pb-DOTA-TOC	+	AR42J	+	2.4	7.0	0.35
	[^{212}Pb]Pb-PSC-TOC	+	AR42J	+	9.2	5.4	1.70
	[^{212}Pb]Pb-PSC-PEG$_2$-TOC	+	AR42J	+	12.7	6.2	2.04
	[^{212}Pb]Pb-PSC-PEG$_2$-TOC	+	AR42J	+	8.7	3.2	2.69
Tafreshi [75]	[^{225}Ac]Ac-DOTATATE	−	N/A	−	N/A	6.8	N/A

3.3. Clinical Applications

An overview of published clinical studies is given in Table 5. Only studies reporting results from a cohort of patients were considered for further analysis, therefore excluding individual case reports.

Table 5. Overview of clinical studies in targeted alpha therapy. QoL = quality of life, PR = partial response, SD = stable disease, PD = progressive disease, TEAE = treatment emerging adverse event, CE-US = contrast enhanced ultrasound, CE-CT = contrast enhanced CT. * n = 14 total, n = 3 ^{213}Bi.

Author	Indication	Radiopharmaceutical	N	Aim	Findings
Ballal [90]	GEP-NETs	[^{225}Ac]Ac-DOTA-TATE	32	Present early results on safety, efficacy, QoL following TAT in patients stable or refractory to [^{177}Lu]Lu-DOTATATE	Morphological response assessed in 24/34 patients, n = 15 PR, n = 9 SD. No disease progression. Therapy was well tolerated in this population.
Ballal [91]	GEP-NETs	[^{225}Ac]Ac-DOTA-TATE	91	Evaluate long-term outcome of TAT in GEP-NET patients in mixed population of PRRT naive and pre-treated.	TAT improved OS, even in patients refractory to prior ^{177}Lu, with transient and acceptable toxicity.
Delpassand [92]	GEP-NETs	[^{212}Pb]Pb-DOTAM-TATE	20	Establish safety of ^{212}Pb-DOTAM-TATE in phase 1 dose-escalation study.	TAT well tolerated, no serious TEAEs related to the study drug. ORR of 80% at 2.50 MBq/kg/cycle, showing potential benefit over approved therapies.
Demirci [93]	NETs	[^{225}Ac]Ac-DOTA-TATE	11	Retrospective study including 11 patients with NETs of different primary sites treated with [^{225}Ac]Ac-DOTA-TATE.	Nine patients had PET/CT follow up. No grade III/IV toxicity, 4/9 partial response, 8/9 disease control. ^{225}Ac is safe and effective in treatment of patients refractory to β-PRRT.

Table 5. Cont.

Author	Indication	Radiopharmaceutical	N	Aim	Findings
Giesel [94]	Hepatic NET mets	[^{213}Bi]Bi-DOTA-TOC	14 *	Investigate the role of contrast enhanced ultrasound in monitoring tumour response to α/β PRRT.	CE-US comparable to CE-CT and suitable for monitoring PRRT response. Decrease in perfusion indicative of tumour response.
Kratochwil [95]	NETs	[^{213}Bi]Bi-DOTA-TOC	8	Report first in-human experience in PRRT pre-treated patients with [^{213}Bi]Bi-DOTA-TOC.	Specific tumour uptake shown on imaging. TAT produced enduring response with moderate nephrotoxicity, is effective against β-refractory disease.
Kratochwil [96]	NETs	[^{225}Ac]Ac-DOTA-TOC	39	Estimate optimal single cycle and cumulative activity for [^{225}Ac]Ac-DOTA-TOC.	~20 MBq/cycle (4-month interval) and cumulative activity ≤ 60–80 MBq avoided acute and chronic grade III/IV haemato-toxicity, some chronic renal toxicity.
Yadav [97]	Metastatic paraganglioma	[^{225}Ac]Ac-DOTA-TATE	9	Evaluate the efficacy and safety of TAT in advanced stage paragangliomas.	50% PR, 37.5% SD, 12.5% PD, with symptoms decreased. No grade III/IV renal or haematological toxicity. Benefit even in patients refractory to β-PRRT.
Zhang [98]	NETs	[^{225}Ac]Ac-DOTA-TOC	10	Discuss experience with first-in-human use of novel radiopharmaceuticals, including [^{225}Ac]Ac-DOTA-TOC, at Bad Berka.	α-PRRT was well tolerated and effective, including in one patient treated intra-arterially.

3.3.1. Clinical Administration Regimen

There is no typical administration regimen for clinical studies of TAT in the published literature. Randomised controlled trials (RCTs) are so far sparse, meaning many patients included in this review were treated according to the local physician's discretion. Typically a fractionated administration regimen was adopted, except in the study of [^{212}Pb]Pb-DOTAMTATE which was initially considered as a single administration before moving to multiple administrations during the study [92]. An overview of the administration regimens used across the included studies is given in Table 6.

Table 6. Summary of clinical administration regimen. Med = median. Amino acids = lysine, arginine. Diuretic = hydrochlorothiazide. Radiosensitiser = capecitabine.

Author	Radiopharmaceutical	Activity/Cycle (MBq)	N Cycles	Interval (Weeks)	Cumulative Activity (MBq)	Co-Admin
Ballal [90]	[^{225}Ac]Ac-DOTA-TATE	0.1/kg (8/80 kg)	1–4	8	23 (8–33)	Amino acid
Ballal [91]	[^{225}Ac]Ac-DOTA-TATE	0.1/kg (8/80 kg)	1–10 (med = 4)	8	36 (22–59)	Amino acid, radiosensitiser
Delpassand [92]	[^{212}Pb]Pb-DOTAMTATE	1.13/kg (90/80 kg)	1	8	84	Amino acid
		1.48/kg (118/80 kg)	1	8	112	Amino acid
		1.92/kg (154/80 kg)	3	8	406	Amino acid
		2.50/kg (200/80 kg)	4	8	791	Amino acid
Demirci [93]	[^{225}Ac]Ac-DOTA-TATE	0.1–0.12/kg (8–9.6/80 kg)	1–3	18	N/A	Amino acid
Giesel [94]	[^{213}Bi]Bi-DOTA-TOC	N/A	N/A	N/A	N/A	N/A
Kratochwil [95]	[^{213}Bi]Bi-DOTA-TOC	1000–10,500	1–5 (med = 4.5)	8	45	Amino acid
Kratochwil [96]	[^{225}Ac]Ac-DOTA-TOC	6–60	1–5 (med = 4.5)	8–52 (med = 16)	15,800 (3300–20,600)	Amino acid, diuretic

Table 6. *Cont.*

Author	Radiopharmaceutical	Activity/Cycle (MBq)	N Cycles	Interval (Weeks)	Cumulative Activity (MBq)	Co-Admin
Yadav [97]	[^{225}Ac]Ac-DOTA-TATE	0.1/kg (8/80 kg)	2–9 (med = 3)	8	42.4 (15.5–86.6)	Amino acid, radiosensitiser
Zhang [98]	[^{225}Ac]Ac-DOTA-TOC	N/A	N/A	N/A	N/A	N/A

3.3.2. Clinical Efficacy

In total, 223 patients were reported across 9 studies. The majority of these patients were treated with [^{225}Ac]Ac-DOTATATE (n = 143). Treatment outcome according to RECIST criteria was reported in 6/9 studies, comprising 146/223 patients.

Combining results from the included studies, the rate of response following TAT was determined and is shown in Figure 6 (left). The objective response rate (ORR), combining complete and partial responses, was 51%. This rate is impressive when compared with the objective tumour response rate reported in the NETTER-1 (complete response 1/101, partial response 17/101) [21].

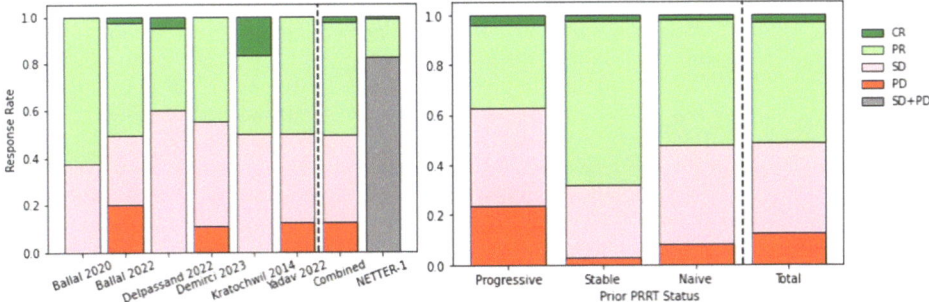

Figure 6. Response following TAT for metastatic NETs (**left**) and stratified by prior PRRT status (**right**) [90–93,95,97]. CR = complete response, PR = partial response, SD = stable disease, PD = progressive disease.

It was also possible to stratify response rate according to the patient's disease status prior to PRRT treatment with a β-emitter, also shown in Figure 6 (right). TAT response in patients with stable disease prior to PRRT treatment is better than for those with progressive disease. However, 38% of patients showed an objective response despite being refractory to β-PRRT, demonstrating the potential of TAT to overcome resistance to agents such as [^{177}Lu]Lu-DOTATATE.

As well as morphologically, response was observed biochemically via a decrease in chromogranin A (CgA) (secreted by functional NETs), and in quality of life, via improvements in Karnofsky performance status (KPS) [91].

Despite impressive results, it is still unclear as to what the optimal activity for each α-emitting radiopharmaceutical is, and no relationship between tumour-absorbed dose and response has been reported. Imaging is feasible, to varying extents, for each of the α-emitters covered in these studies; therefore, image-based dosimetry should be performed in future patients to better understand how absorbed dose and biological effect are related.

3.3.3. Clinical Toxicity

Experience with β-emitters has shown that the incidence and severity of adverse events from PRRT is modest. However, the toxicity that does occur is often associated with the kidneys, acknowledged as the dose-limiting organ in current clinical practice, and the bone marrow [7]. Incidence of grade IV/V renal toxicity was reported as 9.2%

in a series of 1109 patients [99]. Bodei and collaborators [100] demonstrated that in a cohort of 807 patients treated with either [^{177}Lu]Lu-DOTATATE, [^{90}Y]Y-DOTATOC or a combination of both, renal toxicity was least common in patients receiving ^{177}Lu alone. This result may lend itself to speculation that renal toxicity is associated with the range of the β-particle, implying that the lower energy of the ^{177}Lu emission is less damaging to potentially radiosensitive structures in the kidney, for example the glomerulus [101]. This would imply that TAT, with the short range associated with the α-particle (approximately 0.1 mm), may prevent renal toxicity in the same manner. However, damage to the tubular cells, via which radiolabelled peptides are re-absorbed, is a known driver of chronic kidney disease [30]. Given this, and the significant difference in physical parameters such as LET, the toxicities associated with TAT cannot be considered identical to the toxicities associated with β-PRRT.

Of the clinical studies included here, toxicity was reported in 7/9 and was most commonly assessed in accordance with the common criteria for adverse events (CTCAE) framework [102]. Toxicity was generally assessed via routine clinical assessment and blood sampling, though one study did perform renal scintigraphy to assess kidney function post-therapy [96]. The length of follow-up varied from 3 to 60 months.

Concerning nephrotoxicity, Delpassand and collaborators [92] reported three serious treatment emergent adverse events (TEAEs) after [^{212}Pb]Pb-DOTAMTATE (two in single activity escalation cohorts, deemed unrelated, and one in the multiple cycle cohort in a patient with multiple existing risk factors). Kratchowil and collaborators [95] reported moderate chronic kidney toxicity in patients treated with [^{213}Bi]Bi-DOTATOC, evidenced by a 30% decline in glomerular filtration rate (GFR) and a 40% decline in tubular excretion rate (TER) over two years. The same group also reported outcomes in 22 patients treated with [^{225}Ac]Ac-DOTATOC with a median follow up of 57 months [96]. Two patients developed terminal kidney failure after >4 years, though both patients presented with prior risk factors. Analysis showed eGFR loss of 8.4 mL/min/year and a TER decrease of 7.6% in the first 6 months after TAT and 14% in the first 18 months. Otherwise, no incidence of renal toxicity was reported, and no study reported a relationship between treatment activity and toxicity.

Low-grade haematological toxicity was reported as the most common treatment-related side effect in two studies by Ballal and collaborators with [^{225}Ac]Ac-DOTATATE [90,91], and shown by a statistically significant but recoverable drop in lymphocytes after [^{212}Pb]Pb-DOTAMTATE [92]. Treatment with [^{225}Ac]Ac-DOTATOC also resulted in activity-dependent thrombocytopenia and leucopenia, and severe grade III/IV toxicity was observed with activities above 44 kBq given as a single cycle. With repeated administrations, no cumulative toxicity effect was observed when given at 4-month intervals, but at 2-month intervals, additive toxicity was observed. The incidence of high-grade haematological toxicity was modest, with seven grade III/IV adverse events reported across the studies.

A wide range of other adverse events was reported, commonly loss of appetite and transient nausea, although these side effects are also associated with the administration of amino acids for renal protection. There was one report of induced Graves' disease, considered treatment related because thyroid cells may express SSTR$_2$ [94].

When attempting to draw conclusions from these studies, it is noted again that these patient cohorts represent a heterogeneous group, many of which have already received β-PRRT. If TAT were to follow prior therapy with a β-emitter, there are many unanswered questions about how this potentially cumulative absorbed dose to healthy organs would affect toxicity and any possible relationship between absorbed dose and response. No studies in this review reported a relationship between administered activity and toxicity, though the incidence of toxicity was low, with the majority of studies reporting no grade III/IV toxicity. This may imply that there is scope for activity escalation, at least in a sub-cohort of patients, to potentially improve the anti-tumour effect. The understanding of the balance between efficacy and toxicity for TAT would be aided by dosimetry, but no studies to date have calculated absorbed doses in clinical α-PRRT. This should be considered a limitation, given that it is known that administration of fixed activities leads to a wide range of absorbed doses to normal organs [103].

A common point made across several studies was that patients with prior risk factors were more likely to suffer treatment-related adverse events, for example renal toxicity. This implies that some level of patient stratification, as implemented in the phase II ILUMINET trial by applying different absorbed dose limits for patients with and without prior risk factors receiving β-PRRT [104], may be beneficial when attempting to widen the therapeutic window for individual cases.

3.4. Ongoing Clinical Trials

A phase I trial (NCT03466216) of a [^{212}Pb]Pb-DOTAMTATE compound, termed Alphamedix, was sponsored by Radiomedix and completed in 2021. This trial was considered successful and a phase II trial (NCT05153772) of this conjugate is ongoing, with PRRT-naive patients receiving 67.6 μCi/kg *per* cycle. A phase 1/2a dose escalation trial (NCT05636618) of [^{212}Pb]Pb-VMT-α-NET, sponsored by Perspective Therapeutics, began enrolment in July 2023, with an expanded indication to include all NETs. One trial using ^{225}Ac, sponsored by RayzeBio, is currently recruiting (NCT05477576). In phase 1, the safety, pharmacokinetics and recommended phase 3 dose of RYZ101 ([^{225}Ac]Ac-DOTATATE) will be determined in patients who have progressed following ^{177}Lu-SSA. Following this, safety and efficacy will be assessed.

4. Discussion

Targeted therapy with α-emitters has shown excellent promise in the preclinical setting, and this is beginning to be translated to the clinic. Complete responses to therapy are reported extensively in mouse models, and observed at rates beyond those which can be expected from β-PRRT in the limited clinical experience currently published. Anti-tumour efficacy is demonstrated in patients with progressive disease following prior PRRT with a β-emitter, demonstrating the potential potency of α-emitters for this indication.

However, a review of the relevant literature highlights the lack of understanding as to the relationships between activity, absorbed dose and biological end point at all scales. Better understanding of these relationships can provide the basis for treatment optimisation and individualisation, as well as providing insight into the fundamental radiobiology underpinning the effectiveness of high-LET radiation.

One interpretation of optimisation in the context of any targeted therapy would be to maximise anti-tumour efficacy while maintaining the risk of healthy organ toxicity below an acceptable level. In order to implement this, there must be a fundamental understanding of how tumour response and toxicity are related to the quantity of the specific radiation quality administered. This review shows that these relationships are poorly defined for α-emitters, leading to arbitrary choices of therapeutic activity, comparisons between high- and low-LET radiation at activities that are not equitoxic, and the extrapolation of constraints on absorbed dose from external beam radiotherapy that are unlikely to translate to TAT [105].

No clinical estimates of absorbed doses to the tumour or to organs at risk in humans have been published. Dosimetry was performed in a minority of cases in both the in vitro and in vivo settings. Even when absorbed doses were estimated, methodologies differed substantially, potentially reducing the scope for comparison between studies. Uncertainties associated with estimates of absorbed dose were also rarely included, despite their importance for interpretation of the result [106]. It should also be acknowledged that the most common dosimetry methods in the preclinical studies reviewed here are macroscopic and aim at characterising mean organ-absorbed dose. Given the likely heterogeneous distribution of the radiopharmaceutical on the cellular scale, it may be that mean organ-absorbed dose is too crude a measure to correlate with biological endpoint, and alternative approaches including organ sub-unit dosimetry and microdosimetry are necessary [107,108]. Clearly, standardised methods for dosimetry and uncertainty calculation should be included in future work.

Impressive preclinical responses indicate that TAT has a high potential for anti-tumour efficacy in $SSTR_2$-overexpressing cancers. However, clinical imaging studies have demonstrated that uniformly positive receptor expression may not be typical in NET patients [109]. Given the short range of the α-particle, cells with lower receptor expression than neighbour high-expressing cells are less likely to be irradiated due to the crossfire effect. This demonstrates the role of imaging in identifying potentially sub-optimal candidates for TAT, and the potential role of combination therapies in future patients in a so-called 'cocktail approach' [110].

5. Conclusions

In this review, we hope to have highlighted the substantial benefit that TAT could offer patients for whom PRRT is indicated. We have laid out the radiobiological advantages of α-particles over β-particles due to their high-LET and draw attention to impressive results with a moderate toxicity profile in both the preclinical and clinical settings. The ORR of TAT in a population of mixed prior PRRT status was 51%, and efficacy is demonstrated in patients who are refractory to β-PRRT. However, we also demonstrate how research in this area is discordant and treatment remains non-optimised. It is hoped that theragnostic imaging, dosimetry and a better understanding of the relationships between absorbed dose, therapeutic response and toxicity will facilitate this optimisation to provide benefit for future patients.

Author Contributions: Study conception and design: P.M.D.G., M.K.S., G.J.S. and S.Y.A.T., data collection: P.M.D.G., data collection and curation: P.M.D.G., analysis: P.M.D.G., writing (initial draft): P.M.D.G., writing (review and editing): P.M.D.G., M.K.S., G.J.S. and S.Y.A.T., supervision: M.K.S., G.J.S. and S.Y.A.T. All authors have read and agreed to the published version of the manuscript.

Funding: This work was partially supported by the EPSRC Centre for Doctoral Training in Smart Medical Imaging [EP/S022104/1] and Perspective Therapeutics (PG). S.Y.A.T. was supported by MRC Grant [MR/X00841X/1]. G.J.S. would like to thank the MRC [MR/T002573/1] and EPSRC [EP/V027549/1 and EP/T026367/1] for funding. M.K.S. was supported by grants R44CA268314, R44CA250872, R44CA254613, 1R01CA243014, 1P50CA174521 from the NIH/NCI, and is an employee of Perspective Therapeutics.

Institutional Review Board Statement: Not applicable.

Informed Consent Statement: Not applicable.

Data Availability Statement: Authors would be happy to share data upon request.

Acknowledgments: The authors thank Fiorenza Ianzini at Perspective Therapeutics for assisting with the editing and revision of the manuscript.

Conflicts of Interest: Author M.K.S is employed by the company Perspective Therapeutics. The remaining authors declare that the research was conducted in the absence of any commercial or financial relationships that could be construed as a potential conflict of interest.

References

1. Hope, T.A.; Pavel, M.; Bergsland, E.K. Neuroendocrine Tumors and Peptide Receptor Radionuclide Therapy: When Is the Right Time? *J. Clin. Oncol.* **2022**, *40*, 2818. [CrossRef]
2. Rindi, G.; Klimstra, D.S.; Abedi-Ardekani, B.; Asa, S.L.; Bosman, F.T.; Brambilla, E.; Busam, K.J.; Krijger, R.R.d.; Dietel, M.; El-Naggar, A.K.; et al. A common classification framework for neuroendocrine neoplasms: An International Agency for Research on Cancer (IARC) and World Health Organization (WHO) expert consensus proposal. *Mod. Pathol.* **2018**, *31*, 1770–1786. [CrossRef]
3. Modlin, I.M.; Oberg, K.; Chung, D.C.; Jensen, R.T.; de Herder, W.W.; Thakker, R.V.; Caplin, M.; Delle Fave, G.; Kaltsas, G.A.; Krenning, E.P.; et al. Gastroenteropancreatic neuroendocrine tumours. *Lancet Oncol.* **2008**, *9*, 61–72. [CrossRef]
4. Metz, D.C.; Choi, J.; Strosberg, J.; Heaney, A.P.; Howden, C.W.; Klimstra, D.; Yao, J.C. A rationale for multidisciplinary care in treating neuroendocrine tumours. *Curr. Opin. Endocrinol. Diabetes Obes.* **2012**, *19*, 306. [CrossRef] [PubMed]
5. Sorbye, H.; Kong, G.; Grozinsky-Glasberg, S. PRRT in high-grade gastroenteropancreatic neuroendocrine neoplasms (WHO G3). *Endocr.-Relat. Cancer* **2020**, *27*, R67–R77. [CrossRef] [PubMed]

6. Hicks, R.J.; Kwekkeboom, D.J.; Krenning, E.; Bodei, L.; Grozinsky-Glasberg, S.; Arnold, R.; Borbath, I.; Cwikla, J.; Toumpanakis, C.; Kaltsas, G.; et al. ENETS Consensus Guidelines for the Standards of Care in Neuroendocrine Neoplasia: Peptide Receptor Radionuclide Therapy with Radiolabeled Somatostatin Analogues. *Neuroendocrinology* **2017**, *105*, 295–309. [CrossRef] [PubMed]
7. Zaknun, J.J.; Bodei, L.; Mueller-Brand, J.; Pavel, M.E.; Baum, R.P.; Hörsch, D.; O'Dorisio, M.S.; O'Dorisiol, T.M.; Howe, J.R.; Cremonesi, M.; et al. The joint IAEA, EANM, and SNMMI practical guidance on peptide receptor radionuclide therapy (PRRNT) in neuroendocrine tumours. *Eur. J. Nucl. Med. Mol. Imaging* **2013**, *40*, 800–816. [CrossRef]
8. Theodoropoulou, M.; Stalla, G.K. Somatostatin receptors: From signaling to clinical practice. *Front. Neuroendocrinol.* **2013**, *34*, 228–252. [CrossRef] [PubMed]
9. Uhlén, M.; Fagerberg, L.; Hallström, B.M.; Lindskog, C.; Oksvold, P.; Mardinoglu, A.; Sivertsson, Å.; Kampf, C.; Sjöstedt, E.; Asplund, A.; et al. Tissue-based map of the human proteome. *Science* **2015**, *347*, 1260419. [CrossRef]
10. Özgüven, S.; Filizoğlu, N.; Kesim, S.; Öksüzoğlu, K.; Şen, F.; Öneş, T.; İnanır, S.; Turoğlu, H.T.; Erdil, T.Y. Physiological Biodistribution of 68Ga-DOTA-TATE in Normal Subjects. *Mol. Imaging Radionucl. Ther.* **2021**, *30*, 39–46. [CrossRef]
11. Reubi, J.C.; Laissue, J.; Krenning, E.; Lamberts, S.W.J. Somatostatin receptors in human cancer: Incidence, characteristics, functional correlates and clinical implications. *J. Steroid Biochem. Mol. Biol.* **1992**, *43*, 27–35. [CrossRef] [PubMed]
12. Bousquet, C.; Puente, E.; Buscail, L.; Vaysse, N.; Susini, C. Antiproliferative effect of somatostatin and analogs. *Chemotherapy* **2001**, *47* (Suppl. 2), 30–39. [CrossRef]
13. Krenning, E.P.; Bakker, W.H.; Kooij, P.P.M.; Breeman, W.A.P.; Oei, H.Y.; Jong, M.d.; Reubi, J.C.; Visser, T.J.; Bruns, C.; Kwekkeboom, D.J.; et al. Somatostatin Receptor Scintigraphy with Indium-111-DTPA-D-Phe-1-Octreotide in Man: Metabolism, Dosimetry and Comparison with Iodine-123-Tyr-3-Octreotide. *J. Nucl. Med.* **1992**, *33*, 652–658.
14. Krenning, E.P.; Kwekkeboom, D.J.; Bakker, W.H.; Breeman, W.A.; Kooij, P.P.; Oei, H.Y.; van Hagen, M.; Postema, P.T.; de Jong, M.; Reubi, J.C. Somatostatin receptor scintigraphy with [^{111}In-DTPA-D-Phe^1]- and [^{123}I-Tyr^3]-octreotide: The Rotterdam experience with more than 1000 patients. *Eur. J. Nucl. Med.* **1993**, *20*, 716–731. [CrossRef]
15. Krenning, E.P.; Kooij, P.P.; Bakker, W.H.; Breeman, W.A.; Postema, P.T.; Kwekkeboom, D.J.; Oei, H.Y.; de Jong, M.; Visser, T.J.; Reijs, A.E. Radiotherapy with a radiolabeled somatostatin analogue, [^{111}In-DTPA-D-Phe^1]-octreotide. A case history. *Ann. N. Y. Acad. Sci.* **1994**, *733*, 496–506. [CrossRef] [PubMed]
16. Valkema, R.; de Jong, M.; Bakker, W.H.; Breeman, W.A.P.; Kooij, P.P.M.; Lugtenburg, P.J.; de Jong, F.H.; Christiansen, A.; Kam, B.L.R.; de Herder, W.W.; et al. Phase I study of peptide receptor radionuclide therapy with [^{111}In-DTPA^0]octreotide: The rotterdam experience. *Semin. Nucl. Med.* **2002**, *32*, 110–122. [CrossRef]
17. Bodei, L.; Ćwikla, J.B.; Kidd, M.; Modlin, I.M. The role of peptide receptor radionuclide therapy in advanced/metastatic thoracic neuroendocrine tumors. *J. Thorac Dis.* **2017**, *9*, S1511–S1523. [CrossRef]
18. Otte, A.; Jermann, E.; Behe, M.; Goetze, M.; Bucher, H.C.; Roser, H.W.; Heppeler, A.; Mueller-Brand, J.; Maecke, H.R. DOTATOC: A powerful new tool for receptor-mediated radionuclide therapy. *Eur. J. Nucl. Med.* **1997**, *24*, 792–795. [CrossRef]
19. Otte, A.; Mueller-Brand, J.; Dellas, S.; Nitzsche, E.U.; Herrmann, R.; Maecke, H.R. Yttrium-90-labelled somatostatin-analogue for cancer treatment. *Lancet* **1998**, *351*, 417–418. [CrossRef]
20. de Jong, M.; Breeman, W.A.P.; Bakker, W.H.; Kooij, P.P.M.; Bernard, B.F.; Hofland, L.J.; Visser, T.J.; Srinivasan, A.; Schmidt, M.A.; Erion, J.L.; et al. Comparison of 111In-labeled Somatostatin Analogues for Tumor Scintigraphy and Radionuclide Therapy1. *Cancer Res.* **1998**, *58*, 437–441. [PubMed]
21. Strosberg, J.R.; Caplin, M.E.; Kunz, P.L.; Ruszniewski, P.B.; Bodei, L.; Hendifar, A.; Mittra, E.; Wolin, E.M.; Yao, J.C.; Pavel, M.E.; et al. 177Lu-Dotatate plus long-acting octreotide versus high-dose long-acting octreotide in patients with midgut neuroendocrine tumours (NETTER-1): Final overall survival and long-term safety results from an open-label, randomised, controlled, phase 3 trial. *Lancet Oncol.* **2021**, *22*, 1752–1763. [CrossRef]
22. Hennrich, U.; Kopka, K. Lutathera®: The First FDA- and EMA-Approved Radiopharmaceutical for Peptide Receptor Radionuclide Therapy. *Pharmaceuticals* **2019**, *12*, 114. [CrossRef] [PubMed]
23. U.S. Food and Drug Administration. Lutathera Package Insert. Available online: https://www.accessdata.fda.gov/drugsatfda_docs/label/2018/208700s000lbl.pdf (accessed on 22 February 2024).
24. Poty, S.; Francesconi, L.C.; McDevitt, M.R.; Morris, M.J.; Lewis, J.S. α-Emitters for Radiotherapy: From Basic Radiochemistry to Clinical Studies—Part 1. *J. Nucl. Med.* **2018**, *59*, 878–884. [CrossRef]
25. Sgouros, G.; Roeske, J.C.; McDevitt, M.R.; Palm, S.; Allen, B.J.; Fisher, D.R.; Brill, A.B.; Song, H.; Howell, R.W.; Akabani, G. MIRD Pamphlet No. 22 (Abridged): Radiobiology and Dosimetry of α-Particle Emitters for Targeted Radionuclide Therapy. *J. Nucl. Med.* **2010**, *51*, 311–328. [CrossRef] [PubMed]
26. Kassis, A.I. Molecular and cellular radiobiological effects of Auger emitting radionuclides. *Radiat. Prot. Dosim.* **2011**, *143*, 241–247. [CrossRef]
27. Amin, I.K.; Adelstein, S.J. Radiobiologic Principles in Radionuclide Therapy. *J. Nucl. Med.* **2005**, *46*, 4S–12S.
28. Lee, H.; Riad, A.; Martorano, P.; Mansfield, A.; Samanta, M.; Batra, V.; Mach, R.H.; Maris, J.M.; Pryma, D.A.; Makvandi, M. PARP-1-Targeted Auger Emitters Display High-LET Cytotoxic Properties In Vitro but Show Limited Therapeutic Utility in Solid Tumor Models of Human Neuroblastoma. *J. Nucl. Med.* **2020**, *61*, 850–856. [CrossRef] [PubMed]
29. Munro, T.R. The Site of the Target Region for Radiation-Induced Mitotic Delay in Cultured Mammalian Cells. *Radiat. Res.* **1970**, *44*, 748–757. [CrossRef]

30. Liu, B.-C.; Tang, T.-T.; Lv, L.-L.; Lan, H.-Y. Renal tubule injury: A driving force toward chronic kidney disease. *Kidney Int.* **2018**, *93*, 568–579. [CrossRef]
31. Wulbrand, C.; Seidl, C.; Gaertner, F.C.; Bruchertseifer, F.; Morgenstern, A.; Essler, M.; Senekowitsch-Schmidtke, R. Alpha-Particle Emitting 213Bi-Anti-EGFR Immunoconjugates Eradicate Tumor Cells Independent of Oxygenation. *PLoS ONE* **2013**, *8*, e64730. [CrossRef]
32. Barendsen, G.W. Modification of Radiation Damage by Fractionation of the Dose, Anoxia, and Chemical Protectors in Relation to Let. *Ann. N. Y. Acad. Sci.* **1964**, *114*, 96–114. [CrossRef]
33. Feinendegen, L.E.; McClure, J.J. Alpha-Emitters for Medical Therapy: Workshop of the United States Department of Energy: Denver, Colorado, May 30–31, 1996. *Radiat. Res.* **1997**, *148*, 195–201. [CrossRef]
34. Sundlöv, A.; Sjögreen-Gleisner, K. Peptide Receptor Radionuclide Therapy—Prospects for Personalised Treatment. *Clin. Oncol.* **2021**, *33*, 92–97. [CrossRef]
35. Kręcisz, P.; Czarnecka, K.; Królicki, L.; Mikiciuk-Olasik, E.; Szymański, P. Radiolabeled Peptides and Antibodies in Medicine. *Bioconjugate Chem.* **2021**, *32*, 25–42. [CrossRef]
36. Eychenne, R.; Bouvry, C.; Bourgeois, M.; Loyer, P.; Benoist, E.; Lepareur, N. Overview of Radiolabeled Somatostatin Analogs for Cancer Imaging and Therapy. *Molecules* **2020**, *25*, 4012. [CrossRef]
37. McDevitt, M.R.; Ma, D.; Lai, L.T.; Simon, J.; Borchardt, P.; Frank, R.K.; Wu, K.; Pellegrini, V.; Curcio, M.J.; Miederer, M.; et al. Tumor Therapy with Targeted Atomic Nanogenerators. *Science* **2001**, *294*, 1537–1540. [CrossRef]
38. Parker, C.; Nilsson, S.; Heinrich, D.; Helle, S.I.; O'Sullivan, J.M.; Fosså, S.D.; Chodacki, A.; Wiechno, P.; Logue, J.; Seke, M.; et al. Alpha Emitter Radium-223 and Survival in Metastatic Prostate Cancer. *N. Engl. J. Med.* **2013**, *369*, 213–223. [CrossRef]
39. Abou, D.S.; Thiele, N.A.; Gutsche, N.T.; Villmer, A.; Zhang, H.; Woods, J.J.; Baidoo, K.E.; Escorcia, F.E.; Wilson, J.J.; Thorek, D.L.J. Towards the stable chelation of radium for biomedical applications with an 18-membered macrocyclic ligand. *Chem. Sci.* **2021**, *12*, 3733–3742. [CrossRef] [PubMed]
40. Shi, M.; Jakobsson, V.; Greifenstein, L.; Khong, P.-L.; Chen, X.; Baum, R.P.; Zhang, J. Alpha-peptide receptor radionuclide therapy using actinium-225 labeled somatostatin receptor agonists and antagonists. *Front. Med.* **2022**, *9*, 1034315. [CrossRef]
41. Khabibullin, A.R.; Karolak, A.; Budzevich, M.M.; McLaughlin, M.L.; Morse, D.L.; Woods, L.M. Structure and properties of DOTA-chelated radiopharmaceuticals within the (225)Ac decay pathway. *Medchemcomm* **2018**, *9*, 1155–1163. [CrossRef] [PubMed]
42. Schwartz, J.; Jaggi, J.S.; O'Donoghue, J.A.; Ruan, S.; McDevitt, M.; Larson, S.M.; Scheinberg, D.A.; Humm, J.L. Renal uptake of bismuth-213 and its contribution to kidney radiation dose following administration of actinium-225-labeled antibody. *Phys. Med. Biol.* **2011**, *56*, 721. [CrossRef]
43. de Kruijff, R.M.; Wolterbeek, H.T.; Denkova, A.G. A Critical Review of Alpha Radionuclide Therapy—How to Deal with Recoiling Daughters? *Pharmaceuticals* **2015**, *8*, 321–336. [CrossRef]
44. Mirzadeh, S.; Kumar, K.; Gansow, O.A. The Chemical Fate of 212Bi-DOTA Formed by β- Decay of 212Pb(DOTA)2. *Radiochim. Acta* **1993**, *60*, 1–10. [CrossRef]
45. Su, F.M.; Beaumier, P.; Axworthy, D.; Atcher, R.; Fritzberg, A. Pretargeted radioimmunotherapy in tumored mice using an in vivo 212Pb/212Bi generator. *Nucl. Med. Biol.* **2005**, *32*, 741–747. [CrossRef] [PubMed]
46. Lee, D.; Li, M.; Liu, D.; Baumhover, N.J.; Sagastume, E.A.; Marks, B.M.; Rastogi, P.; Pigge, F.C.; Menda, Y.; Johnson, F.L.; et al. Structural modifications toward improved lead-203/lead-212 peptide-based image-guided alpha-particle radiopharmaceutical therapies for neuroendocrine tumors. *Eur. J. Nucl. Med. Mol. Imaging* **2023**, *51*, 1147–1162. [CrossRef]
47. Li, M.; Baumhover, N.J.; Liu, D.; Cagle, B.S.; Boschetti, F.; Paulin, G.; Lee, D.; Dai, Z.; Obot, E.R.; Marks, B.M.; et al. Preclinical Evaluation of a Lead Specific Chelator (PSC) Conjugated to Radiopeptides for 203Pb and 212Pb-Based Theranostics. *Pharmaceutics* **2023**, *15*, 414. [CrossRef] [PubMed]
48. Nelson, B.J.B.; Wilson, J.; Schultz, M.K.; Andersson, J.D.; Wuest, F. High-yield cyclotron production of (203)Pb using a sealed (205)Tl solid target. *Nucl. Med. Biol.* **2023**, *116–117*, 108314. [CrossRef]
49. Pretze, M.; Michler, E.; Runge, R.; Wetzig, K.; Tietze, K.; Brandt, F.; Schultz, M.K.; Kotzerke, J. Influence of the Molar Activity of (203/212)Pb-PSC-PEG(2)-TOC on Somatostatin Receptor Type 2-Binding and Cell Uptake. *Pharmaceuticals* **2023**, *16*, 1605. [CrossRef]
50. Gustafsson, J.; Rodeno, E.; Minguez, P. Feasibility and limitations of quantitative SPECT for (223)Ra. *Phys. Med. Biol.* **2020**, *65*, 085012. [CrossRef]
51. Muller, D.; Herrmann, H.; Schultz, M.K.; Solbach, C.; Ettrich, T.; Prasad, V. 203 Pb-VMT-alpha-NET Scintigraphy of a Patient With Neuroendocrine Tumor. *Clin. Nucl. Med.* **2023**, *48*, 54–55. [CrossRef]
52. Michler, E.; Kastner, D.; Brogsitter, C.; Pretze, M.; Hartmann, H.; Freudenberg, R.; Schultz, M.K.; Kotzerke, J. First-in-human SPECT/CT imaging of [(212)Pb]Pb-VMT-alpha-NET in a patient with metastatic neuroendocrine tumor. *Eur. J. Nucl. Med. Mol. Imaging* **2023**. [CrossRef] [PubMed]
53. Stokke, C.; Gabiña, P.M.; Solný, P.; Cicone, F.; Sandström, M.; Gleisner, K.S.; Chiesa, C.; Spezi, E.; Paphiti, M.; Konijnenberg, M.; et al. Dosimetry-based treatment planning for molecular radiotherapy: A summary of the 2017 report from the Internal Dosimetry Task Force. *EJNMMI Phys.* **2017**, *4*, 27. [CrossRef] [PubMed]
54. McNeil, B.L.; Robertson, A.K.H.; Fu, W.; Yang, H.; Hoehr, C.; Ramogida, C.F.; Schaffer, P. Production, purification, and radiolabeling of the 203Pb/212Pb theranostic pair. *EJNMMI Radiopharm. Chem.* **2021**, *6*, 6. [CrossRef]

55. Kokov, K.V.; Egorova, B.V.; German, M.N.; Klabukov, I.D.; Krasheninnikov, M.E.; Larkin-Kondrov, A.A.; Makoveeva, K.A.; Ovchinnikov, M.V.; Sidorova, M.V.; Chuvilin, D.Y. (212)Pb: Production Approaches and Targeted Therapy Applications. *Pharmaceutics* **2022**, *14*, 189. [CrossRef] [PubMed]
56. Radchenko, V.; Morgenstern, A.; Jalilian, A.R.; Ramogida, C.F.; Cutler, C.; Duchemin, C.; Hoehr, C.; Haddad, F.; Bruchertseifer, F.; Gausemel, H.; et al. Production and Supply of alpha-Particle-Emitting Radionuclides for Targeted alpha-Therapy. *J. Nucl. Med.* **2021**, *62*, 1495–1503. [CrossRef] [PubMed]
57. U.S. Department of Energy Isotope Program 2022 Actinium-225 User Group Meeting. Available online: https://www.isotopes.gov/22UserGroupMeetings (accessed on 22 February 2024).
58. World Nuclear News. CNL Eyes Dramatic Increase in Ac-225 Production. World Nuclear News. 2023. Available online: https://world-nuclear-news.org/Articles/CNL-eyes-dramatic-increase-in-Ac-225-production (accessed on 22 February 2024).
59. Zalutsky, M.R.; Pruszynski, M. Astatine-211: Production and Availability. *Curr. Radiopharm.* **2011**, *4*, 177–185. [CrossRef] [PubMed]
60. Handula, M.; Beekman, S.; Konijnenberg, M.; Stuurman, D.; de Ridder, C.; Bruchertseifer, F.; Morgenstern, A.; Denkova, A.; de Blois, E.; Seimbille, Y. First preclinical evaluation of [(225)Ac]Ac-DOTA-JR11 and comparison with [(177)Lu]Lu-DOTA-JR11, alpha versus beta radionuclide therapy of NETs. *EJNMMI Radiopharm. Chem.* **2023**, *8*, 13. [CrossRef]
61. Chan, H.S.; Konijnenberg, M.W.; de Blois, E.; Koelewijn, S.; Baum, R.P.; Morgenstern, A.; Bruchertseifer, F.; Breeman, W.A.; de Jong, M. Influence of tumour size on the efficacy of targeted alpha therapy with 213Bi-[DOTA0,Tyr3]-octreotate. *EJNMMI Res.* **2016**, *6*, 6. [CrossRef]
62. Chan, H.S.; de Blois, E.; Konijnenberg, M.W.; Morgenstern, A.; Bruchertseifer, F.; Norenberg, J.P.; Verzijlbergen, F.J.; de Jong, M.; Breeman, W.A.P. Optimizing labelling conditions of 213Bi-DOTATATE for preclinical applications of peptide receptor targeted alpha therapy. *EJNMMI Radiopharm. Chem.* **2016**, *1*, 9. [CrossRef]
63. Chan, H.S.; Konijnenberg, M.W.; Daniels, T.; Nysus, M.; Makvandi, M.; de Blois, E.; Breeman, W.A.; Atcher, R.W.; de Jong, M.; Norenberg, J.P. Improved safety and efficacy of 213Bi-DOTATATE-targeted alpha therapy of somatostatin receptor-expressing neuroendocrine tumors in mice pre-treated with l-lysine. *EJNMMI Res.* **2016**, *6*, 83. [CrossRef] [PubMed]
64. Chan, H.S.; de Blois, E.; Morgenstern, A.; Bruchertseifer, F.; de Jong, M.; Breeman, W.; Konijnenberg, M. In Vitro comparison of 213Bi- and 177Lu-radiation for peptide receptor radionuclide therapy. *PLoS ONE* **2017**, *12*, e0181473. [CrossRef]
65. Chapeau, D.; Koustoulidou, S.; Handula, M.; Beekman, S.; de Ridder, C.; Stuurman, D.; de Blois, E.; Buchatskaya, Y.; van der Schilden, K.; de Jong, M.; et al. [(212)Pb]Pb-eSOMA-01: A Promising Radioligand for Targeted Alpha Therapy of Neuroendocrine Tumors. *Pharmaceuticals* **2023**, *16*, 985. [CrossRef]
66. Cieslik, P.; Kubeil, M.; Zarschler, K.; Ullrich, M.; Brandt, F.; Anger, K.; Wadepohl, H.; Kopka, K.; Bachmann, M.; Pietzsch, J.; et al. Toward Personalized Medicine: One Chelator for Imaging and Therapy with Lutetium-177 and Actinium-225. *J. Am. Chem. Soc.* **2022**, *144*, 21555–21567. [CrossRef] [PubMed]
67. Graf, F.; Fahrer, J.; Maus, S.; Morgenstern, A.; Bruchertseifer, F.; Venkatachalam, S.; Fottner, C.; Weber, M.M.; Huelsenbeck, J.; Schreckenberger, M.; et al. DNA Double Strand Breaks as Predictor of Efficacy of the Alpha-Particle Emitter Ac-225 and the Electron Emitter Lu-177 for Somatostatin Receptor Targeted Radiotherapy. *PLoS ONE* **2014**, *9*, e88239. [CrossRef]
68. King, A.P.; Gutsche, N.T.; Raju, N.; Fayn, S.; Baidoo, K.E.; Bell, M.M.; Olkowski, C.S.; Swenson, R.E.; Lin, F.I.; Sadowski, S.M.; et al. 225Ac-Macropatate: A Novel Alpha Particle Peptide Receptor Radionuclide Therapy for Neuroendocrine Tumors. *J. Nucl. Med.* **2022**, *64*, 549–554. [CrossRef]
69. Miederer, M.; Henriksen, G.; Alke, A.; Mossbrugger, I.; Quintanilla-Martinez, L.; Senekowitsch-Schmidtke, R.; Essler, M. Preclinical Evaluation of the α-Particle Generator Nuclide 225Ac for Somatostatin Receptor Radiotherapy of Neuroendocrine Tumors. *Clin. Cancer Res.* **2008**, *14*, 3555–3561. [CrossRef] [PubMed]
70. Müller, C.; Vermeulen, C.; Köster, U.; Johnston, K.; Türler, A.; Schibli, R.; van der Meulen, N.P. Alpha-PET with terbium-149: Evidence and perspectives for radiotheragnostics. *EJNMMI Radiopharm. Chem.* **2016**, *1*, 5. [CrossRef]
71. Nayak, T.K.; Norenberg, J.P.; Anderson, T.L.; Prossnitz, E.R.; Stabin, M.G.; Atcher, R.W. Somatostatin-receptor-targeted α-emitting 213Bi is therapeutically more effective than β−-emitting 177Lu in human pancreatic adenocarcinoma cells. *Nucl. Med. Biol.* **2007**, *34*, 185–193. [CrossRef] [PubMed]
72. Norenberg, J.P.; Krenning, B.J.; Konings, I.R.H.M.; Kusewitt, D.F.; Nayak, T.K.; Anderson, T.L.; de Jong, M.; Garmestani, K.; Brechbiel, M.W.; Kvols, L.K. 213Bi-[DOTA0, Tyr3]Octreotide Peptide Receptor Radionuclide Therapy of Pancreatic Tumors in a Preclinical Animal Model. *Clin. Cancer Res.* **2006**, *12*, 897–903. [CrossRef]
73. Qin, S.; Yang, Y.; Zhang, J.; Yin, Y.; Liu, W.; Zhang, H.; Fan, X.; Yang, M.; Yu, F. Effective Treatment of SSTR2-Positive Small Cell Lung Cancer Using (211)At-Containing Targeted alpha-Particle Therapy Agent Which Promotes Endogenous Antitumor Immune Response. *Mol. Pharm.* **2023**, *20*, 5543–5553. [CrossRef] [PubMed]
74. Stallons, T.A.R.; Saidi, A.; Tworowska, I.; Delpassand, E.S.; Torgue, J.J. Preclinical Investigation of 212Pb-DOTAMTATE for Peptide Receptor Radionuclide Therapy in a Neuroendocrine Tumor Model. *Mol. Cancer Ther.* **2019**, *18*, 1012–1021. [CrossRef] [PubMed]
75. Tafreshi, N.K.; Pandya, D.N.; Tichacek, C.J.; Budzevich, M.M.; Wang, Z.; Reff, J.N.; Engelman, R.W.; Boulware, D.C.; Chiappori, A.A.; Strosberg, J.R.; et al. Preclinical evaluation of [225Ac]Ac-DOTA-TATE for treatment of lung neuroendocrine neoplasms. *Eur. J. Nucl. Med. Mol. Imaging* **2021**, *48*, 3408–3421. [CrossRef] [PubMed]

76. Vaidyanathan, G.; Boskovitz, A.; Shankar, S.; Zalutsky, M.R. Radioiodine and 211At-labeled guanidinomethyl halobenzoyl octreotate conjugates: Potential peptide radiotherapeutics for somatostatin receptor-positive cancers. *Peptides* **2004**, *25*, 2087–2097. [CrossRef]
77. Wharton, L.; Yang, H.; Jaraquemada-Pelaez, M.G.; Merkens, H.; Engudar, G.; Ingham, A.; Koniar, H.; Radchenko, V.; Kunz, P.; Schaffer, P.; et al. Rearmed Bifunctional Chelating Ligand for (225)Ac/(155)Tb Precision-Guided Theranostic Radiopharmaceuticals horizontal line H(4)noneunpaX. *J. Med. Chem.* **2023**, *66*, 13705–13730. [CrossRef]
78. Zhao, B.; Qin, S.; Chai, L.; Lu, G.; Yang, Y.; Cai, H.; Yuan, X.; Fan, S.; Huang, Q.; Yu, F. Evaluation of astatine-211-labeled octreotide as a potential radiotherapeutic agent for NSCLC treatment. *Bioorganic Med. Chem.* **2018**, *26*, 1086–1091. [CrossRef] [PubMed]
79. Hobbs, R.F.; Howell, R.W.; Song, H.; Baechler, S.; Sgouros, G. Redefining Relative Biological Effectiveness in the Context of the EQDX Formalism: Implications for Alpha-Particle Emitter Therapy. *Radiat. Res.* **2014**, *181*, 90–98. [CrossRef]
80. Vaziri, B.; Wu, H.; Dhawan, A.P.; Du, P.; Howell, R.W.; SNMMI MIRD Committee. MIRD Pamphlet No. 25: MIRDcell V2.0 Software Tool for Dosimetric Analysis of Biologic Response of Multicellular Populations. *J. Nucl. Med.* **2014**, *55*, 1557–1564. [CrossRef]
81. Bolch, W.E.; Eckerman, K.F.; Sgouros, G.; Thomas, S.R. MIRD Pamphlet No. 21: A Generalized Schema for Radiopharmaceutical Dosimetry—Standardization of Nomenclature. *J. Nucl. Med.* **2009**, *50*, 477–484. [CrossRef] [PubMed]
82. Lee, D.; Li, M.; Bednarz, B.; Schultz, M.K. Modeling Cell and Tumor-Metastasis Dosimetry with the Particle and Heavy Ion Transport Code System (PHITS) Software for Targeted Alpha-Particle Radionuclide Therapy. *Radiat. Res.* **2018**, *190*, 236–247. [CrossRef]
83. Ladjohounlou, R.; Lozza, C.; Pichard, A.; Constanzo, J.; Karam, J.; Le Fur, P.; Deshayes, E.; Boudousq, V.; Paillas, S.; Busson, M.; et al. Drugs That Modify Cholesterol Metabolism Alter the p38/JNK-Mediated Targeted and Nontargeted Response to Alpha and Auger Radioimmunotherapy. *Clin. Cancer Res.* **2019**, *25*, 4775–4790. [CrossRef] [PubMed]
84. de Jong, M.; Breeman, W.A.P.; Bernard, B.F.; van Gameren, A.; de Bruin, E.; Bakker, W.H.; van der Pluijm, M.E.; Visser, T.J.; Mäcke, H.R.; Krenning, E.P. Tumour uptake of the radiolabelled somatostatin analogue [DOTA0,TYR3]octreotide is dependent on the peptide amount. *Eur. J. Nucl. Med.* **1999**, *26*, 693–698. [CrossRef] [PubMed]
85. Beauregard, J.-M.; Hofman, M.S.; Kong, G.; Hicks, R.J. The tumour sink effect on the biodistribution of 68Ga-DOTA-octreotate: Implications for peptide receptor radionuclide therapy. *Eur. J. Nucl. Med. Mol. Imaging* **2012**, *39*, 50–56. [CrossRef]
86. Li, M.; Robles-Planells, C.; Liu, D.; Graves, S.A.; Vasquez-Martinez, G.; Mayoral-Andrade, G.; Lee, D.; Rastogi, P.; Marks, B.M.; Sagastume, E.A.; et al. Pre-clinical evaluation of biomarkers for the early detection of nephrotoxicity following alpha-particle radioligand therapy. *Eur. J. Nucl. Med. Mol. Imaging* **2023**, 1–14. [CrossRef]
87. de Jong, M.; Krenning, E. New Advances in Peptide Receptor Radionuclide Therapy. *J. Nucl. Med.* **2002**, *43*, 617–620. [PubMed]
88. Strigari, L.; Konijnenberg, M.; Chiesa, C.; Bardies, M.; Du, Y.; Gleisner, K.S.; Lassmann, M.; Flux, G. The evidence base for the use of internal dosimetry in the clinical practice of molecular radiotherapy. *Eur. J. Nucl. Med. Mol. Imaging* **2014**, *41*, 1976–1988. [CrossRef]
89. Bodei, L.; Cremonesi, M.; Ferrari, M.; Pacifici, M.; Grana, C.M.; Bartolomei, M.; Baio, S.M.; Sansovini, M.; Paganelli, G. Long-term evaluation of renal toxicity after peptide receptor radionuclide therapy with 90Y-DOTATOC and 177Lu-DOTATATE: The role of associated risk factors. *Eur. J. Nucl. Med. Mol. Imaging* **2008**, *35*, 1847–1856. [CrossRef]
90. Ballal, S.; Yadav, M.P.; Bal, C.; Sahoo, R.K.; Tripathi, M. Broadening horizons with 225Ac-DOTATATE targeted alpha therapy for gastroenteropancreatic neuroendocrine tumour patients stable or refractory to 177Lu-DOTATATE PRRT: First clinical experience on the efficacy and safety. *Eur. J. Nucl. Med. Mol. Imaging* **2020**, *47*, 934–946. [CrossRef] [PubMed]
91. Ballal, S.; Yadav, M.P.; Tripathi, M.; Sahoo, R.K.; Bal, C. Survival Outcomes in Metastatic Gastroenteropancreatic Neuroendocrine Tumor Patients receiving Concomitant 225Ac-DOTATATE Targeted Alpha Therapy and Capecitabine: A Real-world Scenario Management Based Long-term Outcome Study. *J. Nucl. Med.* **2022**, *64*, 211–218. [CrossRef]
92. Delpassand, E.S.; Tworowska, I.; Esfandiari, R.; Torgue, J.; Hurt, J.; Shafie, A.; Núñez, R. Targeted Alpha-Emitter Therapy With 212Pb-DOTAMTATE for the Treatment of Metastatic SSTR-Expressing Neuroendocrine Tumors: First-in-Human, Dose-Escalation Clinical Trial. *J. Nucl. Med.* **2022**, *63*, 1326–1333. [CrossRef] [PubMed]
93. Demirci, E.; Alan Selcuk, N.; Beydagi, G.; Ocak, M.; Toklu, T.; Akcay, K.; Kabasakal, L. Initial Findings on the Use of [(225)Ac]Ac-DOTATATE Therapy as a Theranostic Application in Patients with Neuroendocrine Tumors. *Mol. Imaging Radionucl. Ther.* **2023**, *32*, 226–232. [CrossRef]
94. Giesel, F.; Wulfert, S.; Zechmann, C.; Kuder, T.; Kauczor, H.-U.; Haberkorn, U.; Kratochwil, C. Monitoring of perfusion changes after systemic versus selective arterial 177Lu/90Y-DOTATOC and 213Bi-DOTATOC radiopeptide therapy using contrast-enhanced ultrasound in liver metastatic neuroendocrine cancer. *J. Nucl. Med.* **2011**, *52*, 1727.
95. Kratochwil, C.; Giesel, F.L.; Bruchertseifer, F.; Mier, W.; Apostolidis, C.; Boll, R.; Murphy, K.; Haberkorn, U.; Morgenstern, A. 213Bi-DOTATOC receptor-targeted alpha-radionuclide therapy induces remission in neuroendocrine tumours refractory to beta radiation: A first-in-human experience. *Eur. J. Nucl. Med. Mol. Imaging* **2014**, *41*, 2106–2119. [CrossRef] [PubMed]
96. Kratochwil, C.; Apostolidis, L.; Rathke, H.; Apostolidis, C.; Bicu, F.; Bruchertseifer, F.; Choyke, P.L.; Haberkorn, U.; Giesel, F.L.; Morgenstern, A. Dosing 225Ac-DOTATOC in patients with somatostatin-receptor-positive solid tumors: 5-year follow-up of hematological and renal toxicity. *Eur. J. Nucl. Med. Mol. Imaging* **2021**, *49*, 54–63. [CrossRef]
97. Yadav, M.P.; Ballal, S.; Sahoo, R.K.; Bal, C. Efficacy and safety of 225Ac-DOTATATE targeted alpha therapy in metastatic paragangliomas: A pilot study. *Eur. J. Nucl. Med. Mol. Imaging* **2022**, *49*, 1595–1606. [CrossRef]

98. Zhang, J.; Singh, A.; Kulkarni, H.R.; Schuchardt, C.; Müller, D.; Wester, H.-J.; Maina, T.; Rösch, F.; van der Meulen, N.P.; Müller, C.; et al. From Bench to Bedside—The Bad Berka Experience With First-in-Human Studies. *Semin. Nucl. Med.* **2019**, *49*, 422–437. [CrossRef] [PubMed]
99. Imhof, A.; Brunner, P.; Marincek, N.; Briel, M.; Schindler, C.; Rasch, H.; Mäcke, H.R.; Rochlitz, C.; Müller-Brand, J.; Walter, M.A. Response, Survival, and Long-Term Toxicity After Therapy With the Radiolabeled Somatostatin Analogue [^{90}Y-DOTA]-TOC in Metastasized Neuroendocrine Cancers. *J. Clin. Oncol.* **2011**, *29*, 2416–2423. [CrossRef] [PubMed]
100. Bodei, L.; Kidd, M.; Paganelli, G.; Grana, C.M.; Drozdov, I.; Cremonesi, M.; Lepensky, C.; Kwekkeboom, D.J.; Baum, R.P.; Krenning, E.P.; et al. Long-term tolerability of PRRT in 807 patients with neuroendocrine tumours: The value and limitations of clinical factors. *Eur. J. Nucl. Med. Mol. Imaging* **2015**, *42*, 5–19. [CrossRef]
101. Sharma, M.; McCarthy, E.T.; Sharma, R.; Fish, B.L.; Savin, V.J.; Cohen, E.P.; Moulder, J.E. Arachidonic Acid Metabolites Mediate the Radiation-Induced Increase in Glomerular Albumin Permeability. *Exp Biol. Med.* **2006**, *231*, 99–106. [CrossRef]
102. U.S. Department of Health and Human Services. *Common Terminology Criteria for Adverse Events (CTCAE) Version 4.0*; National Institutes of Health: New York, NY, USA, 2009; pp. 1–9.
103. Cremonesi, M.; Ferrari, M.E.; Bodei, L.; Chiesa, C.; Sarnelli, A.; Garibaldi, C.; Pacilio, M.; Strigari, L.; Summers, P.E.; Orecchia, R.; et al. Correlation of dose with toxicity and tumour response to 90Y- and 177Lu-PRRT provides the basis for optimization through individualized treatment planning. *Eur. J. Nucl. Med. Mol. Imaging* **2018**, *45*, 2426–2441. [CrossRef]
104. Sundlöv, A.; Gleisner, K.S.; Tennvall, J.; Ljungberg, M.; Warfvinge, C.F.; Holgersson, K.; Hallqvist, A.; Bernhardt, P.; Svensson, J. Phase II trial demonstrates the efficacy and safety of individualized, dosimetry-based 177Lu-DOTATATE treatment of NET patients. *Eur. J. Nucl. Med. Mol. Imaging* **2022**, *49*, 3830–3840. [CrossRef]
105. Strosberg, J.; Hofman, M.S.; Al-Toubah, T.; Hope, T.A. Rethinking Dosimetry: The Perils of Extrapolated External-Beam Radiotherapy Constraints to Radionuclide Therapy. *J. Nucl. Med.* **2024**. [CrossRef]
106. Gear, J.I.; Cox, M.G.; Gustafsson, J.; Gleisner, K.S.; Murray, I.; Glatting, G.; Konijnenberg, M.; Flux, G.D. EANM practical guidance on uncertainty analysis for molecular radiotherapy absorbed dose calculations. *Eur. J. Nucl. Med. Mol. Imaging* **2018**, *45*, 2456–2474. [CrossRef]
107. Geenen, L.; Nonnekens, J.; Konijnenberg, M.; Baatout, S.; De Jong, M.; Aerts, A. Overcoming nephrotoxicity in peptide receptor radionuclide therapy using [(177)Lu]Lu-DOTA-TATE for the treatment of neuroendocrine tumours. *Nucl. Med. Biol.* **2021**, *102–103*, 1–11. [CrossRef]
108. Hofmann, W.; Li, W.B.; Friedland, W.; Miller, B.W.; Madas, B.; Bardies, M.; Balashazy, I. Internal microdosimetry of alpha-emitting radionuclides. *Radiat. Env. BioPhys.* **2020**, *59*, 29–62. [CrossRef]
109. Al-Toubah, T.; Montilla-Soler, J.; El-Haddad, G.; Haider, M.; Strosberg, J. Somatostatin Receptor Expression in Lung Neuroendocrine Tumors: An Analysis of dotatate pet Scans. *J. Nucl. Med.* **2023**, *64*, 1895–1898. [CrossRef]
110. Reubi, J.C.; Maecke, H.R. Approaches to Multireceptor Targeting: Hybrid Radioligands, Radioligand Cocktails, and Sequential Radioligand Applications. *J. Nucl. Med.* **2017**, *58*, 10S–16S. [CrossRef]

Disclaimer/Publisher's Note: The statements, opinions and data contained in all publications are solely those of the individual author(s) and contributor(s) and not of MDPI and/or the editor(s). MDPI and/or the editor(s) disclaim responsibility for any injury to people or property resulting from any ideas, methods, instructions or products referred to in the content.

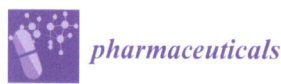 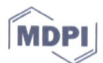

Article

Combining Cisplatin with Different Radiation Qualities—Interpretation of Cytotoxic Effects In Vitro by Isobolographic Analysis

Roswitha Runge [1,*], Falco Reissig [2], Nora Herzog [1], Liane Oehme [1], Claudia Brogsitter [1] and Joerg Kotzerke [1]

[1] Department of Nuclear Medicine, University Hospital Carl Gustav Carus, Technical University Dresden, Fetscherstr. 74, 01307 Dresden, Germany; nora.herzog@uniklinikum-dresden.de (N.H.); claudia.brogsitter@uniklinikum-dresden.de (C.B.); joerg.kotzerke@uniklinikum-dresden.de (J.K.)

[2] Helmholtz-Zentrum Dresden-Rossendorf, Institute of Radiopharmaceutical Cancer Research, Bautzner Landstraße 400, 01328 Dresden, Germany; f.reissig@hzdr.de

* Correspondence: roswitha.runge@uniklinikum-dresden.de; Tel.: +49-351-5481

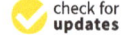

Citation: Runge, R.; Reissig, F.; Herzog, N.; Oehme, L.; Brogsitter, C.; Kotzerke, J. Combining Cisplatin with Different Radiation Qualities—Interpretation of Cytotoxic Effects In Vitro by Isobolographic Analysis. *Pharmaceuticals* **2023**, *16*, 1720. https://doi.org/10.3390/ph16121720

Academic Editor: Hirofumi Hanaoka

Received: 27 October 2023
Revised: 6 December 2023
Accepted: 8 December 2023
Published: 12 December 2023

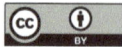

Copyright: © 2023 by the authors. Licensee MDPI, Basel, Switzerland. This article is an open access article distributed under the terms and conditions of the Creative Commons Attribution (CC BY) license (https://creativecommons.org/licenses/by/4.0/).

Abstract: Background: The combination of platinum-containing cytostatic drugs with different radiation qualities has been studied for years. Despite their massive side effects, these drugs still belong to the therapeutic portfolio in cancer treatment. To overcome the disadvantages of cisplatin, our study investigated the cytotoxic effects of combining radionuclides with cisplatin. Methods: FaDu cells were treated with cisplatin (concentration ≈ 2 µM) and additionally irradiated after two hours with the alpha-emitter ^{223}Ra, the beta-emitter ^{188}Re as well as external X-rays using dose ranges of 2–6 Gy. Cell survival was followed by colony formation assays and plotted against cisplatin concentration and radiation dose. The results were interpreted by isobolograms. Results: Isobolographic analyses revealed a supra-additive cytotoxic effect for the combination of cisplatin and ^{223}Ra. A sub-additive effect was observed for the combination of cisplatin and ^{188}Re, whereas a protective effect was found for the combination with X-rays. Conclusions: The combination of cisplatin and ^{223}Ra may have the potential to create a successfully working therapy scheme for various therapy approaches, whereas the combination with ^{188}Re as well as single-dose X-ray treatment did not lead to a detectable radiosensitizing effect. Thus, the combination with alpha-emitters might be advantageous and, therefore, should be followed in future studies when combined with cytostatic drugs.

Keywords: cisplatin; radionuclides; alpha-emitter; cancer therapy; combined treatment; isobolograms

1. Introduction

Cisplatin (cis-diammine-dichloro-platinum (II), CDDP) and its derivatives, carboplatin and oxaliplatin, have been widely used in the treatment of human cancers, such as bladder, head and neck, lung, ovarian, and testicular carcinomas [1]. Their mechanism of action is based on direct interactions of the platinum complexes within the DNA strands, resulting in the inhibition of cell repair mechanisms and thereby reducing tumor volume. In the past, the general use of platinum pharmaceuticals in cancer treatment focused on the rather unselective therapy of different tumor tissues [2,3]. Platinum drugs are used as a first-line treatment for solid tumors when radiation is not an option or as a second-line treatment in combination with other chemotherapeutic agents. The major limitations in the use of cisplatin and its derivatives are the renal side effects as well as the development of resistance in cancer cells [4].

In the past, extensive clinical studies have demonstrated the high efficacy of targeted radionuclide therapies such as ^{177}Lu-PSMA-617 radioligand therapy for metastatic castration-resistant prostate cancer (VISION) [5]; ^{177}Lu-DOTATATE for progressive midgut neuroendocrine tumors (NETTER-1) [6]; and radionuclide therapy with radium-223-dichloride, selectively targeting bone metastases from prostate cancer (ALSYMPCA) [7]. Subsequently, the successful proof of concept for targeted alpha therapy (TAT) has led to further research interest in this area [8,9]. In addition, the clinical applications of TAT are continuously growing, with different radionuclides, such as ^{225}Ac, ^{212}Pb, and ^{227}Th, as promising candidates. Alpha-particles are characterized by high linear energy transfer (LET), leading predominantly to a direct radiation response and impaired DNA repair [10].

To overcome the normal tissue side effects, the focus has been directed on the optimization of commonly used approaches, namely cisplatin-based chemo-radiotherapy. In recent years, several radiosensitizing effects have been reported, providing promising data. In particular, increased DNA damage has been observed in tumor cells after the combination of platinum drugs and external irradiation [11–14]. Numerous clinical studies have been performed on this topic. Marcu et al. proposed techniques to increase the tumor control probability (TCP) of head and neck cancer while protecting normal tissue in a phase II study [15]. In addition, a higher rate of complete pathologic response was observed in patients treated with platinum-based chemo-radiotherapy compared with patients receiving chemotherapy alone [12].

Additionally, the preclinical evaluation of nanoparticle encapsulated cisplatin (BNC-LP-CDDP) as chemo-radiotherapy treatment revealed the elimination of the nephrotoxic properties in vitro and in vivo, and thus, the nanoparticles can improve the local deposition of higher doses in the target region [16]. Sisin et al. found increased efficacy of tumor control for the combination of cisplatin and bismuth oxide nanoparticles (BiONP) on MCF-7 cells under ^{192}Ir-high dose rate brachytherapy [17].

It may be advantageous to combine cytostatics with different radiation qualities, such as beta and alpha radiation, as well as external X-rays. Due to the special physical properties of radionuclides, their low-dose rate of radiation is an important aspect when considering the high-dose rate of X-rays. Thus, the biological effects assessed from radionuclide exposure may, at least in part, underly different signaling pathways than those induced by X-rays.

To date, only a few studies have been performed using radionuclides that are commonly used in nuclear medicine [18–21]. The enhancement of radiobiological effects of radiometals, especially the underlying mechanism of Auger effects, has been reviewed by Kobayashi et al. and Nias et al. [22,23]. Another interesting aspect of platinum is the availability of radioactive platinum isotopes, which would even allow the use of a radiolabeled platinum complex. The DNA-destructive effect of radioactive platinum isotopes has also been reported [22,24,25].

Overall, the growing interest in the use of radiotherapy, especially the TAT approaches, indicates the need for further basic research in this area.

As a consequence, our investigations may contribute to discovering if the chemo-radiotherapeutic approach has the potential for successful application in cancer therapy.

In this particular study, human-derived head and neck cancer cells (FaDu) were incubated with cisplatin and additionally irradiated with ^{233}Ra as alpha-emitter, ^{188}Re as beta-emitter, or external X-rays. Cytotoxicity was measured by observing cell viability using colony formation assays. Results were interpreted by isobolographic analyses to distinguish between supra-additive, additive, or protective effects [26,27].

2. Results

2.1. Dose–Response Curves of Single Cytotoxin Incubations

To evaluate the damaging potential of the cytostatic drug and all radiation qualities, single incubations were performed on FaDu cells, and dose–response relationships were measured via clonogenic cell survival. The dose–response curves are shown in Figure 1.

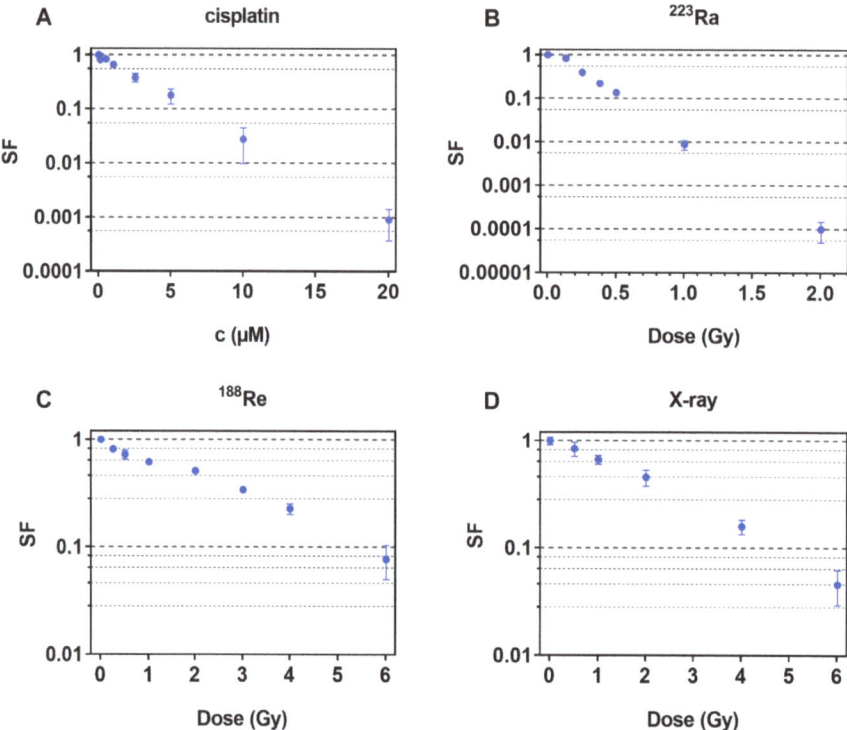

Figure 1. Cell survival fractions of FaDu cells after exposure to cisplatin (**A**), ^{223}Ra (**B**), ^{188}Re (**C**) or X-ray (**D**). Data are expressed as mean and standard deviation (±SD).

A clear dependence of the cell survival on concentration and radiation dose was observed for all different cytotoxins—cisplatin and radionuclides. In particular, the incubation of ^{223}Ra seems to cause more damage compared to ^{188}Re and X-rays at similar doses.

Additionally, the cisplatin concentrations that reduced the survival fractions to 0.37 or 0.50 (C_{37}, C_{50}) and the corresponding radiation doses D_{37} and D_{50} were calculated and are shown in Table 1.

Table 1. Calculated C_{37} and C_{50} as well as D_{37} and D_{50} values for combined treatments of FaDu cells—mean value (95% confidence interval in brackets).

Treatment Conditions	C_{50} (µM)/D_{50} (Gy)	C_{37} (µM)/D_{37} (Gy)
Cisplatin (µM)	1.90 (1.85–1.95)	2.72 (2.65–2.80)
^{223}Ra (Gy)	0.163 (0.156–0.169)	0.232 (0.223–0.242)
^{188}Re (Gy)	1.69 (1.61–1.78)	2.42 (2.31–2.55)
X-ray (Gy)	1.75 (1.66–1.85)	2.39 (2.28–2.50)

Cisplatin, X-rays, and ^{188}Re show similar D_{37} and D_{50} values, whereas about 10-fold-lower D_{37} and D_{50} values were observed for ^{223}Ra.

2.2. Dose–Response Curves of Combined Treatments

To determine the nature of the interaction between cisplatin and radiation, isobolograms were constructed for two survival levels (SF = 0.37 or SF = 0.5). The interactions become supra-additive (radiosensitizing) when the effect of the combined therapy is greater than the sum of the responses of the respective single agents. Mode I represents the simple additivity of responses, while Mode II takes into account dose additivity as described in Section 4.

2.2.1. Combination of Cisplatin and ^{223}Ra

Combination experiments of cisplatin and ^{223}Ra at certain concentration ratios are displayed in Figure 2A. It can be seen that the combined treatment resulted in a significant reduction in the survival fractions. The measured values for ^{223}Ra and the combination were fitted according to the linear–quadratic model (LQ-Fit). The theoretical isoeffective curves for the combination of both agents were calculated for Mode I and II (see Section 4). However, the resulting lines for these two agents are almost indistinguishable. Isobolograms for the interaction of both drugs are shown in Figure 2B,C. According to Figure 2A, the combination of cisplatin and ^{223}Ra caused a small supra-additive effect. It can be assumed that a cisplatin-induced blockade of DNA replication and DNA repair enhances cell death, leading to an increase in irreparable damage to DNA, which in turn causes cell death [28,29]. It is well known that the efficiency of radiation therapy depends on the early induction of cell damage (apoptosis), and thus, the alpha-emitter ^{223}Ra may enhance cell death more efficiently than ^{188}Re or X-rays as radiation characterized by low-LET emitters [30].

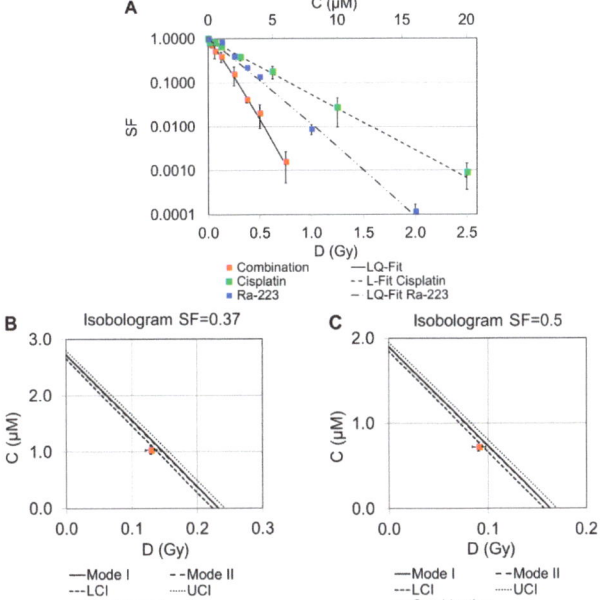

Figure 2. Survival curves of single and combined treatment experiments with cisplatin and ^{223}Ra are displayed, and the measured values are shown as mean ± SD (**A**). Isobolograms are displayed for survival fractions 0.37 (**B**) and 0.50 (**C**). The solid line represents the line of additivity; the dashed lines are the calculated errors with respect to the lower (LCI) and upper (UCI) 95% confidence intervals.

2.2.2. Combination of Cisplatin and ^{188}Re

Combination experiments of cisplatin and ^{188}Re at specific concentration ratios are shown in Figure 3A. The logarithms of the survival were fitted by a linear function (L-Fit) in both cases. Compared to the curves for cisplatin and ^{188}Re alone, the SF values for the combined treatment are significantly smaller. Approximately 2.4 Gy are required to achieve an SF value of 0.37, whereas only about 1.4 Gy is required for the combination with cisplatin. Isobolograms for the interaction of both drugs for a surviving cell fraction of 0.37 or 0.50 are shown in Figure 3B,C.

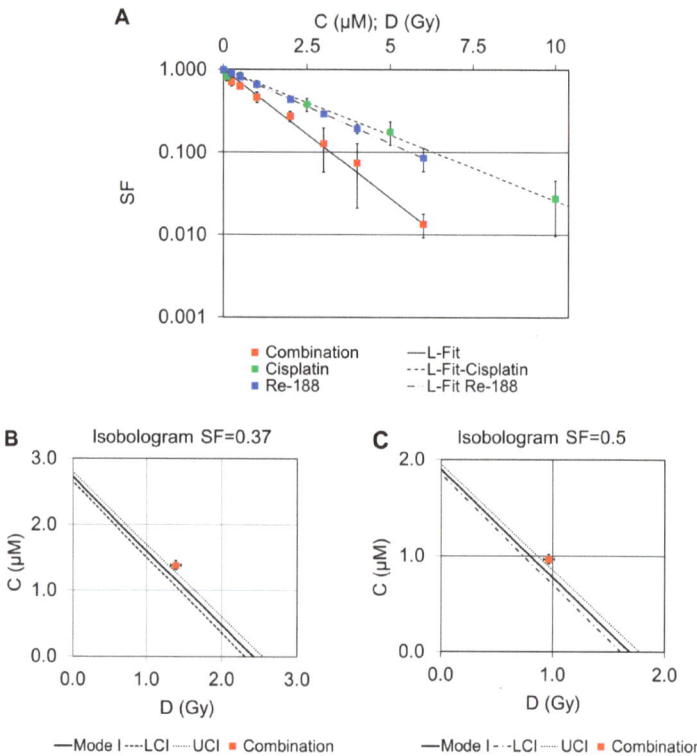

Figure 3. Survival curves of single and combined treatment experiments with cisplatin and [188]Re are displayed, and the measured values are shown as mean ± SD (**A**). Isobolograms show survival fractions of 0.37 (**B**) and 0.50 (**C**). The solid line represents the line of additivity; the dashed lines are the calculated errors in terms of the lower (LCI) and upper (UCI) 95% confidence intervals.

The corresponding survival for the combination of both drugs (red boxes in Figure 3B,C) is slightly above the 95% confidence interval of the cytotoxicity of irradiation and cisplatin alone, indicating that there was a sub-additive effect when cisplatin and [188]Re were combined. Because we assumed linear dose–response curves for both cisplatin and [188]Re, there is no difference between Mode I and II in the calculated lines of additivity in this isobolographic analysis (see Section 4).

2.2.3. Combination of Cisplatin and External X-rays

Combination experiments of cisplatin and external X-ray at specific concentration ratios are shown in Figure 4A. The survival curves for X-ray and the combination were best described by the linear–quadratic model. There are very similar proportions of surviving cells induced by X-rays and cisplatin alone, as well as for their combination at the respective dose points. Isobolograms for the interaction of both drugs are shown in Figure 4B,C. In the isobolograms, the envelope of additivity, i.e., the difference between Mode I and Mode II calculations, is clearly visible.

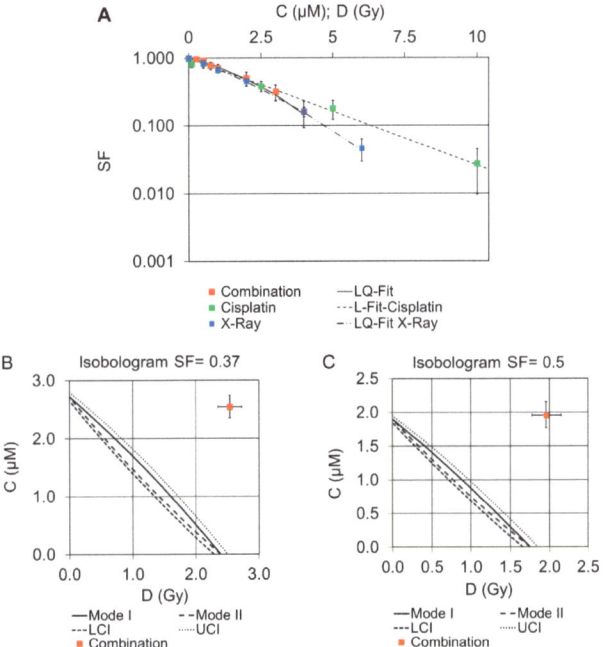

Figure 4. Survival curves of single and combined treatment experiments with cisplatin and X-rays are shown. Measurements are expressed as mean ± SD (**A**). Isobolograms show survival fractions of 0.37 (**B**) and 0.50 (**C**). The solid line represents the line of additivity; the dashed lines are the calculated errors with respect to the lower (LCI) and upper (UCI) 95% confidence intervals.

According to the results shown in Figure 4A, the combination of cisplatin and external X-rays did not lead to an additive effect (Figure 4B,C). In contrast, a clear protective effect was observed by interpreting the isobolograms (red boxes).

3. Discussion

In our study, we investigated the combined treatment using cisplatin and the radionuclides ^{233}Ra, ^{188}Re, as well as external X-rays. Head and neck tumor cells (FaDu) served as biological models. To interpret the results as supra-additive, additive, or protective, the concept of isobolographic analyses was used.

Looking at the results for the single treatment with ^{223}Ra, the survival curve leads to the assumption that the alpha-emitter is more effective in cell eradication compared to ^{188}Re and X-rays at similar doses. Ten times lower D_{37} and D_{50} values were observed for ^{223}Ra compared to ^{188}Re and X-rays. This is primarily due to the different mechanisms of DNA damage induction. While ^{188}Re and X-rays induce strand breaks mainly via indirect effects and the generation of free radical species, ^{223}Ra is capable of inducing direct DNA double-strand breaks (DSB) by emitting high-energy particles. Similar results were found for the alpha-emitter ^{223}Ra compared to ^{188}Re in PCCL3 cells [31]. Recently, our group published a study that investigated the effects of cisplatin in combination with radionuclides using plasmid pUC19 as a biophysical model. No significant increase in the number of DNA strand breaks has been found [32].

A study by Dewey et al. summarized that a significant amount of apoptosis recruits tumor cells into the apoptotic-susceptible fraction between daily external radiation doses [30]. The authors postulated that fractionated radiation therapy increases cell killing by apoptosis more than large single doses. This may be one explanation for the radioprotective effect of cisplatin in combination with a single dose of X-rays in our experiments.

In conclusion, our results of the combinatorial treatments showed a supra-additive effect only for the combination of cisplatin and ^{223}Ra, which again could be caused by the mechanism of action of cisplatin and the already higher effect of ^{223}Ra. In more detail, cisplatin molecules form adducts with nucleophilic sites of DNA, which can block DNA replication, transcription and damage repair [29]. Damage could also result from the emission of Auger electrons and photoelectrons generated by radiation in high-Z atoms such as platinum [22]. Thus, the enhancement of cell death in combined treatments is most likely provoked by the enhancement of irreparable damage to DNA, leading to an increase in initial lesions. Additionally, the high-LET emitter ^{223}Ra may enhance cell death more efficiently than low-LET emitters such as ^{188}Re caused by impaired repair of the DNA damage [28].

Geldof et al. demonstrated supra-additive treatment effects in prostate cancer cells by combining ^{186}Re-HEDP and cisplatin [20]. The combined treatment of HepG2 tumor cells with ^{131}I-NaI as a radiotherapeutic agent and cisplatin also resulted in improved cell death in a supra-additive manner [19], suggesting successful radiosensitizing effects when cisplatin is combined with low-LET emitters.

Recently, a preclinical and a clinical study evaluated combined chemo- and radionuclide therapy approaches. Timin et al. implemented these concepts using radionuclide carriers (^{177}Lu-labeled core-shell particles) and cisplatin to treat metastatic lung cancer in animals [21]. This combination increased the therapeutic efficacy of tumor treatment compared to monotherapy. A clinical trial evaluated the efficacy of ^{90}Y-transarterial radioembolization with cisplatin for the first-line treatment of locally advanced intrahepatic cholangiocarcinoma (iCCA). The authors found this approach to be an effective treatment for iCCA with a high rate of downstaging to tumor resection [18].

Many studies have investigated the combination of external beam radiation and a chemotherapeutic agent. Gorodetsky et al. showed both radiosensitizing and radioprotective effects depending on the chosen treatment sequence of the noxes X-ray and cisplatin [14]. Akudugu and Slabbert investigated the modulation of radiosensitivity by cisplatin in V79 Chinese hamster lung fibroblasts [33]. Their results show that the mode of interaction between cisplatin and gamma irradiation depends on the concentration and exposure time of cisplatin, as well as the timing of irradiation after cisplatin administration. Increased radiosensitivity was found when cisplatin was present in the cells for 8–12 h and 20–24 h. This experimental setting is in contrast to our study, which used a drug incubation interval of 4 h.

Additionally, the importance of different LET values on radiosensitizing effects with cisplatin has been investigated. Shiba et al. found that low-LET carbon–ion irradiation in combination with cisplatin produced higher cytotoxic effects than high-LET carbon–ion irradiation in cervical cancer cells [34]. On the other hand, carbon ion irradiation combined with cisplatin showed superior potential to kill breast cancer cells with irreparable DNA damage [35]. Benzina et al. combined cisplatin as well as oxaliplatin in two different studies with high-LET irradiation by p (65) + Be neutrons (dose rate 0.2 Gy/min) using glioblastoma cells. Their approaches enhanced the cytotoxicity in a more than additive way or caused a marked reduction in tumor growth in nude mice xenografts, respectively [28,36]. In addition, high-LET CIERT was more effective than photon irradiation in preventing the proliferation of HNSCC cell lines [37].

Overall, several studies have shown the improved efficacy of cancer therapy in vitro and in vivo, even when radionuclides are used in combination with cisplatin. Similarly, our in vitro study showed, at least for ^{223}Ra in combination with cisplatin, improved tumor cell eradication, which can be interpreted as a supra-additive effect. We are aware that our results were obtained using the same combination protocol for all experiments. By changing the first and second cytotoxin, as described by some authors [8,14,33], such changes in the cytotoxin sequence could lead to results different from ours. Furthermore, in our experiments, cisplatin and radiotherapy treatments were administered only once, whereas realistic therapies for both cytostatic drugs and external irradiation are likely to be administered in cycles. Thus, it can be expected that the clinical effects of fractionated radiotherapy and chemotherapy applied in cycles may lead to different effects on tumor survival. Overall, experiments using in vitro cell models are only partly applicable to living organisms. Further studies should focus on potential clinical applications in nuclear medicine.

From a biological point of view, other endpoints, such as apoptosis or cell cycle analysis, might be helpful to gain more insights into the cellular response to combined chemo-radiotherapy. A better understanding of the molecular response of cells could lead to research based on treatments that combine pharmacological interventions with ionizing radiation to more specifically target tumor tissue, namely, multiple DNA repair pathways, cell cycle checkpoints, or modulation of signal transduction pathways [38].

For our study, it can be assumed that the radiation qualities other than ^{223}Ra, namely ^{188}Re and X-rays, could have similar effects when different experimental schemes are applied. This is something to be tested in more detail to complement this study, which has demonstrated that the applied statistical methods and settings used are well-suited to detect different drug interactions in this particular area of interest.

4. Materials and Methods

4.1. Radionuclides and X-ray Irradiation

The β-emitter ^{188}Re-perrhenate (^{188}ReO$_4^-$) was obtained by elution of a 40-GBq alumina-based ^{188}W/^{188}Re generator (Isotope Technologies Garching GmbH, Garching Germany). Physical properties of ^{188}Re are half-life $T_{1/2}$ = 17 h and maximum β-energy = 2.1 MeV.

The α-particle emitter ^{223}Ra-radium dichloride (^{223}RaCl$_2$, Xofigo) was provided by Bayer Vital GmbH (Leverkusen, Germany) with an activity concentration of 1000 kBq/mL. ^{223}Ra (half-life 11.4 days) decays through a cascade of short-lived α- and β-particle emitters. Each decay of ^{223}Ra produces four α-particles, resulting in the emission of approximately 28 MeV of energy, with 95% of the energy from the α-emissions.

Each of the radioactive samples was measured with an Isomed 2010 (Nuvia Instruments, Dresden, Germany) dose calibrator.

For the external irradiations at the OncoRay site (National Center for Radiation Research in Oncology, Medical Faculty Dresden, Germany), an X-ray tube (Y.TU 320, Yxlon International, Hamburg, Germany) with 200 kV X-rays (20 mA, dose rate ≈ 1.24 Gy/min, filtered with 0.5 mm Cu) was used.

4.2. Cell Culture

FaDu cells are epithelial, squamous cell carcinoma cells of the pharynx. They were established in 1968 from a biopsy of an undifferentiated human squamous cell carcinoma growing as a monolayer (HTB-43^{TM}, American Type Culture Collection (ATCC®), Manassas, VA, USA) [39]. Our experiments were performed with the sub-cell line FaDu$_{DD}$, kindly provided by the Department of Radiotherapy and Radiation Oncology, Medical Faculty, Technische Universität Dresden. This cell line has been used in cancer research, particularly in radiobiological experiments, since the 1980s. [40]. The cells were maintained in Dulbecco's minimum essential medium (DMEM, Fisher Scientific, Wesel, Germany) containing 2% (v/v) HEPES buffer, 1% (v/v) of non-essential amino acids, 1% (v/v) of sodium pyruvate, and 10% (v/v) of fetal calf serum. All chemicals added to the cell culture medium were purchased from Sigma Aldrich (Sigma Aldrich, Taufkirchen, Germany). Exponentially growing cells were split twice weekly using trypsin (Sigma Aldrich) and cultured in a humidified incubator at 37 °C and 5% CO$_2$. To prevent cell dedifferentiation, the experiments were performed at identical passage numbers. Cells were routinely screened for mycoplasma infection.

4.3. Cisplatin Incubation, Irradiation Procedure, and Colony Formation Assay

To study the cytotoxicity of cisplatin (Merck KGaA, Darmstadt, Germany), X-rays, and the radionuclides ^{188}Re or ^{223}Ra as single agents, 0.5×10^6 FaDu cells were plated in each well of 6-well multititer plates (MTP) one day before the start of the experiment. To investigate the cytotoxic effects of cisplatin (0.01; 0.1; 0.5; 1.0; 2.5; 5.0; 10; and 20 μM), FaDu cells were treated for 4 h. The ^{188}Re-, ^{223}Ra-radioactive solutions, 0.69–16.5 MBq/mL, and 0.008–0.127 MBq/mL, respectively, were added to the cells to achieve doses of 0.25–6.0 Gy. In the case of X-ray irradiation, the cells were exposed to 0.5–6.0 Gy. Untreated control samples were included in each experiment.

After calculating the respective D_{50} and C_{50} values for each of the radionuclides and for cisplatin, the iso-effective doses or concentrations were chosen to establish the relationship between them. For the combined treatment experiments, we decided to use a relation of 1:1 for radionuclide doses and cisplatin concentrations (0.25; 0.5; 1.0; 2.0; 3.0; 4.0; 6.0 Gy or cisplatin in μM, factor 1.0). An exception was necessary for ^{223}Ra due to the D_{50} value of 0.163 Gy. Therefore, the ratio of 0.125 Gy ^{223}Ra to 1 μM cisplatin was used, resulting in a factor of 0.125. After a 2 h preincubation period with cisplatin alone, the ^{188}Re- and ^{223}Ra-radioactive solutions were added to the cells for a further 2 h incubation period to achieve dosages of 0.25–6.0 Gy or 0.25–6.0 μM, respectively. Similarly, for X-ray, cells were preincubated with cisplatin for 2 h and then exposed to 0.5–6.0 Gy (23.5–282 s). To ensure the same 4 h incubation time of cisplatin after X-ray irradiation, the incubation of the cells was continued for the remaining time window.

To determine the cytotoxic effects of the chemo-radio-therapeutic approach, the clonogenic cell survival was analyzed. Colony formation assays were performed as previously described [41]. Following irradiation, the radioactive supernatant was discarded, and the cells were washed with phosphate-buffered saline (PBS, 37 °C) and detached by trypsin. An aliquot of the cell suspension was seeded at a low density for colony formation at respective cell numbers adjusted to the doses or concentrations (200–50,000 cells) into T25 cell culture flasks (Greiner Bio-one, Frickenhausen, Germany) for an incubation period of 10 days. To stop colony formation, the cells were fixed in 80% (v/v) ethanol and stained with crystal violet solution. All chemicals were obtained by Merck KGaA.

Finally, cell colonies (>50 cells) were counted manually under a light microscope. The plating efficiency (PE) was calculated for treated and untreated cells based on the number of seeded cells. The surviving fraction (SF) was calculated as the relative plating efficiency of treated vs. untreated samples [42].

4.4. Isobologram Analysis

The possible interactions between radiation and chemotherapy were defined by Steel and Peckham [43]. For the isoeffective plots, the calculation of the theoretical lines of additivity was performed in two ways: Mode I and Mode II [26,43,44].

In short, Mode I assumes an independent action of the agents; the expected survival is the product of the individual survival for a given combination of concentration (cisplatin) and dose (irradiation). In Mode II, there may be an interaction between the agents, so an isoequivalent approach is performed. The first agent (cisplatin) causes damage, leading to surviving fraction (SF), and the radiation dose that would have had the same effect in an independent treatment is sought. It is then necessary to determine the additional dose that would have been required to achieve the desired level of survival. In the isobologram, the Mode I and II additivity curves are different and form an additivity envelope when the log survival curve is non-linear for at least one agent. In summary, this envelope refers to additive effects, but combined treatment could lead to supra-additive or protective effects.

4.5. Dosimetry

The dose calculation for radioactivity (^{188}Re, ^{223}Ra) was performed with Geant4 simulations for a 10 μm cell monolayer at the bottom of the well (9.6 cm^2) in 2 mL cell culture medium. The dose from a source volume to a target volume is calculated as the product of the time-integrated activity in the source volume and a source-target-specific S value [31]. According to this model, only the extracellular irradiation of the medium was considered [45]. Thus, the applied X-ray radiation (external irradiation) is comparable to the dose of radioactivity generated.

For an effective dose of 1 Gy after 2 h of irradiation, the following activity concentrations were calculated: 5.5 MBq/2 mL ^{188}Re, 0.127 MBq/2 mL ^{223}Ra. The variation of the effective dose was achieved by increasing or decreasing the volume activity at a constant irradiation time of 2 h.

4.6. Statistical Analysis

All experiments were performed in three to four independent experiments. Triplicate samples were prepared for each dose point. The mean values of cell survival, including the calculated standard deviations, are presented against the respective cisplatin concentration or radiation dose. All data were statistically evaluated using the SPSS Statistics 24.0 software (IBM Corporation, Armonk, NY, USA). Curve fitting was performed by linear regression analysis.

In addition to standard statistics, isobolographic analyses were performed to better understand the drug–drug interaction of irradiation and cisplatin. For each treatment condition, the functional relationship between concentration or dose and the measured cell survival was analyzed according to the linear or linear–quadratic model. This curve fitting of log survival as dependent and either concentration or dose (and dose square) as independent variables was performed with the Linear Regression Tool of SPSS. The obtained regression coefficients for each treatment condition allowed the calculation of theoretical values of concentration and dose for a considered level of survival.

The generation of isobolograms was performed in Microsoft EXCEL 2010. The envelope of additivity was calculated according to Section 4.4. from the experiments with single noxes of radiation and cisplatin. The combined treatment, in our case with a fixed ratio of concentration and dose, delivers a single point in the isobologram. Its position in relation to the additivity envelope was visually interpreted. To determine the uncertainties in terms of confidence levels, we repeated the isobolographic calculation using the upper and lower confidence intervals of the predicted values from the regression analyses. Therefore, the presented isobolograms show the effect of the combination experiments to interpret the overall cell survival as a function of these different drugs.

5. Conclusions

It has been shown that a general supra-additive effect is not to be expected after the combination of cisplatin and different radiation qualities. Nevertheless, the combination of ^{223}Ra as a high-LET emitting radionuclide with the cytostatic drug cisplatin resulted in a supra-additive effect that can now be further evaluated. With the development of a well-functioning scheme for therapy at the cellular level, patients may also benefit from more knowledge about these combination approaches, and higher tumor-destroying effects may be achieved with lower radiation or drug doses.

Author Contributions: Conceptualization, J.K. and R.R.; methodology, N.H. and R.R.; software, L.O.; validation, R.R., F.R. and L.O.; formal analysis, N.H.; investigation, N.H.; resources, C.B.; data curation, N.H.; writing—original draft preparation, F.R. and R.R.; writing—review and editing, J.K. and C.B.; visualization, R.R. and L.O.; supervision, J.K.; project administration, C.B. All authors have read and agreed to the published version of the manuscript.

Funding: This research received no external funding.

Institutional Review Board Statement: Not applicable.

Informed Consent Statement: Not applicable.

Data Availability Statement: Data can be requested by contacting the corresponding author.

Acknowledgments: The authors thank Kerstin Wetzig for her technical assistance.

Conflicts of Interest: The authors declare no conflict of interest.

References

1. Dasari, S.; Tchounwou, P.B. Cisplatin in cancer therapy: Molecular mechanisms of action. *Eur. J. Pharmacol.* **2014**, *740*, 364–378. [CrossRef]
2. Brown, A.; Kumar, S.; Tchounwou, P.B. Cisplatin-Based Chemotherapy of Human Cancers. *J. Cancer Sci. Ther.* **2019**, *11*, 97.
3. Makovec, T. Cisplatin and beyond: Molecular mechanisms of action and drug resistance development in cancer chemotherapy. *Radiol. Oncol.* **2019**, *53*, 148–158. [CrossRef]
4. Romani, A.M.P. Cisplatin in cancer treatment. *Biochem. Pharmacol.* **2022**, *206*, 115323. [CrossRef]
5. Sartor, O.; de Bono, J.; Chi, K.N.; Fizazi, K.; Herrmann, K.; Rahbar, K.; Tagawa, S.T.; Nordquist, L.T.; Vaishampayan, N.; El-Haddad, G.; et al. Lutetium-177-PSMA-617 for Metastatic Castration-Resistant Prostate Cancer. *N. Engl. J. Med.* **2021**, *385*, 1091–1103. [CrossRef]
6. Strosberg, J.; El-Haddad, G.; Wolin, E.; Hendifar, A.; Yao, J.; Chasen, B.; Mittra, E.; Kunz, P.L.; Kulke, M.H.; Jacene, H.; et al. Phase 3 Trial of ^{177}Lu-Dotatate for Midgut Neuroendocrine Tumors. *N. Engl. J. Med.* **2017**, *376*, 125–135. [CrossRef]
7. Parker, C.; Nilsson, S.; Heinrich, D.; Helle, S.I.; O'Sullivan, J.M.; Fossa, S.D.; Chodacki, A.; Wiechno, P.; Logue, J.; Seke, M.; et al. Alpha emitter radium-223 and survival in metastatic prostate cancer. *N. Engl. J. Med.* **2013**, *369*, 213–223. [CrossRef]
8. Milenic, D.E.; Kim, Y.S.; Baidoo, K.E.; Wong, K.J.; Barkley, R.; Delgado, J.; Brechbiel, M.W. Exploration of a F(ab')$_2$ Fragment as the Targeting Agent of alpha-Radiation Therapy: A Comparison of the Therapeutic Benefit of Intraperitoneal and Intravenous Administered Radioimmunotherapy. *Cancer Biother. Radiopharm.* **2018**, *33*, 182–193. [CrossRef]
9. Parker, C.C.; James, N.D.; Brawley, C.D.; Clarke, N.W.; Hoyle, A.P.; Ali, A.; Ritchie, A.W.S.; Attard, G.; Chowdhury, S.; Cross, W.; et al. Radiotherapy to the primary tumour for newly diagnosed, metastatic prostate cancer (STAMPEDE): A randomised controlled phase 3 trial. *Lancet* **2018**, *392*, 2353–2366. [CrossRef]
10. Guerra Liberal, F.D.C.; O'Sullivan, J.M.; McMahon, S.J.; Prise, K.M. Targeted Alpha Therapy: Current Clinical Applications. *Cancer Biother. Radiopharm.* **2020**, *35*, 404–417. [CrossRef]
11. Biston, M.C.; Joubert, A.; Adam, J.F.; Elleaume, H.; Bohic, S.; Charvet, A.M.; Esteve, F.; Foray, N.; Balosso, J. Cure of Fisher rats bearing radioresistant F98 glioma treated with cis-platinum and irradiated with monochromatic synchrotron X-rays. *Cancer Res.* **2004**, *64*, 2317–2323. [CrossRef]
12. Candelaria, M.; Chanona-Vilchis, J.; Cetina, L.; Flores-Estrada, D.; Lopez-Graniel, C.; Gonzalez-Enciso, A.; Cantu, D.; Poitevin, A.; Rivera, L.; Hinojosa, J.; et al. Prognostic significance of pathological response after neoadjuvant chemotherapy or chemoradiation for locally advanced cervical carcinoma. *Int. Semin. Surg. Oncol.* **2006**, *3*, 3. [CrossRef]
13. Caney, C.; Singh, G.; Lukka, H.; Rainbow, A.J. Combined gamma-irradiation and subsequent cisplatin treatment in human squamous carcinoma cell lines sensitive and resistant to cisplatin. *Int. J. Radiat. Biol.* **2004**, *80*, 291–299. [CrossRef]
14. Gorodetsky, R.; Levy-Agababa, F.; Mou, X.; Vexler, A.M. Combination of cisplatin and radiation in cell culture: Effect of duration of exposure to drug and timing of irradiation. *Int. J. Cancer* **1998**, *75*, 635–642. [CrossRef]
15. Marcu, L.G. Improving therapeutic ratio in head and neck cancer with adjuvant and cisplatin-based treatments. *Biomed. Res. Int.* **2013**, *2013*, 817279. [CrossRef]
16. Shin, S.H.; Park, S.S.; Lee, K.J.; Ju, E.J.; Park, J.; Ko, E.J.; Jung, J.; Kuroda, S.; Hong, S.M.; Hwang, J.J.; et al. Preclinical evaluation of cisplatin-incorporated bio-nanocapsules as chemo-radiotherapy for human hepatocellular carcinoma. *Oncol. Rep.* **2017**, *38*, 2259–2266. [CrossRef]
17. Sisin, N.N.T.; Abdul Razak, K.; Zainal Abidin, S.; Che Mat, N.F.; Abdullah, R.; Ab Rashid, R.; Khairil Anuar, M.A.; Mohd Zainudin, N.H.; Tagiling, N.; Mat Nawi, N.; et al. Radiosensitization Effects by Bismuth Oxide Nanoparticles in Combination with Cisplatin for High Dose Rate Brachytherapy. *Int. J. Nanomed.* **2019**, *14*, 9941–9954. [CrossRef]
18. Ahmed, O.; Yu, Q.; Patel, M.; Hwang, G.; Pillai, A.; Liao, C.Y.; Fung, J.; Baker, T. Yttrium-90 Radioembolization and Concomitant Systemic Gemcitabine, Cisplatin, and Capecitabine as the First-Line Therapy for Locally Advanced Intrahepatic Cholangiocarcinoma. *J. Vasc. Interv. Radiol.* **2023**, *34*, 702–709. [CrossRef]
19. Chenoufi, N.; Raoul, J.L.; Lescoat, G.; Brissot, P.; Bourguet, P. In vitro demonstration of synergy between radionuclide and chemotherapy. *J. Nucl. Med.* **1998**, *39*, 900–903.
20. Geldof, A.A.; de Rooij, L.; Versteegh, R.T.; Newling, D.W.; Teule, G.J. Combination ^{186}Re-HEDP and cisplatin supra-additive treatment effects in prostate cancer cells. *J. Nucl. Med.* **1999**, *40*, 667–671.
21. Timin, A.S.; Postovalova, A.S.; Karpov, T.E.; Antuganov, D.; Bukreeva, A.S.; Akhmetova, D.R.; Rogova, A.S.; Muslimov, A.R.; Rodimova, S.A.; Kuznetsova, D.S.; et al. Calcium carbonate carriers for combined chemo- and radionuclide therapy of metastatic lung cancer. *J. Control. Release* **2022**, *344*, 1–11. [CrossRef]
22. Kobayashi, K.; Usami, N.; Porcel, E.; Lacombe, S.; Le Sech, C. Enhancement of radiation effect by heavy elements. *Mutat. Res.* **2010**, *704*, 123–131. [CrossRef] [PubMed]
23. Nias, A.H. Radiation and platinum drug interaction. *Int. J. Radiat. Biol. Relat. Stud. Phys. Chem. Med.* **1985**, *48*, 297–314. [CrossRef] [PubMed]
24. Nadar, R.A.; Franssen, G.M.; Van Dijk, N.W.M.; Codee-van der Schilden, K.; de Weijert, M.; Oosterwijk, E.; Iafisco, M.; Margiotta, N.; Heskamp, S.; van den Beucken, J.; et al. Bone tumor-targeted delivery of theranostic ^{195m}Pt-bisphosphonate complexes promotes killing of metastatic tumor cells. *Mater. Today Bio.* **2021**, *9*, 100088. [CrossRef] [PubMed]

25. Obata, H.; Tsuji, A.B.; Sudo, H.; Sugyo, A.; Minegishi, K.; Nagatsu, K.; Ogawa, M.; Zhang, M.R. In Vitro Evaluation of No-Carrier-Added Radiolabeled Cisplatin ([(^{189,191})Pt]cisplatin) Emitting Auger Electrons. *Int. J. Mol. Sci.* **2021**, *22*, 4622. [CrossRef] [PubMed]
26. Tallarida, R.J. An overview of drug combination analysis with isobolograms. *J. Pharmacol. Exp. Ther.* **2006**, *319*, 1–7. [CrossRef] [PubMed]
27. Wilson, G.D.; Bentzen, S.M.; Harari, P.M. Biologic basis for combining drugs with radiation. *Semin. Radiat. Oncol.* **2006**, *16*, 2–9. [CrossRef] [PubMed]
28. Benzina, S.; Fischer, B.; Miternique-Grosse, A.; Dufour, P.; Denis, J.M.; Bergerat, J.P.; Gueulette, J.; Bischoff, P. Cell death induced in a human glioblastoma cell line by p(65) + Be neutrons combined with cisplatin. *Life Sci.* **2006**, *79*, 513–518. [CrossRef] [PubMed]
29. Furuta, T.; Ueda, T.; Aune, G.; Sarasin, A.; Kraemer, K.H.; Pommier, Y. Transcription-coupled nucleotide excision repair as a determinant of cisplatin sensitivity of human cells. *Cancer Res.* **2002**, *62*, 4899–4902.
30. Dewey, W.C.; Ling, C.C.; Meyn, R.E. Radiation-induced apoptosis: Relevance to radiotherapy. *Int. J. Radiat. Oncol. Biol. Phys.* **1995**, *33*, 781–796. [CrossRef]
31. Runge, R.; Oehme, L.; Kotzerke, J.; Freudenberg, R. The effect of dimethyl sulfoxide on the induction of DNA strand breaks in plasmid DNA and colony formation of PC Cl3 mammalian cells by alpha-, beta-, and Auger electron emitters ^{223}Ra, ^{188}Re, and ^{99m}Tc. *EJNMMI Res.* **2016**, *6*, 48. [CrossRef] [PubMed]
32. Reissig, F.; Runge, R.; Naumann, A.; Kotzerke, J. Cisplatin—A more Efficient Drug in Combination with Radionuclides? *Nuklearmedizin* **2022**, *61*, 325–332. [CrossRef] [PubMed]
33. Akudugu, J.M.; Slabbert, J.P. Modulation of radiosensitivity in Chinese hamster lung fibroblasts by cisplatin. *Can. J. Physiol. Pharmacol.* **2008**, *86*, 257–263. [CrossRef] [PubMed]
34. Shiba, S.; Wakatsuki, M.; Ohno, T.; Nakano, T. Differences in Linear Energy Transfer Affect Cell-killing and Radiosensitizing Effects of Spread-out Carbon-ion Beams. *Anticancer Res.* **2020**, *40*, 5497–5502. [CrossRef] [PubMed]
35. Sai, S.; Vares, G.; Kim, E.H.; Karasawa, K.; Wang, B.; Nenoi, M.; Horimoto, Y.; Hayashi, M. Carbon ion beam combined with cisplatin effectively disrupts triple negative breast cancer stem-like cells in vitro. *Mol. Cancer* **2015**, *14*, 166. [CrossRef]
36. Benzina, S.; Altmeyer, A.; Malek, F.; Dufour, P.; Denis, J.M.; Gueulette, J.; Bischoff, P. High-LET radiation combined with oxaliplatin induce autophagy in U-87 glioblastoma cells. *Cancer Lett.* **2008**, *264*, 63–70. [CrossRef]
37. Fang, X.; Sun, P.; Dong, Y.; Huang, Y.; Lu, J.J.; Kong, L. In vitro evaluation of photon and carbon ion radiotherapy in combination with cisplatin in head and neck squamous cell carcinoma cell lines. *Front. Oncol.* **2023**, *13*, 896142. [CrossRef]
38. Begg, A.C. Cisplatin and radiation: Interaction probabilities and therapeutic possibilities. *Int. J. Radiat. Oncol. Biol. Phys.* **1990**, *19*, 1183–1189. [CrossRef]
39. Rangan, S.R. A new human cell line (FaDu) from a hypopharyngeal carcinoma. *Cancer* **1972**, *29*, 117–121. [CrossRef]
40. Eicheler, W.; Zips, D.; Dorfler, A.; Grenman, R.; Baumann, M. Splicing mutations in TP53 in human squamous cell carcinoma lines influence immunohistochemical detection. *J. Histochem. Cytochem.* **2002**, *50*, 197–204. [CrossRef]
41. Maucksch, U.; Runge, R.; Wunderlich, G.; Freudenberg, R.; Naumann, A.; Kotzerke, J. Comparison of the radiotoxicity of the (99m)Tc-labeled compounds (99m)Tc-pertechnetate, (99m)Tc-HMPAO and (99m)Tc-MIBI. *Int. J. Radiat. Biol.* **2016**, *92*, 698–706. [CrossRef] [PubMed]
42. Franken, N.A.; Rodermond, H.M.; Stap, J.; Haveman, J.; van Bree, C. Clonogenic assay of cells in vitro. *Nat. Protoc.* **2006**, *1*, 2315–2319. [CrossRef] [PubMed]
43. Steel, G.G.; Peckham, M.J. Exploitable mechanisms in combined radiotherapy-chemotherapy: The concept of additivity. *Int. J. Radiat. Oncol. Biol. Phys.* **1979**, *5*, 85–91. [CrossRef] [PubMed]
44. Redpath, J.L. Mechanisms in combination therapy: Isobologram analysis and sequencing. *Int. J. Radiat. Biol. Relat. Stud. Phys. Chem. Med.* **1980**, *38*, 355–356. [CrossRef]
45. Freudenberg, R.; Runge, R.; Maucksch, U.; Berger, V.; Kotzerke, J. On the dose calculation at the cellular level and its implications for the RBE of ^{99m}Tc and ^{123}I. *Med. Phys.* **2014**, *41*, 062503. [CrossRef]

Disclaimer/Publisher's Note: The statements, opinions and data contained in all publications are solely those of the individual author(s) and contributor(s) and not of MDPI and/or the editor(s). MDPI and/or the editor(s) disclaim responsibility for any injury to people or property resulting from any ideas, methods, instructions or products referred to in the content.

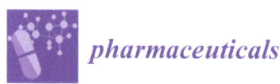 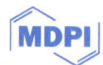

Review

Radiopharmaceuticals for Treatment of Adrenocortical Carcinoma

Kerstin Michalski [1,*], Wiebke Schlötelburg [1], Philipp E. Hartrampf [1], Aleksander Kosmala [1], Andreas K. Buck [1], Stefanie Hahner [2] and Andreas Schirbel [1]

1. Department of Nuclear Medicine, Würzburg University Hospital, University of Würzburg, Oberdürrbacher Straße 6, D-97080 Würzburg, Germany; buck_a@ukw.de (A.K.B.); schirbel_a@ukw.de (A.S.)
2. Division of Endocrinology and Diabetes, Department of Medicine I, Würzburg University Hospital, University of Würzburg, Oberdürrbacher Straße 6, D-97080 Würzburg, Germany; hahner_s@ukw.de
* Correspondence: michalski_k@ukw.de

Abstract: Adrenocortical carcinoma (ACC) represents a rare tumor entity with limited treatment options and usually rapid tumor progression in case of metastatic disease. As further treatment options are needed and ACC metastases are sensitive to external beam radiation, novel theranostic approaches could complement established therapeutic concepts. Recent developments focus on targeting adrenal cortex-specific enzymes like the theranostic twin [$^{123/131}$I]IMAZA that shows a good image quality and a promising therapeutic effect in selected patients. But other established molecular targets in nuclear medicine such as the C-X-C motif chemokine receptor 4 (CXCR4) could possibly enhance the therapeutic regimen as well in a subgroup of patients. The aims of this review are to give an overview of innovative radiopharmaceuticals for the treatment of ACC and to present the different molecular targets, as well as to show future perspectives for further developments since a radiopharmaceutical with a broad application range is still warranted.

Keywords: adrenocortical carcinoma; theranostics; endoradiotherapy; IMAZA

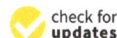

Citation: Michalski, K.; Schlötelburg, W.; Hartrampf, P.E.; Kosmala, A.; Buck, A.K.; Hahner, S.; Schirbel, A. Radiopharmaceuticals for Treatment of Adrenocortical Carcinoma. *Pharmaceuticals* **2024**, *17*, 25. https://doi.org/10.3390/ph17010025

Academic Editor: Gerald Reischl

Received: 14 November 2023
Revised: 20 December 2023
Accepted: 21 December 2023
Published: 23 December 2023

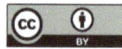

Copyright: © 2023 by the authors. Licensee MDPI, Basel, Switzerland. This article is an open access article distributed under the terms and conditions of the Creative Commons Attribution (CC BY) license (https://creativecommons.org/licenses/by/4.0/).

1. Introduction

Adrenocortical carcinoma (ACC) is a rare tumor entity with an estimated incidence of about 0.5–2 new cases per million people per year [1,2]. ACC occurs at any age and shows a peak incidence between 40 and 60 years, whereby women are more often affected (55–60%) [3]. The tumor arises from the cortex of the adrenal gland and 50–60% of patients with ACC have clinical hormone excess. Treatment options are limited and complete resection is the only means of cure. Still, retrospective studies reported that 40–70% of ACCs eventually recur even after complete resection [4–7]. In general, the prognosis is heterogeneous and the median overall survival of all ACC patients is about 3–4 years. For tumors confined to the adrenal gland five-year survival rates are between 60–80%, for locally advanced disease 35–50%, and much lower in case of metastases with reported survival rates ranging from 0 to 28% [8–14].

Due to the rareness of the disease and the limited resources dedicated to the implementation of new therapeutic options, there is little progress in the medical therapy of ACC [15]. International guidelines recommend to use of adjuvant mitotane in most patients [3,16]. The results of a large phase 3 trial led to a combination treatment of mitotane, etoposide, doxorubicin, and cisplatin as a first-line therapy [11]. Unfortunately, the combination of these chemotherapeutics only led to an objective response rate of 23% with a progression-free survival of only 5.1 months despite severe toxicity. Hence, further therapeutic options for second- and third-line treatment are warranted. ACC used to be considered resistant to radiation [17,18]. However, recent data show a benefit in regards to local tumor control, the palliative treatment of symptomatic cerebral or osseous metastases and in case of vena cava obstruction as well as a reduction of local recurrence after primary resection [19–25]. In this sense, endoradiotherapy is a possible therapeutic option in patients with metastasized ACC after first-line treatment. The concept of endoradiotherapy is based upon theranostic radiopharmaceuticals that can be used for diagnostic and therapeutic purposes, depending on the labeled radionuclide. It is possible to use either the same molecule or a very similar compound. These molecules are radiolabeled with gamma and positron emitters for imaging purposes or beta minus emitters and (rarer) alpha emitters for endoradiotherapy. Some radionuclides, such as iodine-131 and lutetium-177 are beta and gamma emitters and can be used for both imaging and therapy, whereas the gamma emitter iodine-123 can be used only for diagnostics [26]. Other radionuclides for imaging are fluorine-18 or gallium-68 (both positron emitters) and Yttrium-90 (beta minus emitter) for therapy. The use of an image-based patient selection allows for a personalized medicine approach with a possible higher therapeutic efficacy. Furthermore, reduced side effects and high tumor doses can be administered because of the precise radiation deposition and the short tissue penetration of only a few millimeters of beta minus emitters [27].

The present review aims to give an overview of theranostic radiopharmaceuticals for the treatment of ACC, to present various molecular targets and to show future perspectives.

2. Molecular Imaging and Theranostic Approaches in ACC

For molecular imaging of ACC, positron emission tomography (PET)/computed tomography (CT) with [^{18}F]fluorodeoxyglucose (FDG) can be used [28] but is not considered standard of care [3], in contrast to CT or magnetic resonance imaging. Nevertheless, FDG PET/CT is useful for prognostic evaluation as a higher uptake is associated with a shorter survival [29,30]. However, FDG does not provide a theranostic approach. For a detailed description of molecular imaging approaches in ACC, please refer to a recent review of adrenal imaging [31].

Peptide receptor radionuclide therapy targeting the somatostatin receptor (SSTR) using, i.e., [^{177}Lu]Lu-DOTA-0-Tyr3-Octreotate (DOTATATE) is established in the treatment of well-differentiated neuroendocrine midgut tumors [32] and other neuroendocrine tumors [33]. A recent ex vivo study described a heterogeneous SSTR expression in some ACC tissue samples [34]. However, to date, only one study exists that reports the results of a case series of 19 patients with 2 patients receiving either [^{90}Y]Y- or [^{177}Lu]Lu-DOTATOC (DOTA(0)-Phe(1)-Tyr(3))octreotid), which resulted in disease control of 4 and 12 months, respectively [35].

In analogy, endoradiotherapy targeting the prostate-specific membrane antigen (PSMA) is not just a treatment option for metastasized castration-resistant prostate cancer using, i.e., [^{177}Lu]Lu-vipivotide tetraxetan (PSMA-617) [36], but also for other tumor entities. In an ex vivo analysis, PSMA was significantly overexpressed in ACC tissue samples compared to normal adrenal glands and adrenocortical adenomas [37]. To our knowledge, there is no report providing data on PSMA radioligand therapy in ACC. Only one case report describes a patient with ACC having a PSMA expression in tumor sites equal to physiological liver background on [^{68}Ga]Ga-PSMA-11 PET/CT, which was not considered sufficient for PSMA-directed radioligand therapy [38].

C-X-C motif chemokine receptor 4 (CXCR4) is a G-protein coupled receptor that can be found in many hematological malignancies as well as solid tumors and constitutes a possible theranostic target [39]. CXCR4 expression can be found in ACC samples as well [40]. A strong membranous expression of CXCR4 in ACC specimens was found in half of the cases (94 of 187 specimens) in an ex vivo study. Interestingly, immunohistochemical staining of CXCR4 was higher in samples derived from metastases than from primary tumors [41]. A high in vivo CXCR4 expression on CXCR4-directed PET/CT was found in 30 patients with ACC [42]. A possible theranostic application was found by Bluemel et al., who rated 17 (57%) of 30 patients as suitable and 4 patients (13%) as potentially suitable for CXCR4-directed treatment [43]. Of note, CXCR4-directed therapy using, i.e., [^{177}Lu]Lu-/[^{90}Y]Y-anditixafortide (PentixaTher) leads to bone marrow ablation and can only be applied in case of available hematopoietic stem cells which are usually harvested during previous chemotherapeutic protocols [44].

The enzymes CYP11B1 (11β-hydroxylase) and CYP11B2 (aldosterone synthase) are part of the cortisol and aldosterone synthesis in the adrenal gland and can be blocked by imidazole drugs such as etomidate or ketoconazole [45]. As these enzymes are highly specific for the adrenal gland, they are potential targets for molecular imaging [46]. Bergström et al. developed the PET imaging agent [^{11}C]etomidate and its methyl ester [^{11}C]metomidate ([^{11}C]MTO) and showed their potential to specifically visualize the normal adrenal cortex in an animal study [47]. This approach was transferred to a clinical setting and the authors could demonstrate that [^{11}C]MTO PET can distinguish between lesions of adrenocortical and nonadrenocortical origin in a cohort of 15 patients [48], and in another cohort of 173 patients [49]. The latter study included 13 patients with ACC which showed a relatively high tracer uptake.

In order to develop a possible theranostic radiopharmaceutical, the compound [^{123}I]iodometomidate ([^{123}I]IMTO) that inhibits CYP11B1/2 was developed. High imaging quality was shown in animal studies [50–52] and a high and specific tracer uptake of the radiopharmaceutical was found for adrenocortical tissue [51]. These promising results could be transferred into clinical application: [^{123}I]IMTO planar whole-body scans and single photon emission computed tomography (SPECT)/CT images showed high sensitivity and specificity for the differentiation of adrenocortical tumors from lesions of non-adrenocortical origin in case of a lesion size of 2 cm or more [53]. The theranostic counterpart of [^{123}I]IMTO is [^{131}I]IMTO, which can be used in patients with advanced ACC. Disease control was achieved in 6 of 11 patients with ACC treated with [^{131}I]IMTO with a median progression-free survival of 14 months (range 5–33 months) in responders. Of these, 5 patients showed a stable disease on follow-up CT scans, and a partial response was found in one patient [54]. As IMTO shows a rapid metabolic inactivation, the metabolically more stable derivative (R)-1-[1-(4-iodophenyl)ethyl]-1H-imidazole-5-carboxylic acid azetidinyl amide (IMAZA) was developed by replacing the methyl ester in IMTO by a carboxylic amide. IMAZA outperformed IMTO in regards to pharmacokinetic and imaging properties in mice and in a dual tracer approach in three patients [55]. Hahner et al. screened 69 patients with advanced ACC refractory to standard treatments using [^{123}I]IMAZA SPECT/CT and identified 13 patients with intense uptake in all tumor lesions [56]. These patients were treated with a median of 25.7 GBq [^{131}I]IMAZA (range 18.1–30.7 GBq). Response to therapy was assessed according to Response Evaluation Criteria in Solid Tumors (RECIST version 1.1) [57]. Two patients experienced a decrease in RECIST target lesions of up to 26%. A median progression-free survival of 14.3 months (range 8.3–21.9) was noted for five patients with stable disease. Median overall survival in all 13 patients was 14.1 months (4.0–56.5). The treatment was well tolerated by the patients, and no severe toxicities (CTCAE grade $\geq$ 3) were noted. Figure 1 shows a patient who underwent [^{131}I]IMAZA therapy. Figure 2 summarizes the different theranostic targets in ACC and Figure 3 shows the corresponding radiopharmaceuticals.

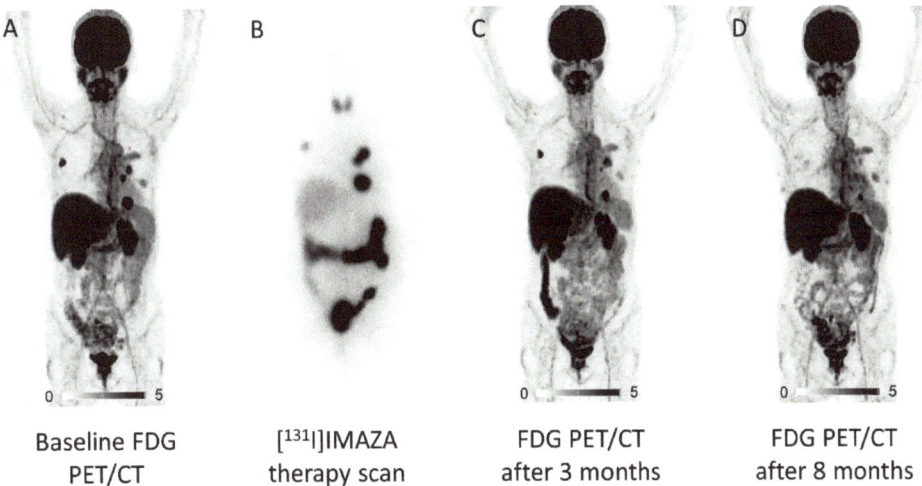

Figure 1. [^{131}I]IMAZA therapy in a 53-year-old patient with metastatic adrenocortical cancer. FDG PET maximum intensity projection (MIP) is shown at baseline (**A**). Post-therapeutic whole-body scintigraphy 2 days after first therapy (**B**) shows concordant tracer accumulation to FDG PET/CT. Response assessment after 3 and 8 months (**C**,**D**) shows a significant decrease in metabolic activity and a reduction in the diameter of the target lesion of 26%. After a progression-free survival of 18 months, a second therapy with [^{131}I]IMAZA was applied. The patient died after an overall survival of 56 months after the first [^{131}I]IMAZA therapy.

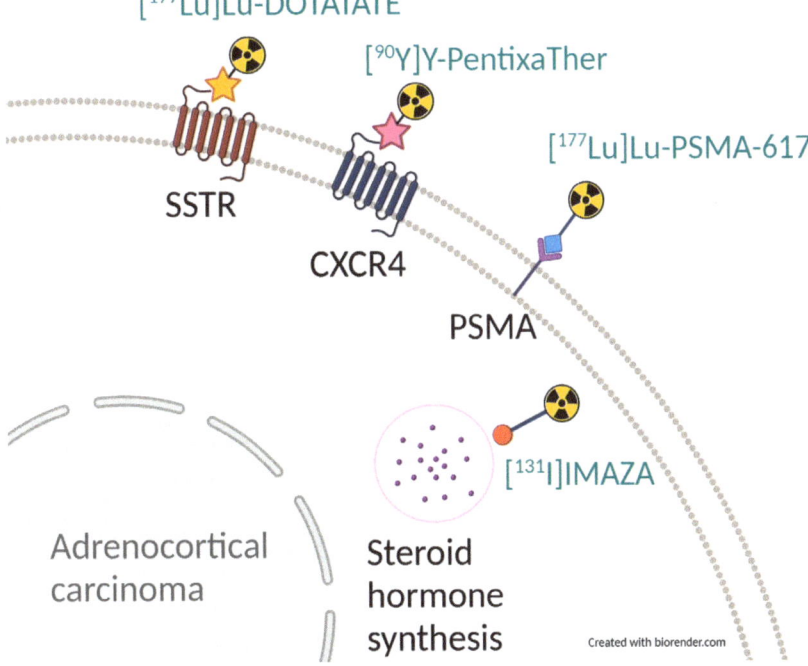

Figure 2. Schematic depiction of possible theranostic targets in adrenocortical carcinoma (black font) and the respective therapeutic radiopharmaceuticals (exemplary, blue font).

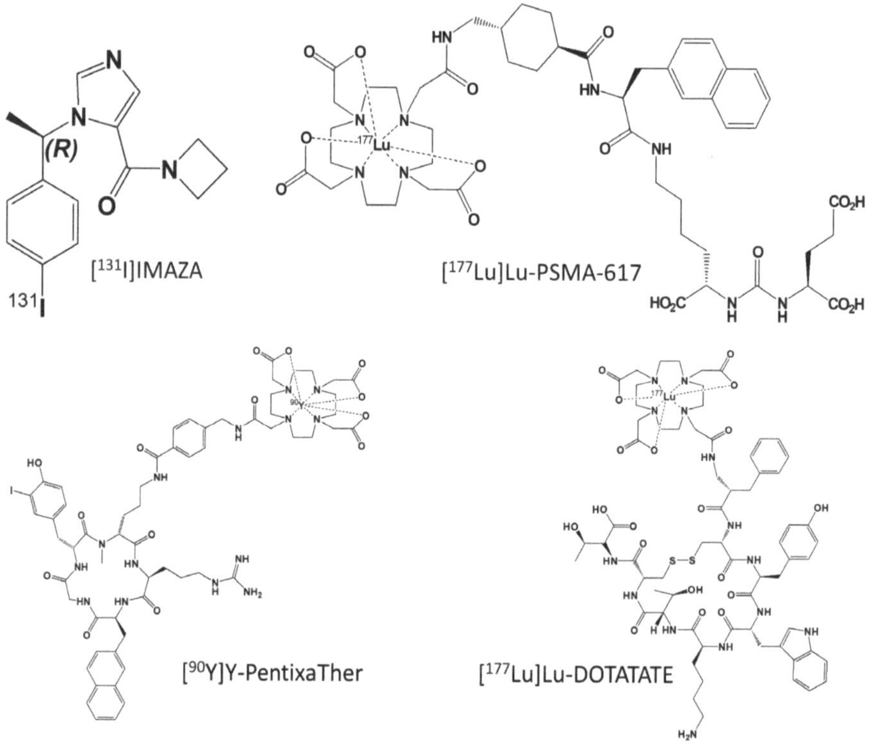

Figure 3. Chemical structure of possible theranostic radiopharmaceuticals for treatment of ACC. To date, [^{131}I]IMAZA is the only compound that has been already used in patients.

3. Radiosynthesis of [^{131}I]IMAZA

The radiosynthesis and quality control of [$^{123/131}$I]IMAZA for scintigraphy, dosimetry and therapy has already been published [55]. Here, destannylation reactions were used for labeling. Since this method yields the labeled products under very mild reaction conditions and with very high radiochemical yields, this method is frequently used and should be easily established in radiochemical laboratories that have experience with radioiodination. However, this does not apply to radioiodinations with > 30 GBq I-131, which are challenging in terms of radiation protection due to the high volatility of radioiodine in combination with the extremely high activity levels and the relatively high gamma energy of 364 keV. Therefore, labeling of [^{131}I]IMAZA for endoradiotherapy had to be performed by an automated synthesis module (custom-made by Scintomics GmbH, Fürstenfeldbruck, Germany) inside a well-ventilated lead cell (see Figure 4).

To the delivery vial in which the [^{131}I]iodide is dissolved in 1 mL 0.01 N NaOH (IBSSO; GE Healthcare, Braunschweig, Germany) were consecutively injected 5 mg trimethylstannylazetidinylamide in 1 mL ethanol, 120 µL 2 N hydrochloric acid and 2.25 mg chloramine T trihydrate in 150 µL water. The reaction solution was allowed to stand for three minutes. Thereafter, the reaction was quenched by adding 135 µL 2 N HCl and a solution of 4.50 mg $Na_2S_2O_5$ in 150 µL water and the mixture was injected directly into the injection valve of the semi-preparative high-performance liquid chromatography system (HPLC) equipped with a RP-18 HPLC column (250 × 8 mm). An ethanol/phosphate buffer (40/60 v/v) mixture served as the HPLC solvent with a flow of 2.0 mL/min. Using typical starting activities of 34 GBq [^{131}I]iodide, reproducibly > 25 GBq [^{131}I]IMAZA were obtained, which were administered to the patients after successful quality control.

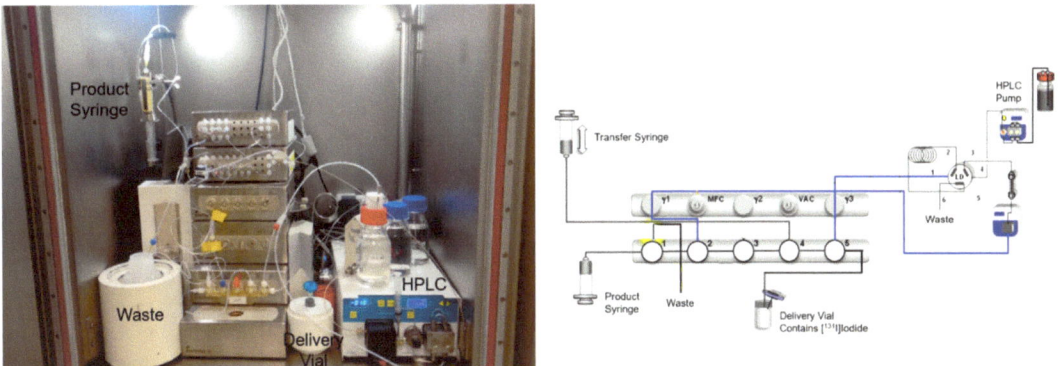

Figure 4. Photo and scheme of module for radiosynthesis of [^{131}I]IMAZA.

For each radiosynthesis, the exhaust air from the lead box was passed through activated carbon filters and checked for possible contamination. The personnel involved were monitored by means of personal dosimeters, finger ring dosimeters and a thyroid monitor. In all cases, only very low levels of contamination were detectable, so that the high-dose endoradiotherapies with [^{131}I]IMAZA could be carried out safely. Regarding the radiosynthesis of the commercially available products [^{177}Lu]Lu-DOTATATE, [^{177}Lu]Lu-/[^{90}Y]Y-PentixaTher and [^{177}Lu]Lu-PSMA-617, please refer to the respective publications [58–61].

4. Future Perspectives

The investigations of patients with metastatic ACC with [^{123}I]IMAZA showed an uptake in all known lesions (metastases and/or primary tumor) in only about 40% of the patients. This is likely due to dedifferentiation of the tumor cells resulting in low or no expression of the target enzymes CYP11B1 and CYP11B2. Therefore, only a minority of patients with high tracer uptake are candidates for subsequent endoradiotherapy with the analog [^{131}I]IMAZA. Currently, alternative enzymatic and non-enzymatic targets with broader expression in ACC tissue are under investigation.

5. Summary

Adrenocortical carcinoma is a rare tumor entity and further therapeutic options in metastatic disease are desperately warranted. Several possible theranostic approaches exist, of which radiopharmaceuticals targeting specific enzymes of the adrenal cortex are currently the most promising and are the only theranostic radiopharmaceuticals ever used in patients to date. The theranostic twin [$^{123/131}$I]IMAZA has shown good image quality and a good therapeutic effect in selected patients with advanced ACC, but cannot be used in all patients with ACC. Therefore, future developments are needed in order to provide a radiopharmaceutical with broader applications.

Funding: This work was supported by the Bavarian Cancer Research Center (personal grant to K.M.) and by the Interdisciplinary Center of Clinical Research (IZKF), University Hospital of Wuerzburg (grant Z-2/91 to W.S.).

Data Availability Statement: Data sharing is not applicable.

Conflicts of Interest: K.M. has received speaker honoraria from Novartis. All other authors declare no conflicts of interest.

References

1. Kerkhofs, T.M.A.; Verhoeven, R.H.A.; Van der Zwan, J.M.; Dieleman, J.; Kerstens, M.N.; Links, T.P.; Van de Poll-Franse, L.V.; Haak, H.R. Adrenocortical carcinoma: A population-based study on incidence and survival in the Netherlands since 1993. *Eur. J. Cancer* **2013**, *49*, 2579–2586. [CrossRef] [PubMed]
2. Kebebew, E.; Reiff, E.; Duh, Q.Y.; Clark, O.H.; McMillan, A. Extent of disease at presentation and outcome for adrenocortical carcinoma: Have we made progress? *World J. Surg.* **2006**, *30*, 872–878. [CrossRef] [PubMed]
3. Fassnacht, M.; Dekkers, O.M.; Else, T.; Baudin, E.; Berruti, A.; de Krijger, R.; Haak, H.R.; Mihai, R.; Assie, G.; Terzolo, M. European Society of Endocrinology Clinical Practice Guidelines on the management of adrenocortical carcinoma in adults, in collaboration with the European Network for the Study of Adrenal Tumors. *Eur. J. Endocrinol.* **2018**, *179*, G1–G46. [CrossRef] [PubMed]
4. Beuschlein, F.; Weigel, J.; Saeger, W.; Kroiss, M.; Wild, V.; Daffara, F.; Libe, R.; Ardito, A.; Al Ghuzlan, A.; Quinkler, M.; et al. Major prognostic role of Ki67 in localized adrenocortical carcinoma after complete resection. *J. Clin. Endocrinol. Metab.* **2015**, *100*, 841–849. [CrossRef] [PubMed]
5. Glenn, J.A.; Else, T.; Hughes, D.T.; Cohen, M.S.; Jolly, S.; Giordano, T.J.; Worden, F.P.; Gauger, P.G.; Hammer, G.D.; Miller, B.S. Longitudinal patterns of recurrence in patients with adrenocortical carcinoma. *Surgery* **2019**, *165*, 186–195. [CrossRef] [PubMed]
6. Liang, J.; Liu, Z.; Zhou, L.; Tang, Y.; Zhou, C.; Wu, K.; Zhang, F.; Zhang, F.; Wei, X.; Lu, Y.; et al. The clinical utility of 'GRAS' parameters in stage I-III adrenocortical carcinomas: Long-term data from a high-volume institution. *Endocrine* **2020**, *67*, 449–456. [CrossRef] [PubMed]
7. Elhassan, Y.S.; Altieri, B.; Berhane, S.; Cosentini, D.; Calabrese, A.; Haissaguerre, M.; Kastelan, D.; Fragoso, M.; Bertherat, J.; Al Ghuzlan, A.; et al. S-GRAS score for prognostic classification of adrenocortical carcinoma: An international, multicenter ENSAT study. *Eur. J. Endocrinol.* **2021**, *186*, 25–36. [CrossRef] [PubMed]
8. Fassnacht, M.; Libe, R.; Kroiss, M.; Allolio, B. Adrenocortical carcinoma: A clinician's update. *Nat. Rev. Endocrinol.* **2011**, *7*, 323–335. [CrossRef]
9. Fassnacht, M.; Johanssen, S.; Fenske, W.; Weismann, D.; Agha, A.; Beuschlein, F.; Fuhrer, D.; Jurowich, C.; Quinkler, M.; Petersenn, S.; et al. Improved Survival in Patients with Stage II Adrenocortical Carcinoma Followed Up Prospectively by Specialized Centers. *J. Clin. Endocr. Metab.* **2010**, *95*, 4925–4932. [CrossRef]
10. Fassnacht, M.; Johanssen, S.; Quinkler, M.; Bucsky, P.; Willenberg, H.S.; Beuschlein, F.; Terzolo, M.; Mueller, H.H.; Hahner, S.; Allolio, B.; et al. Limited Prognostic Value of the 2004 International Union Against Cancer Staging Classification for Adrenocortical Carcinomas. *Cancer* **2009**, *115*, 243–250. [CrossRef]
11. Fassnacht, M.; Terzolo, M.; Allolio, B.; Baudin, E.; Haak, H.; Berruti, A.; Welin, S.; Schade-Brittinger, C.; Lacroix, A.; Jarzab, B.; et al. Combination chemotherapy in advanced adrenocortical carcinoma. *N. Engl. J. Med.* **2012**, *366*, 2189–2197. [CrossRef] [PubMed]
12. Sturgeon, C.; Shen, W.T.; Clark, O.H.; Duh, Q.Y.; Kebebew, E. Risk assessment in 457 adrenal cortical carcinomas: How much does tumor size predict the likelihood of malignancy? *J. Am. Coll. Surg.* **2006**, *202*, 423–430. [CrossRef]
13. Bilimoria, K.Y.; Shen, W.T.; Elaraj, D.; Bentrem, D.J.; Winchester, D.J.; Kebebew, E.; Sturgeon, C. Adrenocortical carcinoma in the United States: Treatment utilization and prognostic factors. *Cancer* **2008**, *113*, 3130–3136. [CrossRef] [PubMed]
14. Kerkhofs, T.M.; Ettaieb, M.H.; Hermsen, I.G.; Haak, H.R. Developing treatment for adrenocortical carcinoma. *Endocr. Relat. Cancer* **2015**, *22*, R325–R338. [CrossRef] [PubMed]
15. Terzolo, M.; Fassnacht, M. Our experience with the management of patients with non-metastatic adrenocortical carcinoma. *Eur. J. Endocrinol.* **2022**, *187*, R27–R40. [CrossRef] [PubMed]
16. Fassnacht, M.; Assie, G.; Baudin, E.; Eisenhofer, G.; de la Fouchardiere, C.; Haak, H.R.; de Krijger, R.; Porpiglia, F.; Terzolo, M.; Berruti, A.; et al. Adrenocortical carcinomas and malignant phaeochromocytomas: ESMO-EURACAN Clinical Practice Guidelines for diagnosis, treatment and follow-up. *Ann. Oncol.* **2020**, *31*, 1476–1490. [CrossRef] [PubMed]
17. Hutter, A.M., Jr.; Kayhoe, D.E. Adrenal cortical carcinoma. Clinical features of 138 patients. *Am. J. Med.* **1966**, *41*, 572–580. [CrossRef] [PubMed]
18. Hajjar, R.A.; Hickey, R.C.; Samaan, N.A. Adrenal cortical carcinoma. A study of 32 patients. *Cancer* **1975**, *35*, 549–554. [CrossRef]
19. Polat, B.; Fassnacht, M.; Pfreundner, L.; Guckenberger, M.; Bratengeier, K.; Johanssen, S.; Kenn, W.; Hahner, S.; Allolio, B.; Flentje, M. Radiotherapy in adrenocortical carcinoma. *Cancer* **2009**, *115*, 2816–2823. [CrossRef]
20. Hermsen, I.G.; Groenen, Y.E.; Dercksen, M.W.; Theuws, J.; Haak, H.R. Response to radiation therapy in adrenocortical carcinoma. *J. Endocrinol. Investig.* **2010**, *33*, 712–714. [CrossRef]
21. Ho, J.; Turkbey, B.; Edgerly, M.; Alimchandani, M.; Quezado, M.; Camphausen, K.; Fojo, T.; Kaushal, A. Role of radiotherapy in adrenocortical carcinoma. *Cancer J.* **2013**, *19*, 288–294. [CrossRef] [PubMed]
22. Fassnacht, M.; Hahner, S.; Polat, B.; Koschker, A.C.; Kenn, W.; Flentje, M.; Allolio, B. Efficacy of adjuvant radiotherapy of the tumor bed on local recurrence of adrenocortical carcinoma. *J. Clin. Endocrinol. Metab.* **2006**, *91*, 4501–4504. [CrossRef] [PubMed]
23. Sabolch, A.; Feng, M.; Griffith, K.; Hammer, G.; Doherty, G.; Ben-Josef, E. Adjuvant and definitive radiotherapy for adrenocortical carcinoma. *Int. J. Radiat. Oncol. Biol. Phys.* **2011**, *80*, 1477–1484. [CrossRef] [PubMed]
24. Zhu, J.; Zheng, Z.; Shen, J.; Lian, X.; Miao, Z.; Shen, J.; Zhang, F. Efficacy of adjuvant radiotherapy for treatment of adrenocortical carcinoma: A retrospective study and an updated meta-analysis. *Radiat. Oncol.* **2020**, *15*, 118. [CrossRef] [PubMed]
25. Gharzai, L.A.; Green, M.D.; Griffith, K.A.; Else, T.; Mayo, C.S.; Hesseltine, E.; Spratt, D.E.; Ben-Josef, E.; Sabolch, A.; Miller, B.S.; et al. Adjuvant Radiation Improves Recurrence-Free Survival and Overall Survival in Adrenocortical Carcinoma. *J. Clin. Endocrinol. Metab.* **2019**, *104*, 3743–3750. [CrossRef] [PubMed]

26. Yordanova, A.; Eppard, E.; Kurpig, S.; Bundschuh, R.A.; Schonberger, S.; Gonzalez-Carmona, M.; Feldmann, G.; Ahmadzadehfar, H.; Essler, M. Theranostics in nuclear medicine practice. *Onco Targets Ther.* **2017**, *10*, 4821–4828. [CrossRef] [PubMed]
27. Kramer-Marek, G.; Capala, J. The role of nuclear medicine in modern therapy of cancer. *Tumour Biol.* **2012**, *33*, 629–640. [CrossRef]
28. Han, S.J.; Kim, T.S.; Jeon, S.W.; Jeong, S.J.; Yun, M.; Rhee, Y.; Kang, E.S.; Cha, B.S.; Lee, E.J.; Lee, H.C.; et al. Analysis of adrenal masses by F-18-FDG positron emission tomography scanning. *Int. J. Clin. Pr.* **2007**, *61*, 802–809. [CrossRef]
29. Leboulleux, S.; Dromain, C.; Bonniaud, G.; Auperin, A.; Caillou, B.; Lumbroso, J.; Sigal, R.; Baudin, E.; Schlumberger, M. Diagnostic and prognostic value of 18-fluorodeoxyglucose positron emission tomography in adrenocortical carcinoma: A prospective comparison with computed tomography. *J. Clin. Endocr. Metab.* **2006**, *91*, 920–925. [CrossRef]
30. Wrenn, S.M.; Moore, A.L.; Shah, H.J.; Barletta, J.A.; Vaidya, A.; Kilbridge, K.L.; Doherty, G.M.; Jacene, H.A.; Nehs, M.A. Higher SUVmax on FDG-PET is associated with shorter survival in adrenocortical carcinoma. *Am. J. Surg.* **2023**, *225*, 309–314. [CrossRef]
31. Werner, R.A.; Hartrampf, P.E.; Schirbel, A.; Hahner, S. Adrenal functional imaging—Which marker for which indication? *Curr. Opin. Urol.* **2022**, *32*, 585–593. [CrossRef] [PubMed]
32. Strosberg, J.; El-Haddad, G.; Wolin, E.; Hendifar, A.; Yao, J.; Chasen, B.; Mittra, E.; Kunz, P.L.; Kulke, M.H.; Jacene, H.; et al. Phase 3 Trial of (177)Lu-Dotatate for Midgut Neuroendocrine Tumors. *N. Engl. J. Med.* **2017**, *376*, 125–135. [CrossRef] [PubMed]
33. Camus, B.; Cottereau, A.S.; Palmieri, L.J.; Dermine, S.; Tenenbaum, F.; Brezault, C.; Coriat, R. Indications of Peptide Receptor Radionuclide Therapy (PRRT) in Gastroenteropancreatic and Pulmonary Neuroendocrine Tumors: An Updated Review. *J. Clin. Med.* **2021**, *10*, 1267. [CrossRef] [PubMed]
34. Germano, A.; Rapa, I.; Duregon, E.; Votta, A.; Giorcelli, J.; Buttigliero, C.; Scagliotti, G.V.; Volante, M.; Terzolo, M.; Papotti, M. Tissue Expression and Pharmacological In Vitro Analyses of mTOR and SSTR Pathways in Adrenocortical Carcinoma. *Endocr. Pathol.* **2017**, *28*, 95–102. [CrossRef] [PubMed]
35. Grisanti, S.; Filice, A.; Basile, V.; Cosentini, D.; Rapa, I.; Albano, D.; Morandi, A.; Lagana, M.; Dalla Volta, A.; Bertagna, F.; et al. Treatment With Y-90/Lu-177-DOTATOC in Patients with Metastatic Adrenocortical Carcinoma Expressing Somatostatin Receptors. *J. Clin. Endocr. Metab.* **2020**, *105*, E1–E5. [CrossRef] [PubMed]
36. Sartor, O.; de Bono, J.; Chi, K.N.; Fizazi, K.; Herrmann, K.; Rahbar, K.; Tagawa, S.T.; Nordquist, L.T.; Vaishampayan, N.; El-Haddad, G.; et al. Lutetium-177-PSMA-617 for Metastatic Castration-Resistant Prostate Cancer. *N. Engl. J. Med.* **2021**, *385*, 1091–1103. [CrossRef] [PubMed]
37. Crowley, M.J.; Scognamiglio, T.; Liu, Y.F.; Kleiman, D.A.; Beninato, T.; Aronova, A.; Liu, H.; Jhanwar, Y.S.; Molina, A.; Tagawa, S.T.; et al. Prostate-Specific Membrane Antigen Is a Potential Antiangiogenic Target in Adrenocortical Carcinoma. *J. Clin. Endocrinol. Metab.* **2016**, *101*, 981–987. [CrossRef]
38. Arora, S.; Damle, N.A.; Aggarwal, S.; Passah, A.; Behera, A.; Arora, G.; Bal, C.; Tripathi, M. Prostate-Specific Membrane Antigen Expression in Adrenocortical Carcinoma on 68Ga-Prostate-Specific Membrane Antigen PET/CT. *Clin. Nucl. Med.* **2018**, *43*, 449–451. [CrossRef] [PubMed]
39. Chatterjee, S.; Behnam Azad, B.; Nimmagadda, S. The intricate role of CXCR4 in cancer. *Adv. Cancer Res.* **2014**, *124*, 31–82. [CrossRef]
40. Weiss, I.D.; Huff, L.M.; Evbuomwan, M.O.; Xu, X.; Dang, H.D.; Velez, D.S.; Singh, S.P.; Zhang, H.W.H.; Gardina, P.J.; Lee, J.H.; et al. Screening of cancer tissue arrays identifies CXCR4 on adrenocortical carcinoma: Correlates with expression and quantification on metastases using Cu-64-plerixafor PET. *Oncotarget* **2017**, *8*, 73387–73406. [CrossRef]
41. Chifu, I.; Heinze, B.; Fuss, C.T.; Lang, K.; Kroiss, M.; Kircher, S.; Ronchi, C.L.; Altieri, B.; Schirbel, A.; Fassnacht, M.; et al. Impact of the Chemokine Receptors CXCR4 and CXCR7 on Clinical Outcome in Adrenocortical Carcinoma. *Front. Endocrinol.* **2020**, *11*, 597878. [CrossRef]
42. Buck, A.K.; Haug, A.; Dreher, N.; Lambertini, A.; Higuchi, T.; Lapa, C.; Weich, A.; Pomper, M.G.; Wester, H.J.; Zehndner, A.; et al. Imaging of C-X-C Motif Chemokine Receptor 4 Expression in 690 Patients with Solid or Hematologic Neoplasms Using (68)Ga-Pentixafor PET. *J. Nucl. Med.* **2022**, *63*, 1687–1692. [CrossRef] [PubMed]
43. Bluemel, C.; Hahner, S.; Heinze, B.; Fassnacht, M.; Kroiss, M.; Bley, T.A.; Wester, H.J.; Kropf, S.; Lapa, C.; Schirbel, A.; et al. Investigating the Chemokine Receptor 4 as Potential Theranostic Target in Adrenocortical Cancer Patients. *Clin. Nucl. Med.* **2017**, *42*, E29–E34. [CrossRef] [PubMed]
44. Buck, A.K.; Serfling, S.E.; Lindner, T.; Hanscheid, H.; Schirbel, A.; Hahner, S.; Fassnacht, M.; Einsele, H.; Werner, R.A. CXCR4-targeted theranostics in oncology. *Eur. J. Nucl. Med. Mol. Imaging* **2022**, *49*, 4133–4144. [CrossRef] [PubMed]
45. Weber, M.M.; Lang, J.; Abedinpour, F.; Zeilberger, K.; Adelmann, B.; Engelhardt, D. Different Inhibitory Effect of Etomidate and Ketoconazole on the Human Adrenal-Steroid Biosynthesis. *Clin. Investig.* **1993**, *71*, 933–938. [CrossRef] [PubMed]
46. Damani, L.A.; Mitterhauser, M.; Zolle, I.; Lin, G.; Oehler, E.; Ho, Y.P. Metabolic and Pharmacokinetic Considerations in the Design of 2-Phenyl Substituted Metyrapone Derivatives—2-Methoxyphenylmetyrapone as a Radioligand for Functional Diagnosis of Adrenal Pathology. *Nucl. Med. Biol.* **1995**, *22*, 1067–1074. [CrossRef] [PubMed]
47. Bergstrom, M.; Bonasera, T.A.; Lu, L.; Bergstrom, E.; Backlin, C.; Juhlin, C.; Langstrom, B. In vitro and in vivo primate evaluation of carbon-11-etomidate and carbon-11-metomidate as potential tracers for PET imaging of the adrenal cortex and its tumors. *J. Nucl. Med.* **1998**, *39*, 982–989. [PubMed]
48. Bergstrom, M.; Juhlin, C.; Bonasera, T.A.; Sundin, A.; Rastad, J.; Akerstrom, G.; Langstrom, B. PET imaging of adrenal cortical tumors with the 11beta-hydroxylase tracer 11C-metomidate. *J. Nucl. Med.* **2000**, *41*, 275–282. [PubMed]

49. Hennings, J.; Lindhe, O.; Bergstrom, M.; Langstrom, B.; Sundin, A.; Hellman, P. [(11)C]metomidate positron emission tomography of adrenocortical tumors in correlation with histopathological findings. *J. Clin. Endocr. Metab.* **2006**, *91*, 1410–1414. [CrossRef]
50. Schirbel, A.; Zolle, I.; Hammerschmidt, F.; Berger, M.L.; Schiller, D.; Kvaternik, H.; Reiners, C. [I-123/131]Iodometomidate as a radioligand for functional diagnosis of adrenal disease: Synthesis, structural requirements and biodistribution. *Radiochim. Acta* **2004**, *92*, 297–303. [CrossRef]
51. Hahner, S.; Stuermer, A.; Kreissl, M.; Reiners, C.; Fassnacht, M.; Haenscheid, H.; Beuschlein, F.; Zink, M.; Lang, K.; Allolio, B.; et al. [^{123}I]Iodometomidate for molecular imaging of adrenocortical cytochrome P450 family 11B enzymes. *J. Clin. Endocrinol. Metab.* **2008**, *93*, 2358–2365. [CrossRef] [PubMed]
52. Zolle, I.M.; Berger, M.L.; Hammerschmidt, F.; Hahner, S.; Schirbel, A.; Peric-Simov, B. New Selective Inhibitors of Steroid 11 beta-Hydroxylation in the Adrenal Cortex. Synthesis and Structure-Activity Relationship of Potent Etomidate Analogues (vol 51, pg 2244, 2008). *J. Med. Chem.* **2008**, *51*, 7652. [CrossRef]
53. Hahner, S.; Kreissl, M.C.; Fassnacht, M.; Haenscheid, H.; Bock, S.; Verburg, F.A.; Knoedler, P.; Lang, K.; Reiners, C.; Buck, A.K.; et al. Functional Characterization of Adrenal Lesions Using [I-123] IMTO-SPECT/CT. *J. Clin. Endocr. Metab.* **2013**, *98*, 1508–1518. [CrossRef] [PubMed]
54. Hahner, S.; Kreissl, M.C.; Fassnacht, M.; Haenscheid, H.; Knoedler, P.; Lang, K.; Buck, A.K.; Reiners, C.; Allolio, B.; Schirbel, A. [I-131]Iodometomidate for Targeted Radionuclide Therapy of Advanced Adrenocortical Carcinoma. *J. Clin. Endocr. Metab.* **2012**, *97*, 914–922. [CrossRef] [PubMed]
55. Heinze, B.; Schirbel, A.; Nannen, L.; Michelmann, D.; Hartrampf, P.E.; Bluemel, C.; Schneider, M.; Herrmann, K.; Haenscheid, H.; Fassnacht, M.; et al. Novel CYP11B-ligand [I-123/131]IMAZA as promising theranostic tool for adrenocortical tumors: Comprehensive preclinical characterization and first clinical experience. *Eur. J. Nucl. Med. Mol. I* **2021**, *49*, 301–310. [CrossRef] [PubMed]
56. Hahner, S.; Hartrampf, P.E.; Mihatsch, P.W.; Nauerz, M.; Heinze, B.; Hanscheid, H.; Fuss, C.T.; Werner, R.A.; Pamporaki, C.; Kroiss, M.; et al. Targeting 11-Beta Hydroxylase With [I-131]IMAZA: A Novel Approach for the Treatment of Advanced Adrenocortical Carcinoma. *J. Clin. Endocr. Metab.* **2022**, *107*, E1348–E1355. [CrossRef] [PubMed]
57. Eisenhauer, E.A.; Therasse, P.; Bogaerts, J.; Schwartz, L.H.; Sargent, D.; Ford, R.; Dancey, J.; Arbuck, S.; Gwyther, S.; Mooney, M.; et al. New response evaluation criteria in solid tumours: Revised RECIST guideline (version 1.1). *Eur. J. Cancer* **2009**, *45*, 228–247. [CrossRef]
58. Aslani, A.; Snowdon, G.M.; Bailey, D.L.; Schembri, G.P.; Bailey, E.A.; Pavlakis, N.; Roach, P.J. Lutetium-177 DOTATATE Production with an Automated Radiopharmaceutical Synthesis System. *Asia Ocean. J. Nucl. Med. Biol.* **2015**, *3*, 107–115.
59. Schottelius, M.; Osl, T.; Poschenrieder, A.; Hoffmann, F.; Beykan, S.; Hanscheid, H.; Schirbel, A.; Buck, A.K.; Kropf, S.; Schwaiger, M.; et al. [(177)Lu]pentixather: Comprehensive Preclinical Characterization of a First CXCR4-directed Endoradiotherapeutic Agent. *Theranostics* **2017**, *7*, 2350–2362. [CrossRef]
60. Hanscheid, H.; Schirbel, A.; Hartrampf, P.; Kraus, S.; Werner, R.A.; Einsele, H.; Wester, H.J.; Lassmann, M.; Kortum, M.; Buck, A.K. Biokinetics and Dosimetry of (177)Lu-Pentixather. *J. Nucl. Med.* **2022**, *63*, 754–760. [CrossRef]
61. Wichmann, C.W.; Ackermann, U.; Poniger, S.; Young, K.; Nguyen, B.; Chan, G.; Sachinidis, J.; Scott, A.M. Automated radiosynthesis of [(68) Ga]Ga-PSMA-11 and (177) Lu]Lu-PSMA-617 on the iPHASE MultiSyn module for clinical applications. *J. Label. Comp. Radiopharm.* **2021**, *64*, 140–146. [CrossRef]

Disclaimer/Publisher's Note: The statements, opinions and data contained in all publications are solely those of the individual author(s) and contributor(s) and not of MDPI and/or the editor(s). MDPI and/or the editor(s) disclaim responsibility for any injury to people or property resulting from any ideas, methods, instructions or products referred to in the content.

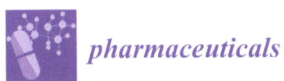

Article

Safety and Efficacy of Selective Internal Radionuclide Therapy with ^{90}Y Glass Microspheres in Patients with Progressive Hepatocellular Carcinoma after the Failure of Repeated Transarterial Chemoembolization

Alexander Bellendorf [1,2,†], Nicolai Mader [3,†], Stefan P. Mueller [1], Samer Ezziddin [4], Andreas Bockisch [1], Hong Grafe [1], Jan Best [5,6], Juliane Goebel [7], Thorsten D. Pöppel [1,8] and Amir Sabet [1,3,*]

1. Department of Nuclear Medicine, University of Duisburg-Essen, Hufelandstr. 55, 45147 Essen, Germany; alexander.bellendorf@ruhrradiologie.de (A.B.); stefan.mueller@uni-due.de (S.P.M.); andreas.bockisch@uk-essen.de (A.B.); hong.grafe@uk-essen.de (H.G.)
2. MVZ Radiologie, Nuklearmedizin und Strahlentherapie Essen GmbH, Rüttenscheider Str. 191, 45131 Essen, Germany
3. Department of Nuclear Medicine, Clinic for Radiology and Nuclear Medicine, University Hospital, Goethe University Frankfurt, Theodor-Stern-Kai 7, 60590 Frankfurt am Main, Germany; n.mader@med.uni-frankfurt.de
4. Department of Nuclear Medicine, Saarland University Medical Center, Kirrberger Straße, 66421 Homburg, Germany; samer.ezziddin@uks.eu
5. Department of Internal Medicine, University Hospital Ruhr-University Bochum, In der Schornau 23-25, 44892 Bochum, Germany; jan.best@kk-bochum.de
6. Department of Internal Medicine, University of Duisburg-Essen, Hufelandstr. 55, 45147 Essen, Germany
7. Department of Diagnostic and Interventional Radiology and Neuroradiology, University of Duisburg-Essen, Hufelandstr. 55, 45147 Essen, Germany; juliane.goebel@uk-essen.de
8. MVZ CDT Strahleninstitut GmbH, Turiner Straße 2, 50668 Cologne, Germany
* Correspondence: sabet@med.uni-frankfurt.de; Tel.: +49-69-63016803
† These authors contributed equally to this work.

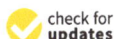

Citation: Bellendorf, A.; Mader, N.; Mueller, S.P.; Ezziddin, S.; Bockisch, A.; Grafe, H.; Best, J.; Goebel, J.; Pöppel, T.D.; Sabet, A. Safety and Efficacy of Selective Internal Radionuclide Therapy with ^{90}Y Glass Microspheres in Patients with Progressive Hepatocellular Carcinoma after the Failure of Repeated Transarterial Chemoembolization. *Pharmaceuticals* **2024**, *17*, 101. https://doi.org/ 10.3390/ph17010101

Academic Editors: Marc Pretze and Jörg Kotzerke

Received: 29 October 2023
Revised: 4 January 2024
Accepted: 8 January 2024
Published: 11 January 2024

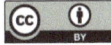

Copyright: © 2024 by the authors. Licensee MDPI, Basel, Switzerland. This article is an open access article distributed under the terms and conditions of the Creative Commons Attribution (CC BY) license (https:// creativecommons.org/licenses/by/ 4.0/).

Abstract: Transarterial chemoembolization (TACE) is currently the standard of care in patients with unresectable hepatocellular carcinoma (HCC), and selective internal radionuclide therapy (SIRT) with ^{90}Y microspheres is mainly used as an alternative modality in patients considered poor candidates for TACE. Treatment with sorafenib is the recommended option for patients with progressive disease after TACE. This study aims to evaluate the safety and efficacy of SIRT with glass microspheres in patients with progressive HCC after repeated TACE who are not eligible for treatment with sorafenib. Forty-seven patients with progressive HCC after a median of three TACE sessions (range 2–14) underwent SIRT (3.5 ± 1.5 GBq; liver target dose 110–120 Gy). Toxicity was recorded 4 and 12 weeks after treatment and reported according to the Common Terminology Criteria for Adverse Events Version 5.0. Treatment response was assessed three months after SIRT using multiphase computed tomography and modified criteria in solid tumors (mRECIST). Survival analyses were performed using Kaplan–Meier curves and a Cox proportional hazards model for uni- and multivariate analyses. Significant but reversible hepatotoxicity (≥grade 3) occurred in five patients (11%). No radioembolization-induced liver disease (REILD) was observed. The number of previous TACE sessions and cumulative administered activity did not predict the incidence of post-SIRT significant hepatotoxicity. Treatment responses consisted of partial responses in 26 (55%), stable disease in 12 (26%), and progressive disease in 9 (19%) patients. The median overall survival (OS) was 11 months (95% confidence interval (CI), 9–13), and objective responses to SIRT were associated with a longer OS ($p = 0.008$). Significant hepatotoxicity (≥grade 3) after SIRT was a contributor to impaired survival (median OS 6 months (95% CI, 4–8) vs. 12 months (95% CI, 10–14), $p < 0.001$). SIRT with glass microspheres is a safe and effective salvage treatment for patients with progressive HCC refractory to TACE who are considered poor candidates for sorafenib treatment.

Keywords: selective internal radionuclide therapy (SIRT); ^{90}Y glass microspheres; hepatocellular carcinoma (HCC); transarterial chemoembolization (TACE)

1. Introduction

The current Practice Guidance by the American Association for the Study of Liver Diseases recommends further diagnostic work-up for hepatocellular carcinoma (HCC) in the presence of a hepatic lesion >1 cm and an increase in alpha-fetoprotein >20 ng/mL in serum. Multiphase CT or MRI are used as imaging modalities, and histological analysis represents the gold standard [1]. In unresectable HCC, palliative liver-directed treatment options like transarterial chemoembolization (TACE) or selective internal radionuclide therapy (SIRT) can significantly reduce hepatic tumor burden and may increase survival in patients with liver-dominant disease [2–4].

TACE is currently the standard treatment for patients with locally advanced HCC without vascular invasion or extrahepatic spread (intermediate stage) [3,5–7]. However, a sufficient response after a single TACE session is rare, and often repeated TACE is required to achieve a good response [8]. Accordingly, at least two TACE sessions should be performed before abandoning the procedure [9]. Despite increasing evidence supporting the favorable efficacy of SIRT with ^{90}Yttrium (^{90}Y) microspheres in patients with intermediate to advanced HCC [10–15], the lack of prospective randomized clinical trials has currently limited its role as an alternative method for patients considered poor candidates for TACE. For patients refractory to repeated TACE, systemic treatment with the multikinase inhibitor sorafenib is recommended, but sometimes with suboptimal tolerability outweighing the survival benefits [16–18]. This leaves SIRT as the only treatment option after failure of TACE in this setting [19,20].

Repeated TACE can be associated with vascular injury and sometimes with liver function deterioration. Furthermore, profound TACE-induced tumor dearterialization may reduce the selective deployment of ^{90}Y microspheres inside the tumor vasculature [21–23]. Therefore, SIRT might be associated with a higher risk of treatment failure and severe hepatic toxicity in patients previously treated with repeated TACE. Conversely, a progressive tumor probably develops new tumor vessels, which might compensate for the TACE-induced devascularization. Thus, this study aims to assess the safety and efficacy of SIRT with glass ^{90}Y microspheres (TheraSphere™, Boston Scientific Corporation, Ottawa, ON, Canada) in patients with progressive HCC refractory to repeated TACE but not eligible for sorafenib treatment.

2. Results

2.1. Toxicity

The mean treatment activity per patient was 3.3 ± 1.5 GBq, and the mean follow-up time was 17 ± 2 months. Three of the 47 patients were still alive at the time of analysis. Recorded acute adverse events were as follows: fatigue in 18 (38%), nausea without vomiting in 10 (21%), fever in 9 (19%), and transient abdominal pain in 5 patients (11%). No patient needed hospitalization due to the reported adverse events, and all symptoms resolved within the first six weeks after SIRT. Prior to the treatment, 24 patients had impaired liver function (grade I: 24, grade II: 7, ≥grade III: 0). Post-SIRT hepatotoxicity was defined as newly impaired liver function (albumin, bilirubin, AST/ALT, INR, ascites) or as deterioration in CTCAE-grading after SIRT. Post-SIRT hepatotoxicity was observed in 36 patients. In 10 patients, liver function parameters deteriorated (grade II), and in 5 patients, a significant new hepatic toxicity of grade III–IV occurred. Detailed information about toxicity after treatment is given in Table 1: 12 patients showed elevated liver transaminase (10 grade I, 2 grade II) within six weeks after treatment, and 20 patients had biliary toxicity (4 grade I; 12 grade II and 4 grade III–IV). Fourteen patients showed relevant hepatic toxicity (grade II) based on both liver transaminase and bilirubin concentrations. Portal vein thrombosis and high hepatic tumor load (≥25%) were the independent contributing factors to treatment-induced significant hepatotoxicity, as depicted in Table 2.

Table 1. Toxicity after SIRT according to the CTCAE v.5.0.

Toxicity (Grade)	Post-SIRT Altered LFT, n (%)			SIRT-Induced Toxicity, n (%)		
	I	II	III–IV	I	II	III–IV
Bilirubin	9 (19)	14 (30)	4 (9)	4 (9)	12 (26)	4 (9)
Albumin	7 (15)	6 (13)	0 (0)	4 (9)	5 (11)	0 (0)
AST/ALT	33 (70)	4 (9)	0 (0)	12 (26)	2 (4)	0 (0)
AST	30 (70)	4 (9)	0 (0)	10 (21)	2 (4)	0 (0)
ALT	24 (51)	0 (0)	0 (0)	12 (26)	0 (0)	0 (0)
INR	13 (28)	3 (6)	0 (0)	9 (19)	3 (6)	0 (0)
Creatinine	0 (0)	0 (0)	3 (6)	0 (0)	0 (0)	2 (4)
Ascites	8 (17)	3 (6)	0 (0)	3 (6)	3 (6)	0 (0)
Toxicity of any kind	22 (47)	14 (30)	7 (15)	21 (45)	10 (21)	5 (11)

SIRT: selective internal radiation therapy; LFT: liver function test; AST: aspartate aminotransferase; ALT: alanine transaminase; INR: International Normalized Ratio.

Table 2. Contributing factors to toxicity after SIRT.

		Statistical Analysis		
		Univariate p Value	Multivariate p Value	(95% CI)
Age	≤65 years	0.402		
	>65 years			
Tumor load	≤25%	0.041	0.029	0.023–0.398
	>25%			
Cumulative activity	<3.5 GBq	0.706		
	≥3.5 GBq			
Tumor spread	Unilobar	0.227		
	Bilobar			
Hepatitis	No	0.256		
	Yes			
BCLC staging	B	0.307		
	C			
Child classification	A	0.559		
	B			
Lymph node involvement	No	0.224		
	Yes			
Hepatitis	No	0.256		
	Yes			
PVT	No	0.074	0.029	0.024–0.420
	Yes			
Altered LFT	Grade 0–I	0.283		
	Grade II–IV			
Pre-treatment	RFA	0.364		
	Resection/LT			
	Embolization/PEI			

BCLC: Barcelona Clinic Liver Cancer; Child classification: Child–Pugh system; PVT: portal vein thrombosis; LFT: liver function test; RFA: radiofrequency ablation; LT: liver transplantation; PEI: percutaneous ethanol ablation.

All five patients with newly induced hepatic toxicity had ≤3 TACE sessions prior to SIRT, and no increase in the incidence of significant toxicity was observed in patients with >3 prior TACE sessions (Figure 1). High cumulative activity (≥3.5 GBq) during SIRT and a higher number of previous TACE sessions was also not associated with increased hepatic toxicity ($p = 0.706$). Significant hepatic toxicity was resolved within 12 weeks in all but one patient who died because of acute renal failure. No severe radioembolization-induced liver disease (REILD) was documented, which was defined as new relevant serum total bilirubin elevation (≥ 3 mg/dL) combined with new ascites 1–2 months after treatment without tumor progression or bile duct obstruction. No radiation-induced pneumonitis, gastroduodenal ulceration, or other organ toxicity was observed.

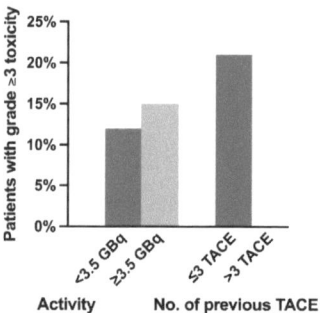

Figure 1. The relation of significant (grade ≥ 3) hepatotoxicity and (1) administered activity and (2) number of previous transarterial chemoembolization (TACE) sessions.

2.2. Response and Survival

Restaging according to mRECIST yielded a partial remission (PR) in 26 (55%), stable disease (SD) in 12 (26%), and progressive disease (PD) in 9 (19%) patients. Complete remission was not observed in our cohort. An example of a patient with a partial response according to mRECIST is displayed in Figure 2.

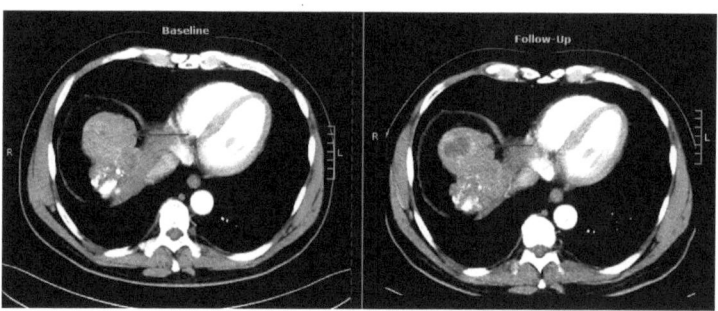

Figure 2. Computer tomography images of a patient showing a partial response after selective internal radiotherapy (red arrow indicates the tumor lesion).

The median time to progression after SIRT was 7 months (95% CI, 6–8) and the median OS was 11 months (95% CI, 9–13). Patients showing objective responses to SIRT (i.e., PR) had a median OS of 14 months (95% CI, 11–17) as opposed to 7 months (95% CI, 5–9) in the remaining patients ($p = 0.008$), as illustrated in Figure 3A. In contrast, progression after SIRT (i.e., PD) was associated with a shorter survival (median OS, 8 months (95% CI, 2–14) versus 12 months (95% CI, 9–15), $p = 0.013$, Figure 3B).

Significant hepatotoxicity ($\geq$grade III) after SIRT was also a contributor to impaired survival (median OS, 6 months (95% CI, 4–8) versus 12 months (95% CI, 10–14), $p < 0.001$, Figure 4A). Patients developing grade II hepatotoxicity showed a trend towards a shorter survival (median OS, 7 months (95% CI, 6–8) versus 14 (95% CI, 11–17), $p = 0.007$, Figure 4B).

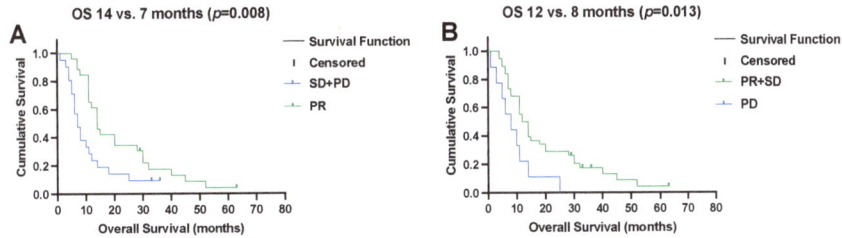

Figure 3. (**A**) Objective remission (partial response (PR)) after selective internal radiotherapy prolongs overall survival (OS), and (**B**) early progressive disease (PD) impairs overall survival.

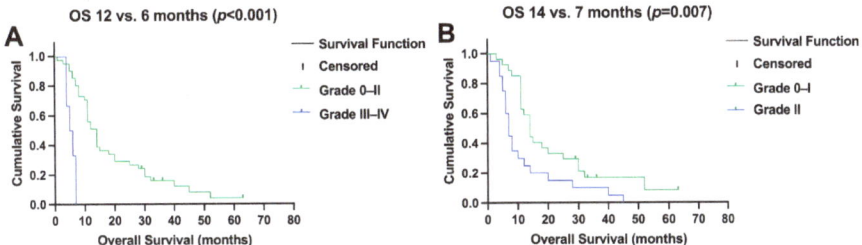

Figure 4. (**A**) Significant (grade ≥ 3) toxicity after selective internal radiotherapy reduced survival, and (**B**) moderate changes in liver function (CTC II) impaired overall survival (OS).

Among the baseline characteristics, a relevant decrease in hepatic functional reserve (≥grade II) was the only independent predictor of survival, as depicted by the multivariate analysis (HR; 95% CI, 5.5 (1.5–19.9), p = 0.009). The analysis of various baseline factors for potential contribution to OS is shown in Table 3.

Table 3. Contributing factors to survival after SIRT.

		Survival Analysis		Statistical Analysis	
		Median OS	HR (95% CI)	Univariate p Value	Multivariate HR (95% CI), p Value
Age	≤65 years	14	11–17	0.685	
	>65 years	14	5–23		
Tumor load	≤25%	14	10–18	0.518	
	>25%	14	11–17		
Cumulative activity	<3.5 GBq	14	8–20	0.323	
	≥3.5 GBq	14	13–15		
Tumor spread	Unilobar	14	6–22	0.620	
	Bilobar	14	12–16		
Hepatitis	No	15	10–20	0.247	
	Yes	11	3–19		
BCLC staging	B	13	11–15	0.389	
	C	8	3–14		
Child classification	A	12	10–15	0.736	
	B	10	6–14		

Table 3. Cont.

		Survival Analysis		Statistical Analysis	
		Median OS	HR (95% CI)	Univariate p Value	Multivariate HR (95% CI), p Value
Lymph node involvement	No	11	9–13	0.686	
	Yes	11	0–39		
Hepatitis	No	12	9–15	0.288	
	Yes	10	4–16		
PVT	No	13	11–15	0.352	
	Yes	7	3–11		
Altered LFT	Grade 0–I	12	10–14	0.002	5.5 (1.5–19.9) 0.009
	Grade II–IV	6	5–8		
Toxicity after SIRT	Grade 0–II	14	12–17	<0.001	
	Grade III–IV	6	5–7		

OS: overall survival; HR: hazard ratio; CI: confidence interval; BCLC: Barcelona Clinic Liver Cancer; Child classification: Child–Pugh system; PVT: portal vein thrombosis; LFT: liver function test; SIRT: selective internal radiation therapy.

3. Discussion

This retrospective study provides the first results regarding the risk factors for the hepatotoxicity of SIRT with glass-based ^{90}Y microspheres (TheraSphere™) in a well-characterized patient cohort (n = 47) with unresectable HCC failing repeated TACE. In clinical practice, previous TACE is considered a major risk factor for serious SIRT-induced toxicity. Fitting to this, the detected rate of significant hepatotoxicity in our cohort (11%) was higher than the previously reported rate of 4–9% in treatment-naive patients or heterogeneous cohorts regarding previous treatment modalities [2,24–33]. However, treatment-induced hepatotoxicity was almost always reversible, and liver function parameters returned to pre-treatment levels in all but one patient.

Portal vein thrombosis (PVT) is an absolute contraindication for TACE. On the contrary, SIRT with glass microspheres has a very low embolic tendency and can be safely applied to patients with PVT [34–36]. Although PVT was associated with a higher incidence of moderate hepatotoxicity in our cohort, the survival outcome of patients who had developed PVT under TACE did not differ from patients without PVT. Among all other analyzed baseline characteristics, only a hepatic tumor load of >25% was a risk factor for significant hepatotoxicity. This observation is in line with the reported data after treatment with ^{90}Y resin microspheres in a large prospective observational study (CIRT study). In a recent study on 1027 patients in a heterogenous patient cohort with various liver tumors, including HCC in 422 patients, a tumor load of >20% was a significant predictor of increased hepatotoxicity (p = 0.0283) [37]. Notably, the number of previous TACE sessions was not a predictor of hepatotoxicity in our cohort, encouraging the consideration of SIRT in patients heavily pre-treated with TACE, similar to previous findings in a smaller patient group (n = 29), indicating the suitability of SIRT after TACE not to be limited by increased risk of toxicity [38].

Achievement of disease control in 81% is promising and compares favorably with the other treatment modalities. Sorafenib, as the recommended agent for TACE-refractory HCC lesions [16,17,39,40], is commonly associated with adverse effects leading to treatment interruption or even permanent drug discontinuation [16,17,39]. Moreover, an objective radiological response is rarely observed after treatment with sorafenib. The reported overall survival in the main clinical phase III trial of sorafenib (SHARP trial) was 10.7 months [17]. Although comparing our retrospective data with results from prospective trials is of limited validity, the objective response rate (ORR) of 55% and median OS of 11 months (CI 95%,

9–13) in our patients ineligible for treatment with sorafenib is very encouraging. Furthermore, responders (i.e., PR) had a significantly longer survival in our cohort (median OS 14 versus 7 months, $p = 0.008$), underlining the impact of ORR on the survival outcomes of HCC patients after SIRT [15]. The rate of hepatotoxicity in our study was lower than the reported rate after sorafenib treatment. Johnson et al. analyzed the efficacy and safety of SIRT as a salvage therapy after ≥ 1 TACE, resulting in a slightly inferior OS of 8.4 months; however, BCLC stage C was more prevalent in their cohort (72.5% vs. 47%) [38]. Fitting to this, in a study by Reeves et al., a subgroup of BCLC stage B patients with 1–7 TACE before SIRT ($n = 7$) reached an OS of 14.8 months [41].

In addition to tumor progression, therapy-induced hepatotoxicity may affect the survival of patients with HCC [15,17]. In a retrospective study, grade II toxicity has been suggested as a risk factor for poor survival outcomes. Correspondingly, relevant hepatotoxicity impaired the survival outcome in our cohort ($p < 0.007$). Significant hyperbilirubinemia (grade III/IV), as a hallmark of REILD, has been reported in 14% of patients undergoing ^{90}Y glass microsphere SIRT [24]. Although 9% of our cohort developed grade III transient biliary toxicity, no REILD was observed in our cohort.

Our findings support the application of SIRT with glass microspheres after undergoing repeated TACE who are ineligible for treatment with sorafenib. SIRT could induce disease stabilization in most patients, leading to an improved survival outcome. Hepatotoxicity was reversible and the number of previous TACE was not a risk factor. However, the retrospective design and small patient group limit the statistical power and ability to generalize from our results regarding the subgroup analysis and baseline factors with a potential impact on survival. Furthermore, pathological data were, unfortunately, not available to be included in this clinical observational study. It would be interesting to analyze pathological parameters and the treatment efficacy, which might be the subject of further studies.

4. Materials and Methods

4.1. Patient Characteristics

Forty-seven patients with TACE-refractory HCC (38 men, 9 women; age range: 40–85 years; mean age: 69 years) treated with SIRT in the Department of Nuclear Medicine, University Duisburg-Essen, were included in this retrospective analysis [42]. The decision to perform SIRT was based on interdisciplinary consent after discussion in a multidisciplinary tumor board. All patients had progressive liver tumors despite repeated TACE procedures (median: 3, range 2–14) and were not suitable for sorafenib treatment. Apart from repeated TACE, previous treatments were comprised of radiofrequency ablation ($n = 9$), surgical resection ($n = 7$), liver transplantation ($n = 4$), and transarterial embolization or ethanol injection ($n = 2$). All patients fulfilled the general inclusion criteria for radioembolization [43,44]. Twenty-three patients presented with a unilobar, and 24 patients with a bilobar hepatic tumor spread. At the time of SIRT, 25 patients were classified as stage B and 22 as stage C according to the Barcelona Clinic Liver Cancer (BCLC) staging classification. In 39 patients, HCC was confined to the liver, while 8 patients showed a liver-dominant disease with extrahepatic metastases. In these eight patients, the tumor board identified the extrahepatic metastases as not predominately prognostically relevant regarding survival, size, quantity, and localization of the metastases. The baseline patient characteristics are presented in Table 4. The local committee on ethics approved this retrospective study, and all subjects signed a written informed consent to treatment prior to evaluation and radioembolization session.

Table 4. Baseline patient characteristics.

	All Patients ($n = 47$)
Age	
>65 years	32 (68)
$\leq$65 years	15 (32)

Table 4. *Cont.*

	All Patients (*n* = 47)
Hepatic tumor load	
>25%	23 (49)
≤25%	24 (51)
Cumulative applied activity during SIRT session(s)	
≥3.5 GBq	21 (45)
<3.5 GBq	26 (55)
Hepatic tumor spread	
Bilobar	24 (51)
Unilobar	23 (49)
BCLC staging	
Stage C	22 (47)
Stage B	25 (53)
Child classification	
Child B	21 (45)
Child A	26 (55)
Extrahepatic lymph node metastasis	
No	39 (83)
Yes	8 (17)
Hepatitis	
Yes	21 (45)
No	26 (55)
Etiology of hepatitis	
Alcohol-related	6 (13)
NASH	12 (26)
Viral	18 (38)
Cryptogenic	11 (23)
PVT	
Yes	16 (33)
No	31 (66)
Pre-treatment	
RFA	9 (19)
Embolization/PEI	2 (4)
Resection/LT	11 (24)
LFT in all patients	
Total bilirubin (mg/dL, normal range: 0.3–1.0)	1.0 ± 0.5
Albumin (g/dL, normal range: 3.4–5.4)	3.9 ± 0.5
AST (U/L, normal range: 5–40)	77.6 ± 62.4
ALT (U/L, normal range: 7–56)	59.5 ± 41.1
INR (normal range: 0.8–1.1)	1.1 ± 0.1
Altered LFT (CTC I)	
Total bilirubin (>ULN–1.5 × ULN, mg/dL)	16 (34)
Albumin (<LLN–3 g/dL)	6 (13)
AST/ALT (>ULN–3 × ULN, U/L)	26 (55)
INR (>1.2–1.5 × baseline)	4 (9)
Ascites	5 (11)
Altered LFT (CTC II)	
Total bilirubin (>1.5–3.0 × ULN, mg/dL)	2 (4)
Albumin (3–2 g/dL)	2 (4)
AST/ALT (>3–5 × ULN, U/L)	2 (4)
INR (>1.5–2.5)	0 (0)
Ascites	0 (0)

Data presented as *n* (%). SIRT: selective internal radiotherapy; GBq: gigabecquerel; BCLC: Barcelona Clinic Liver Cancer; Child classification: Child–Pugh system; NASH: non-alcoholic steatohepatitis; PVT: portal vein thrombosis; RFA: radiofrequency ablation; PEI: percutaneous ethanol ablation; LT: liver transplantation; LFT: liver function test; CTC: Common Terminology for Common Adverse Events (v.5.0); ULN: upper limit of normal; LLN: lower limit of normal; AST: aspartate aminotransferase; ALT: alanine transaminase; INR: International Normalized Ratio.

4.2. Radioembolization Procedure

Intra-abdominal and excessive pulmonary (lung-shunt fraction) deposition were excluded prior to radioembolization by a pre-treatment diagnostic angiogram with planar and SPECT/CT ^{99m}Technetium-HSA (human serum albumin microspheres) imaging after an intra-arterial injection of 150 MBq of ^{99m}Tc-HSA [45]. Radioembolization was performed within an interval of 1–4 weeks following diagnostic angiography using glass-based ^{90}Y microspheres (TheraSphere™). The prescription of activity was derived from the MIRD-based dose calculation method provided by the manufacturer (Boston Scientific Corporation, Marlborough, MA, USA, former BTG plc, London, UK, former Nordion Inc., Ottawa, ON, Canada) to achieve a standard target dose of 100–120 Gy. The liver was treated in a single session (unilobar, $n = 23$, whole liver, $n = 1$) or in a sequential lobar fashion ($n = 23$ patients). Post-treatment ^{90}Y bremsstrahlung imaging was performed to document target accumulation. Parameters for liver function (albumin, bilirubin, AST/ALT, INR, ascites) were determined before as well as 4 and 12 weeks after each SIRT. Hepatic toxicity was classified according to the Common Terminology Criteria for Adverse Events Version 5.0 (CTCAE v.5.0). Morphological response to SIRT was assessed using contrast-agent-enhanced computed tomography (CT, early arterial and venous phase) 3 months after SIRT using modified response criteria in solid tumors (mRECIST) [46,47].

4.3. Statistical Analysis

Statistical analyses were performed using the SPSS software package version 29.0 (IBM, Armonk, NY, USA). Graph-Pad Prism version 10.1 (GraphPad Software, San Diego, CA, USA) was used to plot graphs. The results were presented as mean ± standard deviation for continuous variables; categorical variables are presented as frequencies with respective percentages. The association of treatment-induced hepatic toxicity (grade I–IV) with the baseline characteristics of the study population, number of previous TACE sessions, and administered activity were examined, applying non-parametric tests for independent samples as well as multiple regression analysis. Survival assessment from the start of radioembolization was performed using the Kaplan–Meier method. Overall survival (OS) was assessed from the first radioembolization session, and the death of patients was considered as an event for OS irrespective of the cause. Survival outcomes were stratified by various variables and compared using the log-rank test. Multivariate analysis (Cox proportional hazards model) was performed with those variables showing at least a trend ($p < 0.1$) of influence on the univariate analysis (log-rank test). A p value < 0.05 was considered significant.

5. Conclusions

SIRT with glass microspheres is an effective salvage treatment in patients with progressive HCC refractory to TACE who are ineligible for treatment with sorafenib. SIRT provides disease stabilization and improves survival. The rate of significant hepatotoxicity was acceptable, considering the lack of alternative treatment options. Furthermore, the number of previous TACE sessions should not preclude the consideration of SIRT in heavily pre-treated patients fulfilling the established prerequisites.

Author Contributions: Conceptualization, A.S.; methodology, A.S., A.B. (Alexander Bellendorf) and N.M.; validation, S.P.M., S.E. and A.B. (Andreas Bockisch); formal analysis, A.B. (Alexander Bellendorf), N.M. and A.S.; investigation, A.B. (Alexander Bellendorf), T.D.P., H.G. and A.S.; resources, S.P.M., J.G., J.B. and A.B. (Andreas Bockisch); data curation, A.B. (Alexander Bellendorf) and H.G.; writing—original draft preparation, A.B. (Alexander Bellendorf) and N.M.; writing—review and editing, S.E., S.P.M., A.B. (Andreas Bockisch) and A.S.; visualization, A.B. (Alexander Bellendorf) and N.M.; supervision, A.S. and S.P.M. All authors have read and agreed to the published version of the manuscript.

Funding: This research received no external funding.

Institutional Review Board Statement: This retrospective study was approved by the institutional review board.

Informed Consent Statement: Informed consent was obtained from all subjects involved in the study.

Data Availability Statement: The datasets analyzed and/or analyzed during the current study are available from the corresponding author on reasonable request.

Conflicts of Interest: The authors declare no conflicts of interest.

References

1. Marrero, J.A.; Kulik, L.M.; Sirlin, C.B.; Zhu, A.X.; Finn, R.S.; Abecassis, M.M.; Roberts, L.R.; Heimbach, J.K. Diagnosis, Staging, and Management of Hepatocellular Carcinoma: 2018 Practice Guidance by the American Association for the Study of Liver Diseases. *Hepatology* **2018**, *68*, 723–750. [CrossRef] [PubMed]
2. Salem, R.; Lewandowski, R.J.; Mulcahy, M.F.; Riaz, A.; Ryu, R.K.; Ibrahim, S.; Atassi, B.; Baker, T.; Gates, V.; Miller, F.H.; et al. Radioembolization for hepatocellular carcinoma using Yttrium-90 microspheres: A comprehensive report of long-term outcomes. *Gastroenterology* **2010**, *138*, 52–64. [CrossRef]
3. Cammà, C.; Schepis, F.; Orlando, A.; Albanese, M.; Shahied, L.; Trevisani, F.; Andreone, P.; Craxì, A.; Cottone, M. Transarterial chemoembolization for unresectable hepatocellular carcinoma: Meta-analysis of randomized controlled trials. *Radiology* **2002**, *224*, 47–54. [CrossRef]
4. Brown, Z.J.; Tsilimigras, D.I.; Ruff, S.M.; Mohseni, A.; Kamel, I.R.; Cloyd, J.M.; Pawlik, T.M. Management of Hepatocellular Carcinoma: A Review. *JAMA Surg.* **2023**, *158*, 410–420. [CrossRef] [PubMed]
5. Llovet, J.M.; Bruix, J. Systematic review of randomized trials for unresectable hepatocellular carcinoma: Chemoembolization improves survival. *Hepatology* **2003**, *37*, 429–442. [CrossRef]
6. Dalzell, C.G.; Taylor, A.C.; White, S.B. New Insights on Liver-Directed Therapies in Hepatocellular Carcinoma. *Cancers* **2023**, *15*, 5749. [CrossRef]
7. Vogl, T.J.; Naguib, N.N.; Nour-Eldin, N.E.; Rao, P.; Emami, A.H.; Zangos, S.; Nabil, M.; Abdelkader, A. Review on transarterial chemoembolization in hepatocellular carcinoma: Palliative, combined, neoadjuvant, bridging, and symptomatic indications. *Eur. J. Radiol.* **2009**, *72*, 505–516. [CrossRef] [PubMed]
8. Terzi, E.; Golfieri, R.; Piscaglia, F.; Galassi, M.; Dazzi, A.; Leoni, S.; Giampalma, E.; Renzulli, M.; Bolondi, L. Response rate and clinical outcome of HCC after first and repeated cTACE performed "on demand". *J. Hepatol.* **2012**, *57*, 1258–1267. [CrossRef]
9. Georgiades, C.; Geschwind, J.F.; Harrison, N.; Hines-Peralta, A.; Liapi, E.; Hong, K.; Wu, Z.; Kamel, I.; Frangakis, C. Lack of response after initial chemoembolization for hepatocellular carcinoma: Does it predict failure of subsequent treatment? *Radiology* **2012**, *265*, 115–123. [CrossRef]
10. Lance, C.; McLennan, G.; Obuchowski, N.; Cheah, G.; Levitin, A.; Sands, M.; Spain, J.; Srinivas, S.; Shrikanthan, S.; Aucejo, F.N.; et al. Comparative analysis of the safety and efficacy of transcatheter arterial chemoembolization and yttrium-90 radioembolization in patients with unresectable hepatocellular carcinoma. *J. Vasc. Interv. Radiol.* **2011**, *22*, 1697–1705. [CrossRef]
11. Salem, R.; Lewandowski, R.J.; Kulik, L.; Wang, E.; Riaz, A.; Ryu, R.K.; Sato, K.T.; Gupta, R.; Nikolaidis, P.; Miller, F.H.; et al. Radioembolization results in longer time-to-progression and reduced toxicity compared with chemoembolization in patients with hepatocellular carcinoma. *Gastroenterology* **2011**, *140*, 497–507.e492. [CrossRef]
12. Sangro, B.; Salem, R. Transarterial chemoembolization and radioembolization. *Semin. Liver Dis.* **2014**, *34*, 435–443. [CrossRef] [PubMed]
13. Lewandowski, R.J.; Kulik, L.M.; Riaz, A.; Senthilnathan, S.; Mulcahy, M.F.; Ryu, R.K.; Ibrahim, S.M.; Sato, K.T.; Baker, T.; Miller, F.H.; et al. A comparative analysis of transarterial downstaging for hepatocellular carcinoma: Chemoembolization versus radioembolization. *Am. J. Transplant.* **2009**, *9*, 1920–1928. [CrossRef] [PubMed]
14. Memon, K.; Lewandowski, R.J.; Riaz, A.; Salem, R. Yttrium 90 microspheres for the treatment of hepatocellular carcinoma. *Recent Results Cancer Res.* **2013**, *190*, 207–224. [CrossRef]
15. Mazzaferro, V.; Sposito, C.; Bhoori, S.; Romito, R.; Chiesa, C.; Morosi, C.; Maccauro, M.; Marchianò, A.; Bongini, M.; Lanocita, R.; et al. Yttrium-90 radioembolization for intermediate-advanced hepatocellular carcinoma: A phase 2 study. *Hepatology* **2013**, *57*, 1826–1837. [CrossRef] [PubMed]
16. Cheng, A.L.; Kang, Y.K.; Chen, Z.; Tsao, C.J.; Qin, S.; Kim, J.S.; Luo, R.; Feng, J.; Ye, S.; Yang, T.S.; et al. Efficacy and safety of sorafenib in patients in the Asia-Pacific region with advanced hepatocellular carcinoma: A phase III randomised, double-blind, placebo-controlled trial. *Lancet Oncol.* **2009**, *10*, 25–34. [CrossRef]
17. Llovet, J.M.; Ricci, S.; Mazzaferro, V.; Hilgard, P.; Gane, E.; Blanc, J.F.; de Oliveira, A.C.; Santoro, A.; Raoul, J.L.; Forner, A.; et al. Sorafenib in advanced hepatocellular carcinoma. *N. Engl. J. Med.* **2008**, *359*, 378–390. [CrossRef] [PubMed]
18. Keating, G.M. Sorafenib: A Review in Hepatocellular Carcinoma. *Target. Oncol.* **2017**, *12*, 243–253. [CrossRef]
19. Vilgrain, V.; Pereira, H.; Assenat, E.; Guiu, B.; Ilonca, A.D.; Pageaux, G.P.; Sibert, A.; Bouattour, M.; Lebtahi, R.; Allaham, W.; et al. Efficacy and safety of selective internal radiotherapy with yttrium-90 resin microspheres compared with sorafenib in locally advanced and inoperable hepatocellular carcinoma (SARAH): An open-label randomised controlled phase 3 trial. *Lancet Oncol.* **2017**, *18*, 1624–1636. [CrossRef]

20. Chow, P.K.H.; Gandhi, M.; Tan, S.B.; Khin, M.W.; Khasbazar, A.; Ong, J.; Choo, S.P.; Cheow, P.C.; Chotipanich, C.; Lim, K.; et al. SIRveNIB: Selective Internal Radiation Therapy Versus Sorafenib in Asia-Pacific Patients with Hepatocellular Carcinoma. *J. Clin. Oncol.* **2018**, *36*, 1913–1921. [CrossRef]
21. Clark, T.W. Complications of hepatic chemoembolization. *Semin. Intervent Radiol.* **2006**, *23*, 119–125. [CrossRef] [PubMed]
22. Sun, Z.; Li, G.; Ai, X.; Luo, B.; Wen, Y.; Zhao, Z.; Dong, S.; Guan, J. Hepatic and biliary damage after transarterial chemoembolization for malignant hepatic tumors: Incidence, diagnosis, treatment, outcome and mechanism. *Crit. Rev. Oncol. Hematol.* **2011**, *79*, 164–174. [CrossRef]
23. Binzaqr, S.; Debordeaux, F.; Blanc, J.F.; Papadopoulos, P.; Hindie, E.; Lapouyade, B.; Pinaquy, J.B. Efficacy of Selective Internal Radiation Therapy for Hepatocellular Carcinoma Post-Incomplete Response to Chemoembolization. *Pharmaceuticals* **2023**, *16*, 1676. [CrossRef] [PubMed]
24. Sangro, B.; Gil-Alzugaray, B.; Rodriguez, J.; Sola, I.; Martinez-Cuesta, A.; Viudez, A.; Chopitea, A.; Inarrairaegui, M.; Arbizu, J.; Bilbao, J.I. Liver disease induced by radioembolization of liver tumors: Description and possible risk factors. *Cancer* **2008**, *112*, 1538–1546. [CrossRef] [PubMed]
25. Kennedy, A.S.; McNeillie, P.; Dezarn, W.A.; Nutting, C.; Sangro, B.; Wertman, D.; Garafalo, M.; Liu, D.; Coldwell, D.; Savin, M.; et al. Treatment parameters and outcome in 680 treatments of internal radiation with resin 90Y-microspheres for unresectable hepatic tumors. *Int. J. Radiat. Oncol. Biol. Phys.* **2009**, *74*, 1494–1500. [CrossRef] [PubMed]
26. Atassi, B.; Bangash, A.K.; Lewandowski, R.J.; Ibrahim, S.; Kulik, L.; Mulcahy, M.F.; Murthy, R.; Ryu, R.K.; Sato, K.T.; Miller, F.H.; et al. Biliary sequelae following radioembolization with Yttrium-90 microspheres. *J. Vasc. Interv. Radiol.* **2008**, *19*, 691–697. [CrossRef] [PubMed]
27. Piana, P.M.; Gonsalves, C.F.; Sato, T.; Anne, P.R.; McCann, J.W.; Bar Ad, V.; Eschelman, D.J.; Parker, L.; Doyle, L.A.; Brown, D.B. Toxicities after radioembolization with yttrium-90 SIR-spheres: Incidence and contributing risk factors at a single center. *J. Vasc. Interv. Radiol.* **2011**, *22*, 1373–1379. [CrossRef] [PubMed]
28. Lewandowski, R.J.; Minocha, J.; Memon, K.; Riaz, A.; Gates, V.L.; Ryu, R.K.; Sato, K.T.; Omary, R.; Salem, R. Sustained safety and efficacy of extended-shelf-life (90)Y glass microspheres: Long-term follow-up in a 134-patient cohort. *Eur. J. Nucl. Med. Mol. Imaging* **2014**, *41*, 486–493. [CrossRef]
29. Salem, R.; Lewandowski, R.J.; Atassi, B.; Gordon, S.C.; Gates, V.L.; Barakat, O.; Sergie, Z.; Wong, C.Y.; Thurston, K.G. Treatment of unresectable hepatocellular carcinoma with use of 90Y microspheres (TheraSphere): Safety, tumor response, and survival. *J. Vasc. Interv. Radiol.* **2005**, *16*, 1627–1639. [CrossRef]
30. Carr, B.I. Hepatic arterial 90Yttrium glass microspheres (Therasphere) for unresectable hepatocellular carcinoma: Interim safety and survival data on 65 patients. *Liver Transpl.* **2004**, *10*, S107–S110. [CrossRef]
31. Goin, J.E.; Salem, R.; Carr, B.I.; Dancey, J.E.; Soulen, M.C.; Geschwind, J.F.; Goin, K.; Van Buskirk, M.; Thurston, K. Treatment of unresectable hepatocellular carcinoma with intrahepatic yttrium 90 microspheres: Factors associated with liver toxicities. *J. Vasc. Interv. Radiol.* **2005**, *16*, 205–213. [CrossRef]
32. Hilgard, P.; Hamami, M.; Fouly, A.E.; Scherag, A.; Muller, S.; Ertle, J.; Heusner, T.; Cicinnati, V.R.; Paul, A.; Bockisch, A.; et al. Radioembolization with yttrium-90 glass microspheres in hepatocellular carcinoma: European experience on safety and long-term survival. *Hepatology* **2010**, *52*, 1741–1749. [CrossRef]
33. Szyszko, T.; Al-Nahhas, A.; Tait, P.; Rubello, D.; Canelo, R.; Habib, N.; Jiao, L.; Wasan, H.; Bansi, D.; Thillainayagam, A.; et al. Management and prevention of adverse effects related to treatment of liver tumours with ^{90}Y microspheres. *Nucl. Med. Commun.* **2007**, *28*, 21–24. [CrossRef] [PubMed]
34. Kulik, L.M.; Carr, B.I.; Mulcahy, M.F.; Lewandowski, R.J.; Atassi, B.; Ryu, R.K.; Sato, K.T.; Benson, A., 3rd; Nemcek, A.A., Jr.; Gates, V.L.; et al. Safety and efficacy of ^{90}Y radiotherapy for hepatocellular carcinoma with and without portal vein thrombosis. *Hepatology* **2008**, *47*, 71–81. [CrossRef] [PubMed]
35. Memon, K.; Kulik, L.; Lewandowski, R.J.; Mulcahy, M.F.; Benson, A.B.; Ganger, D.; Riaz, A.; Gupta, R.; Vouche, M.; Gates, V.L.; et al. Radioembolization for hepatocellular carcinoma with portal vein thrombosis: Impact of liver function on systemic treatment options at disease progression. *J. Hepatol.* **2013**, *58*, 73–80. [CrossRef] [PubMed]
36. Salem, R.; Lewandowski, R.; Roberts, C.; Goin, J.; Thurston, K.; Abouljoud, M.; Courtney, A. Use of Yttrium-90 glass microspheres (TheraSphere) for the treatment of unresectable hepatocellular carcinoma in patients with portal vein thrombosis. *J. Vasc. Interv. Radiol.* **2004**, *15*, 335–345. [CrossRef]
37. Maleux, G.; Albrecht, T.; Arnold, D.; Bargellini, I.; Cianni, R.; Helmberger, T.; Kolligs, F.; Munneke, G.; Peynircioglu, B.; Sangro, B.; et al. Predictive Factors for Adverse Event Outcomes After Transarterial Radioembolization with Yttrium-90 Resin Microspheres in Europe: Results from the Prospective Observational CIRT Study. *Cardiovasc. Intervent Radiol.* **2023**, *46*, 852–867. [CrossRef]
38. Johnson, G.E.; Monsky, W.L.; Valji, K.; Hippe, D.S.; Padia, S.A. Yttrium-90 Radioembolization as a Salvage Treatment following Chemoembolization for Hepatocellular Carcinoma. *J. Vasc. Interv. Radiol.* **2016**, *27*, 1123–1129. [CrossRef]
39. Iavarone, M.; Cabibbo, G.; Piscaglia, F.; Zavaglia, C.; Grieco, A.; Villa, E.; Camma, C.; Colombo, M.; on behalf of the SOFIA (SOraFenib Italian Assessment) Study Group. Field-practice study of sorafenib therapy for hepatocellular carcinoma: A prospective multicenter study in Italy. *Hepatology* **2011**, *54*, 2055–2063. [CrossRef]
40. Bruix, J.; Sherman, M.; American Association for the Study of Liver, D. Management of hepatocellular carcinoma: An update. *Hepatology* **2011**, *53*, 1020–1022. [CrossRef]

41. Reeves, H.L.; Reicher, J.; Priona, G.; Manas, D.M.; Littler, P. Selective internal radiation therapy (SIRT) for hepatocellular carcinoma (HCC): Informing clinical practice for multidisciplinary teams in England. *Frontline Gastroenterol.* **2023**, *14*, 45–51. [CrossRef]
42. Bruix, J.; Sherman, M.; Llovet, J.M.; Beaugrand, M.; Lencioni, R.; Burroughs, A.K.; Christensen, E.; Pagliaro, L.; Colombo, M.; Rodés, J. Clinical management of hepatocellular carcinoma. Conclusions of the Barcelona-2000 EASL conference. European Association for the Study of the Liver. *J. Hepatol.* **2001**, *35*, 421–430. [CrossRef] [PubMed]
43. Salem, R.; Thurston, K.G. Radioembolization with 90Yttrium microspheres: A state-of-the-art brachytherapy treatment for primary and secondary liver malignancies. Part 1: Technical and methodologic considerations. *J. Vasc. Interv. Radiol.* **2006**, *17*, 1251–1278. [CrossRef] [PubMed]
44. Kennedy, A.; Nag, S.; Salem, R.; Murthy, R.; McEwan, A.J.; Nutting, C.; Benson, A., 3rd; Espat, J.; Bilbao, J.I.; Sharma, R.A.; et al. Recommendations for radioembolization of hepatic malignancies using yttrium-90 microsphere brachytherapy: A consensus panel report from the radioembolization brachytherapy oncology consortium. *Int. J. Radiat. Oncol. Biol. Phys.* **2007**, *68*, 13–23. [CrossRef] [PubMed]
45. Sabet, A.; Ahmadzadehfar, H.; Muckle, M.; Haslerud, T.; Wilhelm, K.; Biersack, H.J.; Ezziddin, S. Significance of oral administration of sodium perchlorate in planning liver-directed radioembolization. *J. Nucl. Med.* **2011**, *52*, 1063–1067. [CrossRef]
46. Lencioni, R.; Llovet, J.M. Modified RECIST (mRECIST) assessment for hepatocellular carcinoma. *Semin. Liver Dis.* **2010**, *30*, 52–60. [CrossRef]
47. Bruix, J.; Sherman, M. Management of hepatocellular carcinoma. *Hepatology* **2005**, *42*, 1208–1236. [CrossRef]

Disclaimer/Publisher's Note: The statements, opinions and data contained in all publications are solely those of the individual author(s) and contributor(s) and not of MDPI and/or the editor(s). MDPI and/or the editor(s) disclaim responsibility for any injury to people or property resulting from any ideas, methods, instructions or products referred to in the content.

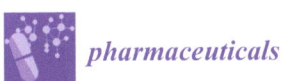

Article

The Importance of Uncertainty Analysis and Traceable Measurements in Routine Quantitative ^{90}Y-PET Molecular Radiotherapy: A Multicenter Experience

Marco D'Arienzo [1,2,†], Emilio Mezzenga [3,†], Amedeo Capotosti [4,*], Oreste Bagni [5], Luca Filippi [5], Marco Capogni [6], Luca Indovina [4] and Anna Sarnelli [3]

1. Medical Physics Section, ASL Roma 6, Borgo Garibaldi 12, 00041 Rome, Italy; marco.darienzo@aslroma6.it
2. UniCamillus International Medical University, 00131 Rome, Italy
3. Medical Physics Unit, IRCCS Istituto Romagnolo per lo Studio dei Tumori (IRST) "Dino Amadori", 47014 Meldola, Italy; emilio.mezzenga@irst.emr.it (E.M.); anna.sarnelli@irst.emr.it (A.S.)
4. Fondazione Policlinico Universitario A. Gemelli IRCCS, 00168 Roma, Italy; luca.indovina@policlinicogemelli.it
5. Nuclear Medicine Department, Santa Maria Goretti Hospital, 04100 Latina, Italy; obagni1@gmail.com (O.B.); l.filippi@ausl.latina.it (L.F.)
6. ENEA, Italian National Institute of Ionizing Radiation Metrology, Via Anguillarese 301, 00123 Rome, Italy; marco.capogni@enea.it
* Correspondence: amedeo.capotosti@policlinicogemelli.it
† These authors contributed equally to this work.

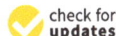

Abstract: Molecular Radiation Therapy (MRT) is a valid therapeutic option for a wide range of malignancies, such as neuroendocrine tumors and liver cancers. In its practice, it is generally acknowledged that there is a need to evaluate the influence of different factors affecting the accuracy of dose estimates and to define the actions necessary to maintain treatment uncertainties at acceptable levels. The present study addresses the problem of uncertainty propagation in ^{90}Y-PET quantification. We assessed the quantitative accuracy in reference conditions of three PET scanners (namely, Siemens Biograph mCT, Siemens Biograph mCT flow, and GE Discovery DST) available at three different Italian Nuclear Medicine centers. Specific aspects of uncertainty within the quantification chain have been addressed, including the uncertainty in the calibration procedure. A framework based on the Guide to the Expression of Uncertainty in Measurement (GUM) approach is proposed for modeling the uncertainty in the quantification processes, and ultimately, an estimation of the uncertainty achievable in clinical conditions is reported.

Keywords: ^{90}Y; PET; dosimetry; radionuclide therapy; quantitative accuracy; uncertainty analysis; MRT; scanner; multicenter

Citation: D'Arienzo, M.; Mezzenga, E.; Capotosti, A.; Bagni, O.; Filippi, L.; Capogni, M.; Indovina, L.; Sarnelli, A. The Importance of Uncertainty Analysis and Traceable Measurements in Routine Quantitative ^{90}Y-PET Molecular Radiotherapy: A Multicenter Experience. *Pharmaceuticals* **2023**, *16*, 1142. https://doi.org/10.3390/ph16081142

Academic Editors: Marc Pretze and Jörg Kotzerke

Received: 17 June 2023
Revised: 1 August 2023
Accepted: 3 August 2023
Published: 11 August 2023

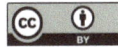

Copyright: © 2023 by the authors. Licensee MDPI, Basel, Switzerland. This article is an open access article distributed under the terms and conditions of the Creative Commons Attribution (CC BY) license (https:// creativecommons.org/licenses/by/ 4.0/).

1. Introduction

Over the last two decades, there has been a massive increase in the development and use of radiopharmaceuticals for treating cancer, and the number of Molecular Radiation Therapy (MRT) treatments worldwide is soaring at an unprecedented rate [1]. Despite growing awareness of the expansion rate of MRT practice, it is generally recognized that quantitative imaging in MRT suffers from considerable inaccuracy and that dosimetry is significantly affected by uncertainties at every step of the dosimetric workflow [2–5]. As a consequence, when compared with conventional external beam radiotherapy, in which there are internationally agreed requirements for dose accuracy (<3% of a reference value), dosimetry in MRT still needs collaborative efforts to bring dosimetry practice to an acceptable standard.

In past years, two major international collaborative EURopean Association on national METrology institutes (EURAMET) projects have addressed the issues of traceability, accuracy, and uncertainties in MRT practice, developing some innovative solutions and proposing new approaches to the problem. The Metrology for Molecular Radiation Therapy (MetroMRT) project [6], concluded in 2015, aimed to develop the background metrology to support routine individual MRT patient dosimetry. The project identified major sources of error in the metrological processes involved in the evaluation of the absorbed dose and assessed uncertainty budgets in the dosimetric workflow. The following Metrology for Clinical Implementation of Dosimetry in Molecular Radiotherapy (MRTDosimetry) project [7] built on the results and outputs from the preceding MetroMRT project and ran for three years, finishing on 31 May 2019. These pan-European initiatives brought together expertise in metrology and nuclear medicine research to address the problem of the clinical implementation of dosimetry in molecular radiotherapy. With this in mind, both projects assessed the major processes and variables within the dose calculation procedure, evaluating their potential effect on the output result.

Quantitative ^{90}Y-PET imaging has received much attention in the past decade [8–12], and the assessment of uncertainties in relation to the dose measurement chain (i.e., from a primary standard to a dosimetry calculation platform) has become a central issue for the evaluation of the efficacy and toxicity of Transarterial Radioembolization (TARE) [13–17]. Of note, one of the specific objectives of the MRTDosimetry project was to assess the internal pair production branching ratio and emission probabilities of ^{90}Y, with the aim to enable improved quantitative imaging accuracy and dose estimation. The reason is that an accurate determination of the branching ratio for pair production is essential for accurate quantification and dosimetry.

Furthermore, recent studies carried out in the context of the above-mentioned EURAMET projects have addressed the issue of assessing an accurate uncertainty propagation schema in the quantification process [3] and in the dosimetry workflow [2]. D'Arienzo and Cox [3] performed uncertainty analysis in the calibration of an emission tomography system for quantitative imaging. In their study, using the general formula given in the Guide to the Expression of Uncertainty in Measurement (GUM) [18,19] for aggregating uncertainty components, the authors derived a practical relation to assess the combined standard uncertainty for the calibration factor of an emission tomography system. In another study, Gears and colleagues [2] proposed a comprehensive and accurate uncertainty propagation schema to evaluate the standard uncertainty in absorbed dose to a target. The paper has been published as an EANM guideline on uncertainty analysis for MRT absorbed dose calculations.

The aim of the present study is twofold. Firstly, it attempts to identify and describe a traceable validation procedure for ^{90}Y-PET quantitative imaging in reference conditions. Secondly, the present research focuses on the problem of uncertainty propagation in the quantification workflow. As uncertainties propagate along each step of the quantification process, establishing a reliable scanner calibration procedure is essential to accurate activity quantification. With this in mind, we assessed the quantitative accuracy in reference conditions (cylindrical uniform geometry) of three PET scanners available at three different Italian Nuclear Medicine centers (namely, TOF Siemens Biograph mCT, TOF Siemens Biograph mCT flow, and GE Discovery DST). Specific aspects of uncertainty within the quantification chain have been addressed, including the uncertainty in the calibration procedure.

In the present paper, the three centers are referred to as indicated in Table 1. The workflow was organized as follows:

1. Three PET scanners available at three Italian centers were calibrated with the aim to recover the ^{90}Y activity from ^{90}Y-PET images. For all the PET scanners, the calibration procedure was performed using a water phantom uniformly filled with a known concentration of ^{18}F-FDG to correlate the count rate to the phantom activity (Section 2.1).
2. After the calibration, for each scanner, a uniform cylindrical phantom containing ^{90}Y was prepared with the aim to assess the quantitative accuracy of the scanner in reference conditions. Each uniform phantom was prepared following a traceable calibration methodology (Section 2.2). For the first two centers (GH, IRST), accurate activity concentration measurements of a stock ^{90}Y radionuclidic solution were performed

directly at the hospital using the ENEA-INMRI portable Triple-to-Double-Coincidence Ratio (TDCR). For one center (SMG), the activity concentration of the stock solution was measured using the on-site dose calibrator, traceable to a primary standard (Section 2.3).

3. Finally, the ability of each scanner to recover the activity concentration on the uniform phantom was assessed taking into account all possible correction factors (Section 2.4) and sources of uncertainty in the quantification processes (Section 2.5). The two TOF PET scanners available at the GH and IRST sites directly supported ^{90}Y as a viable PET radionuclide, while ^{90}Y was not present in the list of radionuclides accepted by the PET scanner available at the SMG center.
4. Ultimately, a framework is proposed for modeling the uncertainty in the quantification processes, along with an estimation of the uncertainty achievable in clinical conditions (Section 4).

In this study, the quantitative accuracy of ^{90}Y-PET/CT was assessed on the following scanners (Table 1):

- Siemens Biograph mCT Flow: TOF PET/CT scanner (Siemens Medical Solutions, USA) available at IRCCS—Istituto Scientifico Romagnolo per lo Studio dei Tumori (IRST) "Dino Amadori" (Meldola, Italy);
- Siemens Biograph mCT: TOF PET/CT scanner (Siemens Medical Solutions USA) available at Fondazione Policlinino Universitario Agostino Gemelli IRCCS (Rome,Italy)
- GE Discovery DST BGO scanner (General Electric, Milwaukee, WI, USA) available at Ospedale Santa Maria Goretti (Latina, Italy)

Table 1. Italian centers participating in the study, along with their scanners and related calibration source.

Site	Scanner Model	^{90}Y-Supported	PET Calibration Source
Santa Maria Goretti Hospital (SMG), Latina [†]	GE Discovery DST (General Electric, Milwaukee, WI, USA)	No	Cylindrical phantom, ^{18}F solution (2% uncertainty, k = 1)
Gemelli Hospital (GH), Rome [‡]	TOF Siemens Biograph mCT (Siemens Medical Solutions USA)	Yes	Cylindrical phantom, ^{18}F solution (1.7% uncertainty, k = 1)
IRST Tumor Center (IRST), Meldola [‡]	TOF Siemens Biograph mCT Flow (Siemens Medical Solutions USA)	Yes	Cylindrical phantom, ^{18}F solution (1.7% uncertainty, k = 1)

[†] The GE Discovery DST scanner used in the present study does not provide an option for specifying imaging-related parameters for the ^{90}Y radionuclide. [‡] Siemens Biograph mCT scanners support ^{90}Y as a viable radionuclide option (i.e., ^{90}Y is available from the scanner console's radionuclide list).

2. Materials and Methods

2.1. Absolute Scanner Calibration

Absolute activity calibration factors are required to convert voxel values into a measure of absolute activity per voxel. A standard source configuration is generally recommended consisting of a phantom containing a known homogeneous activity concentration. The latter can be measured with the on-site dose calibrator. Traceability to the national standards laboratory for the geometry being measured is essential for activity determination and for uncertainty reduction. However, if activity is determined by a national laboratory, the final uncertainty can be reduced significantly.

Generally, all manufacturers have a standard procedure for the acquisition of radioactivity concentration calibration data, and PET absolute activity calibration is referred to in different terms by different manufacturers (e.g., well-counter calibration, radioactivity calibration factors, or SUV calibration). All PET scanners reported in Table 1 were calibrated using a traceable cylindrical phantom filled with a known amount of ^{18}F (10 min-long scan for each calibration procedure).

The decay-corrected scanner calibration factor, f, can be defined as in Equation (1) [20]:

$$f = \frac{R_c [\text{counts}]}{A_c \left[\frac{\text{kBq}}{\text{mL}}\right]} \quad (1)$$

with R_c representing the total counts inside a given Volume Of Interest (VOI) of the calibration phantom and A_c the decay-corrected activity concentration in the calibration phantom, given by [21]:

$$A_c = \frac{A_0}{V_{ph}} \exp\left(\frac{T_{cal} - T_0}{T_{1/2}} \ln 2\right) \left(\frac{T_{1/2}}{\ln 2}\right) \left[1 - \exp\left(-\frac{T_{acq}}{T_{1/2}} \ln 2\right)\right] \quad (2)$$

where

A_0 is the radionuclide activity used in the calibration procedure,
V_{ph} is the volume of the phantom used in the calibration procedure,
T_0 is the acquisition start time,
T_{cal} is the reference calibration time,
$T_{1/2}$ is the radionuclide physical half-life, and
T_{acq} is the acquisition duration.

Equation (2) shows that accurate and precise activity measurements of the quantity A_0 are an essential pre-requisite of quantitative imaging and dosimetry. The ^{18}F activity (A_0 in Equation (2)) was measured using on-site dose calibrators, traceable to primary standards. Activity concentration measurements were performed with an accuracy within 1.7% (at k = 1 level) for the GH and IRST center and 2% (at k = 1 level) for the SMG center (Table 1).

2.2. Preparation of a Traceable Phantom for ^{90}Y-PET Studies

Quantitative imaging studies rely on phantoms containing a traceable amount of activity concentration. As a general rule, the preparation of a calibrated phantom may be prone to a number of uncertainties. However, the preparation of reference phantoms with a metrological approach provides traceability to measurement results.

In the present study, Diethylenetriaminepentaacetic Acid (DTPA) at a concentration of about 50 µg/g was used to prevent radioactive ^{90}Y from sticking to the phantom walls and to guarantee a homogeneous radionuclide solution. A cylindrical uniform phantom (without any insert) was pre-filled with this carrier solution 12 h prior to the addition of $^{90}YCl_3$, thereby contributing to sealing the phantom's inner walls and reducing sticking or plating activity.

The knowledge of the ^{90}Y activity concentration is required to assess the calibration factor (f) through Equation (1). Therefore, accurate volume measurements were required for accurate activity concentration estimates. The volume V of a liquid solution can be conveniently assessed from mass measurements using a calibrated balance and then introducing the liquid density ρ as follows:

$$V = \frac{m}{\rho} \quad (3)$$

where m is the mass of the radionuclide solution. In the present study, we assumed $\rho = 1$ g/cm^3. In order to minimize weighing uncertainties, small masses were measured using a digital four-decimal place balance provided with a draft shield to prevent air turbulence. Phantom volumes were assessed by the difference, weighing the phantom prior to and after its filling.

As a general rule, the significant factors that contribute to measurement uncertainty across the weighing range are repeatability, eccentricity (the error associated with not placing the weight in the center of the weighing pan), nonlinearity (the error due to the nonlinear behavior of the balance upon increasing the load on the weighing pan), and sensitivity (i.e., systematic deviation). If analytic balances are used for the measurements of small masses, uncertainties below 0.001% can be achieved.

2.3. ^{90}Y Activity Concentration Measurements

For the two centers (GH and IRST) using the Siemens Biograph mCT and Siemens Biograph mCT Flow system, accurate activity concentration measurements of the ^{90}Y radionuclidic solution were performed on-site using the ENEA-INMRI portable TDCR. The TDCR method is a primary absolute activity measurement technique specially developed for pure beta- and pure EC-emitters' activity determination [22]. The activity concentration of the stock ^{90}Y solution was determined with an uncertainty of $\pm 1\%$ (at k = 1 level). For the center SMG, the activity concentration of the stock ^{90}Y solution was measured using the on-site dose calibrator, traceable to a primary standard. In this case, activity concentration measurements were performed with an accuracy within $\pm 2.5\%$ (at k = 1 level).

2.4. Quantitative Imaging on ^{90}Y Clinical Acquisitions

In order to validate the calibration procedure, the uniform ^{90}Y cylindrical phantom (see Section 2.2 for details on the preparation) was imaged, and PET/CT phantom images acquired by each center were reconstructed as reported in Table 2. Each dataset was analyzed using the PMOD software (Version 3.9, PMOD Technologies Ltd., Switzerland). A cylindrical VOI was coaxially outlined at the center of the phantom. To minimize edge effects, the cylindrical VOI was selected excluding the inner boundaries of the phantom (3 cm distance from the edges).

Considering that quantification for different positron-emitting radionuclides by PET systems can be performed with a simple rescaling of pixel values based on (i) the half-life and (ii) the branching ratio for positron emission of the investigated/injected radionuclide, the counts within the VOI need to be corrected as described below.

Table 2. PET/CT image acquisition and reconstruction parameters used by the centers.

Site	True ^{90}Y Activity	Reconstruction Algorithm	Applied Corrections	CT Scan Parameters
SMG—Latina (GE Discovery DST), 16 h scan	273 kBq/mL	3D OSEM (15 subsets, 2 iterations)	Uniformity, attenuation scatter, decay, dead-time, and randomness	120 kV, 60 mAs
GH—Rome (TOF Siemens Biograph mCT), 10 h scan	213 kBq/mL	3D TOF-OSEM (21 subsets, 1 iteration)	Uniformity, attenuation scatter, decay, dead-time, and randomness	120 kV, 50 mAs
IRST—Meldola (TOF Siemens Biograph mCT Flow), 10 h scan	308 kBq/mL	3D TOF-OSEM (21 subsets, 1 iteration)	Uniformity, attenuation scatter, decay, dead-time, and randomness	120 kV, 80 mAs

2.4.1. Half-Life Correction

In the case of ^{90}Y clinical imaging, an adjusted decay constant must be introduced in the system in order to account for the different half-lives of the radionuclide used in the calibration procedure and that of ^{90}Y. This correction is generally performed by the PET scanner. If the scanner does not support this option, a Decay Correction Factor (DCF) must be applied to the reconstructed data using the surrogate radionuclide X reported in Equation (4) [23]:

$$DCF(X \to {}^{90}Y) = \frac{T_{1/2}(X)}{T_{1/2}({}^{90}Y)} \cdot \frac{1 - exp\left[-ln(2) \cdot \frac{T_{acq}}{T_{1/2}(X)}\right]}{1 - exp\left[-ln(2) \cdot \frac{T_{acq}}{T_{1/2}({}^{90}Y)}\right]} \quad (4)$$

$T_{1/2}(X)$ being the physical half-life of the radionuclide X and T_{acq} the PET acquisition duration.

2.4.2. Branching Ratio Correction

In addition, the number of counts needs to be rescaled by the ratio of the β^+ emission probability of the surrogate radionuclide and that of ^{90}Y. In order to obtain the ^{90}Y activity concentration in terms of kBq/mL, the total number of counts in the selected VOI (R) needs to be ultimately rescaled by the ratio of the β^+ emission probability of the used radionuclide ($w_{\beta^+}^X$) and that of ^{90}Y ($w_{\beta^+}^{^{90}Y}$) as:

$$R_{90Y} = \frac{R \cdot (w_{\beta^+}^X)}{(w_{\beta^+}^{^{90}Y})} \text{[counts]} \quad (5)$$

where R_{90Y} is the number of counts of ^{90}Y assessed on the VOI. For scanners that do not support ^{90}Y as a viable radionuclide option, a number of surrogate radionuclides have been used in the published literature. The GE Discovery DST scanner used in the present study does not provide an option for specifying imaging-related parameters for the ^{90}Y isotope, while both Siemens Biograph mCT scanners support ^{90}Y as a viable radionuclide option (i.e., ^{90}Y is available from the scanner console's radionuclide list).

2.4.3. ^{90}Y Quantification

Once the PET scanner has been properly calibrated and ^{90}Y images have been acquired, the absolute ^{90}Y activity concentration in any clinical setting, A_c^{clin}, can be assessed combining Equations (1), (2), and (5):

$$A_c^{clin} = \frac{R_{90Y}}{f} = \frac{R}{R_c} \frac{(w_{\beta^+}^X)}{(w_{\beta^+}^{^{90}Y})} \cdot \frac{A_0}{V_{ph}} exp\left(\frac{T_{cal} - T_0}{T_{1/2}} ln\, 2\right) \left(\frac{T_{1/2}}{ln\, 2}\right) \left[1 - exp\left(-\frac{T_{acq}}{T_{1/2}} ln\, 2\right)\right] \quad (6)$$

2.5. Evaluation of Uncertainty

The Guide to the Expression of Uncertainty in Measurement (GUM) [19] is the standard for the evaluation of measurement uncertainty in metrology. Let $Q_1, Q_2, \ldots, Q_n$ denote a set of n "input" quantities and Y an "output" quantity or measurand. The GUM considers the generic measurement model:

$$Y = f(Q_1, Q_2, \ldots, Q_n),$$

that is a known functional relationship between the input and the output quantities. Given estimates $q_1, q_2, \ldots, q_n$ of the input quantities, the GUM uses

$$y = f(q_1, q_2, \ldots, q_n)$$

as the corresponding estimate of Y. Further, given standard uncertainties $u(q_1), u(q_2), \ldots, u(q_n)$ associated with $q_1, q_2, \ldots, q_n$, the GUM applies the Law of Propagation of Uncertainty (LPU) to evaluate the combined standard uncertainty $u(y)$ associated with y. For independent input quantities, the LPU is described by the following expression:

$$u^2(y) = \left(\frac{\partial f}{\partial q_1}\right)^2 u^2(q_1) + \left(\frac{\partial f}{\partial q_2}\right)^2 u^2(q_2) + \cdots + \left(\frac{\partial f}{\partial q_n}\right)^2 u^2(q_n), \quad (7)$$

in which $\partial f/\partial q_i$ denotes $\partial f/\partial Q_i$ evaluated at $q_1, q_2, \ldots, q_n$.

Equation (7) was used in the present study to assess the relative uncertainty in the activity concentration, $u(A_c^{clin})$, as determined by Equation (6).

3. Results

Equation (7) gives the general form for the relative standard uncertainty associated with y. By applying this relation to Equation (6), the combined standard uncertainty in the final activity concentration, $u(A_c^{clin})$, can be obtained. D'Arienzo and Cox [3] have demonstrated that if the acquisition time is much smaller than the radionuclide half-life (i.e., $T_{acq} \ll T_{1/2}$, as it is for ^{90}Y), in terms of relative standard uncertainties, the uncertainty in the calibration factor, f, reduces to:

$$u_{rel}^2(f) \approx u_{rel}^2(R) + u_{rel}^2(V_{p_h}) + u_{rel}^2(A_0)$$
$$+ \left[\frac{(T_0 - T_{cal})\ln 2}{T_{1/2}}\right]^2 \left[u_{rel}^2(T_0 - T_{cal}) + u_{rel}^2(T_{1/2})\right] + u_{rel}^2(T_{acq}). \quad (8)$$

where $u_{rel}(R)$ is the relative uncertainty in the detected counts, $u_{rel}(V_{ph})$ the relative standard uncertainty associated with the volume measurement (which typically translates into weighing of masses) and $u_{rel}(A_0)$ the relative uncertainty in the calibration activity. The quantity $u_{rel}(T_0 - T_{cal})$ in Equation (8) is the relative standard uncertainty associated with the time difference between the acquisition start time T_0 and the reference calibration time T_{cal}. The relative time offset between the two clocks used to determine T_0 and T_{cal} can be considered representative of $u_{rel}(T_0 - T_{cal})$. Ultimately, $u_{rel}(T_{1/2})$ and $u_{rel}(T_{acq})$ represent the uncertainty in the radionuclide half-life and the acquisition time, respectively.

The final combined relative uncertainty in the activity concentration, $u_{rel}(A_c^{clin})$, can be obtained by adding in quadrature the relative uncertainties of the branching ratios $u_{rel}(w_{\beta^+}^X)$, $u_{rel}(w_{\beta^+}^{90Y})$ and the relative uncertainty on the total detected ^{90}Y counts, $u_{rel}(R_c)$, as:

$$u_{rel}^2(A_c^{clin}) \approx u_{rel}^2(R) + u_{rel}^2(V_{p_h}) + u_{rel}^2(A_0)$$
$$+ \left[\frac{(T_0 - T_{cal})\ln 2}{T_{1/2}}\right]^2 \left[u_{rel}^2(T_0 - T_{cal}) + u_{rel}^2(T_{1/2})\right] + u_{rel}^2(T_{acq})$$
$$+ u_{rel}^2(w_{\beta^+}^X) + u_{rel}^2(w_{\beta^+}^{90Y}) + u_{rel}^2(R_c). \quad (9)$$

Following the above-mentioned procedure, we validated the vendor calibration procedure assessing the ability of each PET scanner to accurately recover the ^{90}Y activity concentration in the uniform ^{90}Y phantom. Overnight PET acquisitions of the uniform phantoms (Figure 1) were performed.

Table 3 compares the reconstructed ^{90}Y activity concentrations versus the measured values for each center, while Table 4 reports the relative uncertainties computed for each center, together with the relative activity uncertainty based on Equation (9).

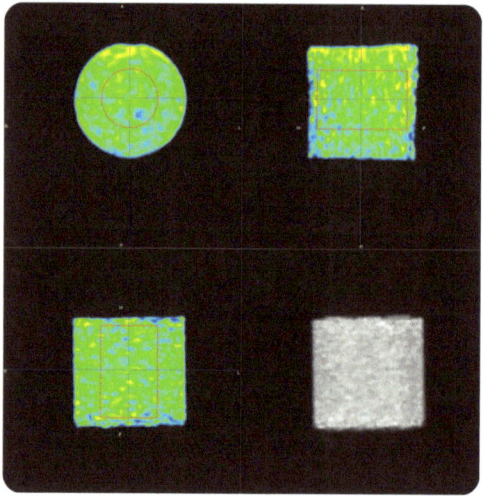

Figure 1. ^{90}Y-PET acquisition of the uniform phantom on the Siemens Biograph mCT Flow.

Table 3. ^{90}Y-PET quantitative accuracy for each center. The ^{90}Y true phantom activity concentration was measured with the on-site dose calibrator for the SMG hospital and with the portable ENEA TDCR for both the IRST and GH centers. Uncertainties in the true phantom activity are reported with a coverage factor of k = 1.

	GE Discovery DST (SMG)	Siemens Biograph mCT Flow (IRST)	Siemens Biograph mCT (GH)
True phantom A_c	(273 ± 7) kBq/mL	(308 ± 3) kBq/mL	(213 ± 2) kBq/mL
Recovered A_c	(257 ± 17) kBq/mL	(325 ± 24) kBq/mL	(207 ± 12) kBq/mL
Deviation	−5.9%	+5.5%	−2.8%

Table 4. ^{90}Y-PET quantitative accuracy in the uniform cylindrical phantom. Relative uncertainties evaluated for each center and variables considered in this study.

Uncertainty Component	GE Discovery DST (SMG)	Siemens Biograph mCT Flow (IRST)	Siemens Biograph mCT (GH)
$u_{\text{rel}}(R_c)$	0.5%	0.5%	0.5%
$u_{\text{rel}}(R)$	6.2%	7.0%	5.5%
$u_{\text{rel}}(V_{ph})$	0.5%	0.5%	0.5%
$u_{\text{rel}}(A_0)$	2.0%	1.7%	1.7%
$u_{\text{rel}}(T_0)$	0.1%	0.1%	0.1%
$u_{\text{rel}}(T_{cal})$	0.1%	0.1%	0.1%
$u_{\text{rel}}(T_{1/2})$	0.1%	0.1%	0.1%
$u_{\text{rel}}(T_{acq})$	0.1%	0.1%	0.1%
$u_{\text{rel}}(w_{\beta^+}^{90Y})$	1.2%	1.2%	1.2%
$u_{\text{rel}}(w_{\beta^+}^{X})$	0.2%	0.2%	0.2%
Acquisition time	16 h	10 h	10 h
$u_{rel}(A_c^{clin})$	**6.6%**	**7.3%**	**5.9%**

The uncertainty in the number of counts, $u(R)$, can be determined with different approaches, depending on the counting statistics. Assuming that the process is dominated by Poisson distributed noise, the uncertainty on the total detected counts can be considered equal to the square root of the total number of detected counts (i.e., $u(R) = \sqrt{R}$). As a general rule, ^{18}F-PET imaging is well described by a Poisson-like distribution. Therefore, in this study, the relative uncertainty in the total counts inside a given VOI of the calibration phantom was determined as $u_{rel}(R_c) = \sqrt{R_c}/R_c$. In particular, $u_{rel}(R_c)$ was conservatively estimated to be about 0.5% for all centers. In fact, the calibration procedure is generally performed using ^{18}F and collecting at least 10^6 counts in the VOI. However, this approach should be used with caution for low counting statistics, as in the case of ^{90}Y-PET, where extremely low count rates are generally observed especially during clinical acquisitions. In the present study, the uncertainty in the ^{90}Y reconstructed images, $u_{rel}(R)$, was determined in terms of the Coefficient Of Variation (COV) (i.e., the ratio of the standard deviation (sd) to the mean value, i.e., $u_{rel}(R) = sd/R$. The uncertainty in the volume of the phantom used in the calibration procedure, $u_{rel}(V_{ph})$, was estimated to be about 0.5%. The uncertainty in the calibration activity, $u_{rel}(A_0)$, was determined to be 2.0% (k = 1) for the SMG center and 1.7% (k = 1) for IRST and GH. All participating centers measured the calibration activity using the on-site radionuclide dose calibrator traceable to national laboratories. Methods to determine dose calibrator uncertainty are extensively described by Gadd et al. [24]. With a conservative approach, the uncertainty in $u_{rel}(T_{cal})$, $u_{rel}(T_0)$, $u_{rel}(T_{acq})$, and $u_{rel}(T_{1/2})$ was assumed to be in the order of 0.1%. Ultimately, the uncertainty in the decay branching ratio of $u_{rel}(w_{\beta^+}^{90Y})$ and $u_{rel}(w_{\beta^+}^{X})$ was assumed to be 1.2% [25] and 0.2% [26], respectively.

The relative difference in the reconstructed activity concentration varied from −5.9% (SMG) to +5.5% (IRST). Of note, the two centers (GH and IRST) operating with the same PET scanner used different post-reconstruction Gaussian filter sizes (i.e., 6 mm for GH and 2 mm for IRST). Most likely, the lower uncertainty in the counts associated with the GH center ($u_R = 5.5\%$) can be attributed to the use of a larger Gaussian filter, responsible for a greater smoothing of the image. This ultimately resulted in an overall lower uncertainty on the recovered activity, $u_{rel}(A_c^{clin})$ (5.9% vs. 7.3%; Figure 2 and Table 4).

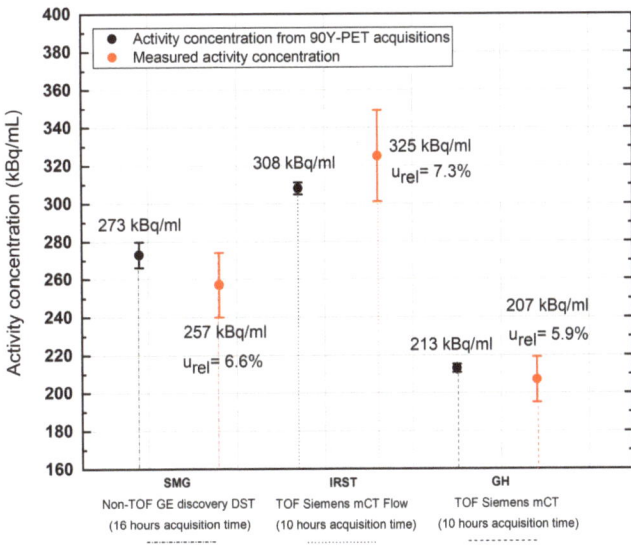

Figure 2. Comparison of recovered activity concentration values in the uniform phantom versus true activity concentration values at the three Italian sites. Acquisition time: 16 h for SMG; 10 h for IRST and GH.

Figure 3 compares the activity concentration recovered with the PMOD 3.9 software ($A_{c,PMOD}$) in the uniform phantom imaged at the GH center with the activity concentration provided by the supplier (±5% uncertainty at the k = 1 level ($A_{c,suppl}$)) and the activity concentration measured with the ENEA-INMRI portable TDCR system (±1.0% at the k = 1 level ($A_{c,TDCR}$)). For the same center, Figure 4 shows the relative standard deviation in the recovered activity concentration as a function of the acquisition time. A total of thirteen acquisitions were performed: from 30 min to 4 h (increasing each new acquisition by 30 min) and from 4 h to 10 h (increasing each new acquisition by 1 h). Of note, for typical clinical acquisitions (±30 min), the COV is in the order of 30% due to the extremely low counts and high random fraction associated with ^{90}Y-β^+ decay. This may possibly introduce a relevant source of uncertainty in patient dosimetry.

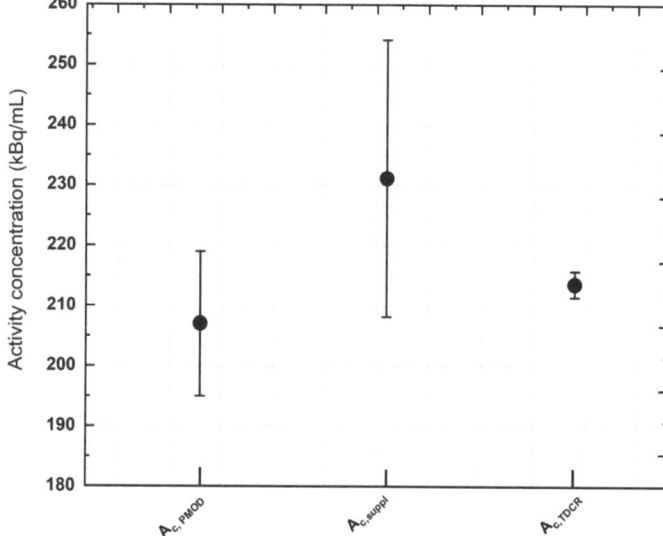

Figure 3. An example of activity concentration assessment performed during the study. The activity concentration recovered with the PMOD 3.9 software ($A_{c,PMOD}$) in the uniform phantom imaged at GH was compared with the activity concentration provided by the supplier ($A_{c,suppl}$) (±5% uncertainty, coverage factor of k = 1) and the activity concentration measured with the ENEA-INMRI portable TDCR portable system ($A_{c,TDCR}$) (±1.0%, coverage factor of k = 1). All activity concentration values lie within the stated uncertainties, with the latter method (TDCR) providing the most-accurate measurement.

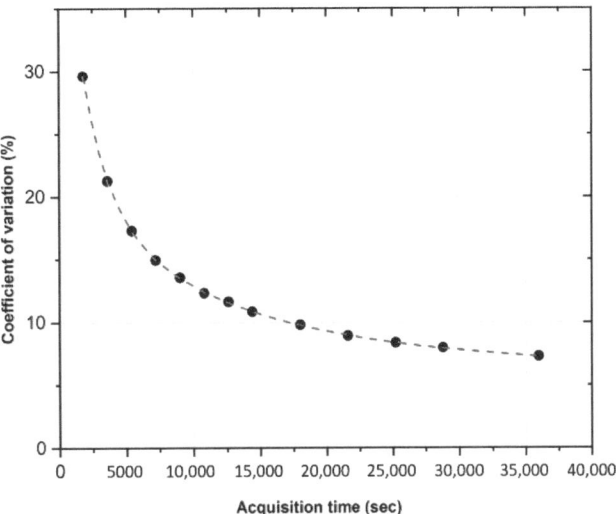

Figure 4. COV evaluation of the activity concentration versus PET acquisition time. Acquisition on the cylindrical phantom uniformly filled with ^{90}Y.

4. Discussion

The determination of the absorbed dose in MRT practice is an essential part of the management of the treatment of each individual patient. In fact, it is a requirement in EC Directive 97/43 Euratom, which states that, for radiotherapeutic purposes, *"exposures of target volumes shall be individually planned"*. The purpose of this study is to establish a traceable workflow for accurate quantitative ^{90}Y-PET imaging with the intention of relating the uncertainty of the output quantity (recovered activity concentration) to the uncertainty of the input data. In fact, in clinical practice, quantitative data are used for radiation dose assessment; therefore, uncertainties in the initial quantities propagate directly into the dose calculation.

The issue of the role and involvement of metrology institutes in quantitative imaging and the entire dosimetric process is not new and has been addressed by several authors in past [4,6,7] and recent [27] research. In conventional External Beam Radiotherapy (EBRT), individual patient dosimetry is mandatory, strictly controlled according to agreed protocols, and there is full traceability to primary standards. In contrast, for nuclear medicine, the role of the metrology institutes is less clear and the calculation of the administered absorbed doses is not traceable in the same manner as EBRT [27]. The need for metrology support is particularly true for difficult-to-measure radionuclides such as ^{90}Y [27].

In the present study, the low counting statistics related to ^{90}Y-PET acquisitions ($u_{rel}(R)$), the uncertainty of the source activity used in the PET system calibration ($u_{rel}(A_0)$), and the uncertainty in the ^{90}Y internal pair production branching ratio ($u_{rel}(w_{\beta^+}^{^{90}Y})$) are the main factors contributing to the final uncertainty of the recovered activity concentration.

The issue of poor image quality related to the low counting statistics associated with the ^{90}Y internal pair production has already been addressed in several literature works and will not be covered here. The reader is referred to [28–31] for further insights

Past research [32] showed the measurement of the calibration factor as being one of the major sources of uncertainties in the dose measurements (together with the uncertainty related to the positive bias due to the intrinsic radioactivity of scanner's crystals). In this work, thanks to the long acquisition time, the relative uncertainties in the recovered ^{90}Y activity concentration were found to be in the range of $\simeq$6–7% depending on the scanner model and, most importantly, on the availability of the TOF technology. It should be noted that, in the present study, the overnight phantom acquisition reflected a relatively uniform image, thereby providing a coefficient of variation in the counting statistics ($u_{rel}(R)$) (Equation (9)) in the order of 5.5–7%. In clinical conditions, a shorter acquisition time is likely to produce larger uncertainties, which may impair both qualitative and quantitative results.

Most notably, few researchers have addressed the importance of phantom preparation. In a past study, Sunderland and colleagues [33] demonstrated that technical error in phantom filling is one of the primary reasons for the exclusion of PET/CT scanners from clinical trials. In addition, the adsorption of radionuclides on the inner walls of plastic phantoms may lead to an inhomogeneous radionuclide distribution, which can negatively affect quantitative imaging studies [34]. Therefore, the preparation of a carrier solution is recommended. The use of tap water should be avoided as minerals and other chemical impurities might stick to the phantom walls or combine with the radiopharmaceuticals, changing the radionuclide distribution. For ^{90}Y-PET studies, ^{90}YCl$_3$ in an aqueous solution of 0.1 mol/dm^3 hydrochloric acid also containing inactive Yttrium at a concentration of about 50 µg/g can be used as a carrier solution. Alternatively, Diethylenetriaminepentaacetic Acid (DTPA) or Ethylenediaminetetraacetic Acid (ETPA) at a concentration of about 50 µg/g can be used to prevent radioactive ^{90}Y from sticking to the phantom walls and to guarantee a homogeneous radionuclide solution. It is recommended that all containers be pre-filled with the carrier 12 h prior to the addition of radioactive ^{90}YCl$_3$. This will help to "seal" the surface and reduce sticking or plating activity. All containers should be emptied, dried, and the used carrier discarded before activity is added. As a general rule, the preparation of a stock solution is recommended. Radioactive ^{90}Y provided by the supplier should be diluted using the carrier solution to the desired volume and concentration. The activity concentration should be determined by measuring an aliquot of the stock solution in terms of the activity per unit mass (or volume). This can then be used to determine the activity of all subsequent sources produced from this stock solution. Filling of the phantoms should be performed using a calibrated (preferably four decimal places) analytic scientific scale and with routine double or triple weighting of the sources. The overall uncertainty in the activity concentration determined using this method is dependent on the precision of the scale being used, as well as the accuracy of the method used to determine the activity concentration of the solution. Radioactivity should be dispensed using calibrated pipette devices or syringes and ensuring that no air bubbles remain in the phantom. If large background volumes are used for calibration purposes, the phantom can be filled with non-radioactive water to measure the fillable volume (and to confirm the phantom is watertight with no leaks). When filling large phantom volumes, a funnel should be used. When the phantom is nearly full, the funnel can be removed and a syringe used to complete the filling process, thereby preventing spillage of radioactive water from the background compartment.

One of the major drawbacks of quantitative imaging with ^{90}Y microspheres is related to the quick microsphere sedimentation over time. Therefore, in order to have a homogeneous solution, phantom calibration studies need to be performed with ^{90}Y chloride (^{90}YCl$_3$) instead of ^{90}Y microspheres. The instrument typically used to measure the administered activity to patients in nuclear medicine procedures is the radionuclide dose calibrator. Recent [35–37] and previous [38] findings reported difficulties of measuring ^{90}Y chloride and other beta emitters using clinically available ionization chambers. This is because dose calibrators available in the clinical nuclear medicine contextperform activity measurements of beta-emitting radionuclides indirectly, by detecting bremsstrahlung emissions. Bremsstrahlung production is highly dependent on the source material, its container, and the calibrator chamber wall. The ionization current also depends on the probability of electron detection within the chamber, which varies with electron energy and individual dose calibrator construction. Moreover, slight variations in the container wall thickness, solution volume, or location within the well can lead to an increase in the overall assay uncertainty when using the manufacturer-supplied calibration factor, which is typically traceable to national standards. For activity measurements of ^{90}YCl$_3$ at a clinical level, it is expected that radionuclide dose calibrators provide accuracy within ±5% (at k = 2 level) [24,39]. However, if the activity is determined by a national metrology institute, uncertainty on the activity concentration can be reduced dramatically. Primary activity standards for ^{90}Y are widely available, and measurement uncertainties below 1% can be achieved [40,41].

Ultimately, another key factor impacting the achievable quantitative accuracy is the uncertainty in the ^{90}Y branching ratio. In 2007, Selwyn et al. [42] determined the branching ratio related to β^+/β^- pair production during ^{90}Y decay to be $(31.86 \pm 0.47) \times 10^{-6}$, following de-excitation from the 0^+ excited state of ^{90}Zr. Recently, the internal pair production branching ratio of ^{90}Y was experimentally determined by the Czech Metrology Institute (CMI) and the National Institute of Standards and Technology (NIST). Dryák and Šolc [25] provided a branching ratio of $(32.6 \pm 0.4) \times 10^{-6}$. Along the same lines, Pibida and colleagues [43] estimated the internal pair production branching ratio to be $(32 \pm 1.5) \times 10^{-6}$ (k = 1), resulting in being within one standard uncertainty with the recommended value of $(32.6 \pm 0.7) \times 10^{-6}$ (k = 1) from the Decay Data Evaluation Project (DDEP) database [26].

Accurate determination of the absorbed dose from ^{90}Y-PET requires accurate evaluation of the radiopharmaceutical localization, adding considerable additional complexity to the dosimetry workflow. The translation of ^{90}Y-PET quantitative data into an accurate dose distribution within the patient is complex, and at present, there is no clear understanding or quantification of the uncertainty involved in ^{90}Y-PET image-based dosimetry in clinical conditions. For clinical reasons, an overall uncertainty below 10% is desirable, and future research should be devoted to identifying major sources of error in the processes involved in the measurement of the absorbed dose and quantify them in terms of the modeling and uncertainty analysis.

5. Conclusions

In this study, we have proposed a workflow for ^{90}Y-PET validation, along with a procedure to assess the uncertainty in the recovered activity, based on the law of propagation of uncertainties (GUM uncertainty approach). In this work, the relative standard uncertainty in the recovered activity was in the range $\simeq$6–7%. However, the shorter acquisition time generally used during clinical acquisition is likely to produce larger uncertainties, which may impair both qualitative and quantitative results. More generally, the low counting statistics related to ^{90}Y-PET acquisitions, the uncertainty of the source activity used in the PET system calibration, and the uncertainty in the ^{90}Y internal pair production branching ratio appear to be the main factors contributing to the final uncertainty of the recovered activity concentration.

Author Contributions: Conceptualization, M.D., E.M. and A.S.; methodology, O.B.; software, A.C. and M.D. validation, O.B. and L.F.; formal analysis, M.D., E.M. and M.C.; investigation, M.D. and E.M.; resources, M.C.; data curation, M.D., E.M., A.C. and L.I.; writing—original draft preparation, M.D. and E.M.; writing—review and editing, M.D., E.M., A.S. and A.C.; supervision, L.I. and A.S.. All authors have read and agreed to the published version of the manuscript.

Funding: This work was partly supported thanks to the contribution of Ricerca Corrente by the Italian Ministry of Health within the research line "Innovative therapies, phase I–III clinical trials and therapeutic strategy trials based on preclinical models, onco-immunological mechanisms and nanovectors".

Institutional Review Board Statement: Not applicable.

Informed Consent Statement: Not applicable.

Data Availability Statement: Not applicable.

Acknowledgments: The authors are grateful to Paola Chiaramida (Product Clinical Specialist in Molecular Imaging, GE Healthcare) and Jacopo Anghilieri (Molecular Imaging Product Sales Expert Marketing, Siemens Healthineers) for their support and valuable suggestions related to the PET systems.

Conflicts of Interest: The authors declare no conflict of interest.

Abbreviations

The following abbreviations are used in this manuscript:

MRT	Molecular Radiation Therapy
MetroMRT	Metrology for Molecular Radiation Therapy
MRTDosimetry	Molecular Radiation Therapy Dosimetry
TARE	Transarterial Radioembolization
GUM	Guide to the Expression of Uncertainty in Measurements
EANM	European Association of Nuclear Medicine
TDCR	Triple-to-Double-Coincidence Ratio
DTPA	Diethylenetriaminepentaacetic Acid
PET	Positron Emission Tomography
TOF	Time Of Flight

References

1. Sgouros, G.; Bodei, L.; McDevitt, M.R.; Nedrow, J.R. Radiopharmaceutical therapy in cancer: Clinical advances and challenges. *Nat. Rev. Drug Discov.* **2020**, *19*, 589–608. [CrossRef]
2. Gear, J.I.; Cox, M.G.; Gustafsson, J.; Gleisner, K.S.; Murray, I.; Glatting, G.; Konijnenberg, M. EANM practical guidance on uncertainty analysis for molecular ra-diotherapy absorbed dose calculations. *Eur. J. Nucl. Med. Mol. Imaging* **2018**, *45*, 2456–2474. [CrossRef]
3. D'Arienzo, M.; Cox, M. Uncertainty analysis in the calibration of an emission tomography system for quantitative imaging. *Comput. Math. Methods Med.* **2017**, *2017*, 9830386. [CrossRef]
4. D'Arienzo, M.; Capogni, M.; Smyth, V.; Cox, M.; Johansson, L.; Solc, J.; Bobin, C.; Rabus, H.; Joulaeizadeh, L. Metrological Issues in Molecular Radiotherapy. *EPJ Web Conf.* **2014**, *77*, 22. [CrossRef]
5. Tran-Gia, J.; Salas-Ramirez, M.; Lassmann, M. What you see is not what you get: On the accuracy of voxel-based dosimetry in molecular radiotherapy. *J. Nucl. Med.* **2020**, *61*, 1178–1186. [CrossRef]
6. MetroMRT—Metrology for Molecular Radiation Therapy. Available online: http://projects.npl.co.uk/metromrt/ (accessed on 11 July 2023).
7. MRTDosimetry. Available online: https://osf.io/69nge/ (accessed on 11 July 2023).
8. Pasciak, A.S.; Bourgeois, A.C.; McKinney, J.M.; Chang, T.T.; Osborne, D.R.; Acuff, S.N.; Bradley, Y.C. Radioembolization and the dynamic role of 90Y-PET/CT. *Front. Oncol.* **2014**, *4*, 38. [CrossRef]
9. Ungania, S.; D'Arienzo, M.; Mezzenga, E.; Pizzi, G.; Vallati, G.; Ianiro, A.; Rea, S.; Sciuto, R.; Soriani, A.; Strigari, L. A Workflow for Dosimetry of 90Y Radio-embolization Based on Quantitative 99mTc-MAA SPECT/CT Imaging and a 3D-Printed Phantom. *Appl. Sci.* **2022**, *12*, 10541. [CrossRef]
10. Willowson, K.P.; Tapner, M.; QUEST Investigator Team; Bailey, D.L. A multicenter comparison of quantitative 90 Y-PET/CT for dosimetric purposes after radioembolization with resin microspheres: The QUEST phantom study. *Eur. J. Nucl. Med. Mol. Imaging* **2015**, *42*, 1202–1222. [CrossRef]
11. Gates, V.L.; Esmail, A.A.; Marshall, K.; Spies, S.; Salem, R. Internal pair production of 90Y permits hepatic localization of microspheres using routine PET: Proof of concept. *J. Nucl. Med.* **2011**, *52*, 72–76. [CrossRef]
12. D'Arienzo, M. Emission of β+ Particles Via Internal Pair Production in the 0+ − 0+ Transition of 90Zr: Historical Background and Current Applications in Nuclear Medicine Imaging. *Atoms* **2013**, *1*, 2–12. [CrossRef]
13. Spreafico, C.; Maccauro, M.; Mazzaferro, V.; Chiesa, C. The dosimetric importance of the number of 90 Y microspheres in liver transarterial radioembolization (TARE). *Eur. J. Nucl. Med. Mol. Imaging* **2014**, *41*, 634–638. [CrossRef]
14. Hardy-Abeloos, C.; Lazarev, S.; Ru, M.; Kim, E.; Fischman, A.; Moshier, E.; Rosenzweig, K.; Buckstein, M. Safety and efficacy of liver stereotactic body radiation therapy for hepatocellular carcinoma after segmental transarterial radioembolization. *Int. J. Radiat. Oncol. Biol. Phys.* **2019**, *105*, 968–976. [CrossRef]
15. Tomozawa, Y.; Jahangiri, Y.; Pathak, P.; Kolbeck, K.J.; Schenning, R.C.; Kaufman, J.A.; Farsad, K. Long-term toxicity after transarterial radioembolization with yttrium-90 using resin microspheres for neuroendocrine tumor liver metastases. *J. Vasc. Interv. Radiol.* **2018**, *29*, 858–865. [CrossRef]
16. Milano, A.; Gil, A.V.; Fabrizi, E.; Cremonesi, M.; Veronese, I.; Gallo, S.; Lanconelli, N.; Faccini, R.; Pacilio, M. In Silico Validation of MCID Platform for Monte Carlo-Based Voxel Dosimetry Applied to 90Y-Radioembolization of Liver Malignancies. *Appl. Sci.* **2021**, *11*, 1939. [CrossRef]
17. Pistone, D.; Italiano, A.; Auditore, L.; Mandaglio, G.; Campenní, A.; Baldari, S.; Amato, E. Relevance of artefacts in99mTc-MAA SPECT scans on pre-therapy pa-tient-specific90Y TARE internal dosimetry: A GATE Monte Carlo study. *Phys. Med. Biol.* **2022**, *67*, 115002. [CrossRef]

18. JCGM Joint Committee for Guides in Metrology. *Evaluation of Measurement Data—Guide to the Expression of Uncertainty in Measurement*; JCM 100:2008. Available online: https://www.bipm.org/documents/20126/2071204/JCGM_100_2008_E.pdf (accessed on 11 July 2023).
19. van der Veen, A.M.; Cox, M.G.; Possolo, A. GUM guidance on developing and using measurement models. *Accredit. Qual. Assur.* **2022**, *27*, 295–297. [CrossRef]
20. Cherry, S.; Sorenson, J.; Phelps, M. *Physics in Nuclear Medicine*; Elsevier/Saunders: Philadelphia, PA, USA, 2012.
21. National Electrical Manufacturers Association. *Performance Measurements of Gamma Cameras*; NEMA NU 1-2007; National Electrical Manufacturers Association: Rosslyn, VA, USA, 2007.
22. Capogni, M.; De Felice, P.A. Prototype of a portable TDCR system at ENEA. *Appl. Radiat. Isot.* **2014**, *93*, 45–51. [CrossRef]
23. Goedicke, A.; Berker, Y.; Verburg, F.; Behrendt, F.; Winz, O.; Mottaghy, F. Study-Parameter Impact in Quantitative 90-Yttrium PET Imaging for Radioembolization Treatment Monitoring and Dosimetry. *IEEE Trans. Med. Imaging* **2013**, *32*, 485–492. [CrossRef]
24. Gadd, R.; Baker, M.; Nijran, K.S.; Owens, S.; Thomas, W.; Woods, M.J.; Zananiri, F. *Measurement Good Practice Guide No. 93: Protocol for Establishing and Maintaining the Calibration of Medical Radionuclide Calibrators and Their Quality Control*; National Physical Laboratory: Teddington, UK, 2006.
25. Dryák, P.; Šolc, J. Measurement of the branching ratio related to the internal pair production of Y-90. *Appl. Radiat. Isot.* **2020**, *156*, 108942. [CrossRef]
26. Decay Data Evaluation Project (DDEP) Database. Available online: http://www.lnhb.fr/ddep_wg/ (accessed on 22 April 2023).
27. Fenwick, A.J.; Wevrett, J.L.; Ferreira, K.M.; Denis-Bacelar, A.M.; Robinson, A.P. Quantitative imaging, dosimetry and metrology; Where do National Metrology Institutes fit in? *Appl. Radiat. Isot.* **2018**, *134*, 74–78. [CrossRef]
28. Carlier, T.; Willowson, K.P.; Fourkal, E.; Bailey, D.L.; Doss, M.; Conti, M. (90)Y -PET imaging: Exploring limitations and accuracy under conditions of low counts and high random fraction. *Med. Phys.* **2015**, *42*, 4295–4309. [CrossRef]
29. Strydhorst, J.; Carlier, T.; Dieudonné, A.; Conti, M.; Buvat, I. A gate evaluation of the sources of error in quantitative 90Y-PET. *Med. Phys.* **2016**, *43*, 5320. [CrossRef]
30. Capotosti, A.; Moretti, R.; Milano, A.; Nardini, M.; Cusumano, D.; Annunziata, S.; Capogni, M.; D'Arienzo, M.; Placidi, L.; Indovina, L. Up-to-Date Optimization of the 90Y-PET/CT Reconstruction Protocol for Volumetric Quantification in Trans-Arterial Ra-dioEmbolization (TARE) Procedures in the Era of Theranostics. *Appl. Sci.* **2022**, *12*, 8418. [CrossRef]
31. Tapp, K.N.; Lea, W.B.; Johnson, M.S.; Tann, M.; Fletcher, J.W.; Hutchins, G.D. The impact of image reconstruction bias on PET/CT 90Y dosimetry after radioembolization. *J. Nucl. Med. Off. Publ. Soc. Nucl. Med.* **2014**, *55*, 1452–1458. [CrossRef]
32. Fourkal, E.; Veltchev, I.; Lin, M.; Koren, S.; Meyer, J.; Doss, M.; Yu, J.Q. 3D inpatient dose reconstruction from the PET-CT imaging of 90Y microspheres for metastatic cancer to the liver: Feasibility study. *Med. Phys.* **2013**, *40*, 081702. [CrossRef]
33. Sunderland, J.; Christian, P.; Kiss, T. (2015) PET/CT scanner validation for clinical trials-reasons for failure, recipes for success: The Clinical Trials Network (CTN) experience. *J. Nucl. Med.* **2015**, *56*, 1737.
34. Park, M.A.; Mahmood, A.; Zimmerman, R.E.; Limpa-Amara, N.; Makrigiorgos, G.M.; Moore, S.C. Adsorption of metallic radionuclides on plastic phantom walls. *Med. Phys.* **2008**, *35*, 1606–1610. [CrossRef]
35. Fenwick, A.; Baker, M.; Ferreira, K.; Keightley, J. Comparison of Y-90 Measurements in UK Hospitals, NPL Report IR 20. 2011. Available online: https://eprintspublications.npl.co.uk/5213/1/IR20.pdf (accessed on 11 July 2023).
36. Ferreira, K.; Fenwick, A.; Arinc, A.; Johansson, L. Standardisation of 90Y and determination of calibration factors for 90Y microspheres (resin) for the NPL secondary ionisation chamber and a Capintec CRC-25R. *Appl. Radiat. Isot.* **2015**, *109*, 226–230.
37. Kossert, K.; Bokeloh, K.; Ehlers, M.; Nähle, O.; Scheibe, O.; Schwarz, U.; Thieme, K. Comparison of 90Y activity measurements in nuclear medicine in Germany. *Appl. Radiat. Isot.* **2015**, *109*, 247–249. [CrossRef]
38. Woods, M.; Munster, A.; Sephton, J.; Lucas, S.; Walsh, C. Calibration of the NPL secondary standard radionuclide calibrator for 32P, 89Sr and 90Y. *Nucl. Instrum. Methods Phys. Res. Sect. A Accel. Spectrometers Detect. Assoc. Equip.* **1996**, *369*, 698–702. [CrossRef]
39. AAPM Task Group 181, The Selection, Use, Calibration, and Quality Assurance of Radionuclide Calibrators Used in Nuclear Medicine (2012) Report of AAPM Task Group 181. Available online: https://www.aapm.org/pubs/reports/rpt_181.pdf (accessed on 11 July 2023).
40. Zimmerman, B.; Ratel, G. Report of the CIPM Key Comparison CCRI(II)-K2 Y-90. Metrologia 42, 06001. 2005. Available online: https://iopscience.iop.org/article/10.1088/0026-1394/42/1A/06001/meta (accessed on 11 July 2023).
41. Dezarn, W.; Kennedy, A. SU-FF-T-380: Significant differences exist across institutions in 90Y activities compared to reference standard. *Med. Phys.* **2007**, *34*, 2489. [CrossRef]
42. Selwyn, R.G.; Nicles, R.J.; Thomadsen, B.R.; DeWerd, L.A.; Micka, J.A. A new internal pair production branching ratio of 90Y: The development of a non-destructive assay for 90Y and 90Sr. *Appl. Radiat. Isot.* **2007**, *65*, 318–327 [CrossRef] [PubMed]
43. Pibida, L.; Zimmerman, B.E.; King, L.; Fitzgerald, R.; Bergeron, D.E.; Napoli, E.; Cessna, J.T. Determination of the internal pair production branching ratio of 90Y. *Appl. Radiat. Isot. Incl. Data Instrum. Methods Use Agric. Ind. Med.* **2020**, *156*, 108943. [CrossRef]

Disclaimer/Publisher's Note: The statements, opinions and data contained in all publications are solely those of the individual author(s) and contributor(s) and not of MDPI and/or the editor(s). MDPI and/or the editor(s) disclaim responsibility for any injury to people or property resulting from any ideas, methods, instructions or products referred to in the content.

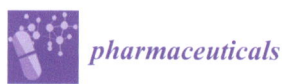

Article

Image-Based Dosimetry in Dogs and Cross-Reactivity with Human Tissues of IGF2R-Targeting Human Antibody

Kevin J. H. Allen [1,†], Ohyun Kwon [2,†], Matthew R. Hutcheson [3], Joseph J. Grudzinski [4], Stuart M. Cain [5], Frederic A. Cruz [5], Remitha M. Vinayakamoorthy [5], Ying S. Sun [5], Lindsay Fairley [5], Chandra B. Prabaharan [6], Ryan Dickinson [7], Valerie MacDonald-Dickinson [8], Maruti Uppalapati [6], Bryan P. Bednarz [2] and Ekaterina Dadachova [1,*]

[1] College of Pharmacy and Nutrition, University of Saskatchewan, Saskatoon, SK S7N 5E5, Canada; kja782@mail.usask.ca
[2] Department of Medical Physics, University of Wisconsin-Madison, Madison, WI 53705, USA; okwon25@wisc.edu (O.K.); bbednarz2@wisc.edu (B.P.B.)
[3] Safety Resources, University of Saskatchewan, Saskatoon, SK S7N 5E5, Canada; matt.hutcheson@usask.ca
[4] Department of Radiology, University of Wisconsin-Madison, Madison, WI 53705, USA; grudzinski@wisc.edu
[5] adMare BioInnovations, Vancouver, BC V6T 1Z3, Canada; scain@admarebio.com (S.M.C.); ecruz@admarebio.com (F.A.C.); remithaaa@gmail.com (R.M.V.); ssun@admarebio.com (Y.S.S.); lfairley@admarebio.com (L.F.)
[6] Department of Pathology and Laboratory Medicine, College of Medicine, University of Saskatchewan, Saskatoon, SK S7N 5E5, Canada; chp347@mail.usask.ca (C.B.P.); maruti.uppalapati@usask.ca (M.U.)
[7] Department of Veterinary Pathology, Western College of Veterinary Medicine, University of Saskatchewan, Saskatoon, SK S7N 5B4, Canada; ryan.dickinson@usask.ca
[8] Department of Small Animal Clinical Sciences, Western College of Veterinary Medicine, University of Saskatchewan, Saskatoon, SK S7N 5B4, Canada; valerie.macdonald@usask.ca
* Correspondence: ekaterina.dadachova@usask.ca
† These authors have contributed equally to this work.

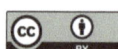

Abstract: Background: Osteosarcoma (OS) represents the most common primary bone tumor in humans and in companion dogs, being practically phenotypically identical. There is a need for effective treatments to extend the survival of patients with OS. Here, we examine the dosimetry in beagle dogs and cross-reactivity with human tissues of a novel human antibody, IF3, that targets the insulin growth factor receptor type 2 (IGF2R), which is overexpressed on OS cells, making it a candidate for radioimmunotherapy of OS. Methods: [^{89}Zr]Zr-DFO-IF3 was injected into three healthy beagle dogs. PET/CT was conducted at 4, 24, 48, and 72 h. RAPID analysis was used to determine the dosimetry of [^{177}Lu]Lu-CHXA''-IF3 for a clinical trial in companion dogs with OS. IF3 antibody was biotinylated, and a multitude of human tissues were assessed with immunohistochemistry. Results: PET/CT revealed that only the liver, bone marrow, and adrenal glands had high uptake. Clearance was initially through renal and hepatobiliary excretion in the first 72 h followed by primarily physical decay. RAPID analysis showed bone marrow to be the dose-limiting organ with a therapeutic range for ^{177}Lu calculated to be 0.487–0.583 GBq. Immunohistochemistry demonstrated the absence of IGF2R expression on the surface of healthy human cells, thus suggesting that radioimmunotherapy with [^{177}Lu]Lu-CHXA''-IF3 will be well tolerated. Conclusions: Image-based dosimetry has defined a safe therapeutic range for canine clinical trials, while immunohistochemistry has suggested that the antibody will not cross-react with healthy human tissues.

Keywords: IGF2R; osteosarcoma; image-based dosimetry RAPID; ^{89}Zr; ^{177}Lu; tissue cross-reactivity; PET/CT

1. Introduction

Osteosarcoma (OS) represents the most common malignant primary bone tumor in dogs and humans and is responsible for 85–98% of malignancies forming in the skeleton in dogs [1] and 55% in children and adolescents [2]. Canine OS carries a poor prognosis with approximately 90% of affected dogs developing pulmonary metastases. The median survival time of dogs treated with amputation alone is only 4 months [3]. In human patients, the overall survival has similarly plateaued at approximately 70% with no meaningful improvement achieved within the last 25 years [2]. Thus, new therapeutic approaches to treating OS are urgently needed for both human and canine patients. The significance of the current study is the evaluation of a human antibody as a potential radioimmunotherapy agent for OS in vivo in canines and in vitro in human tissues.

A decade ago, insulin growth factor receptor type 2 (IGF2R) was identified as being overexpressed on the surface of all commercially available and human patient-derived OS cells [4]. These findings were later expanded to 34 consecutive cases of dogs with OS with all of them displaying some degree of IGF2R expression in the majority of the neoplastic osteoblasts [5]. As murine antibodies are not suitable for clinical trials in human patients because of immunogenicity issues, we created and molecularly characterized novel human antibodies to IGF2R that bind to human, canine, and murine forms of IGF2R [6]. The binding of these human antibodies to murine IGF2R would enable the initial evaluation of RIT efficacy and safety in mice with human OS xenografts, while the binding to canine IGF2R would afford a comparative oncology approach by treating OS-afflicted companion dogs with RIT. We have subsequently evaluated one of these antibodies, IF3, in severe combined immunodeficiency (SCID) mice bearing canine OS xenografts. In vivo single photon emission computed tomography/computed tomography (SPECT/CT) imaging revealed uptake of the IF3 antibody in the neoplastic cells of these xenografts [7]. When radiolabeled with therapeutic radionuclide ^{177}Lu, the IF3 antibody significantly slowed down the growth of the xenograft tumors [7]. However, the biodistribution of IF3 in a larger animal model such as dogs and its potential cross-reactivity with human tissues remained to be investigated.

It is critical to study the safety and efficacy of theranostic agents that deliver therapeutic agents near organs at risk, particularly lymphoid organs (bone marrow, spleen, thymus, draining lymphatics). Furthermore, dosimetry calculations using canines should be more reliable for extrapolation to humans than mouse models. Here, we addressed the need for biodistribution and dosimetry data as well as for antibody cross-reactivity by performing image-based dosimetry estimations for [^{177}Lu]Lu-CHXA"-IF3 antibody derived from the positron emission tomography/computed tomography (PET/CT) imaging of healthy beagle dogs with [^{89}Zr]Zr-DFO-IF3 using PET/CT as well as tissue cross-reactivity evaluation of IF3 antibody with normal human tissues.

2. Results

2.1. [^{89}Zr]Zr-DFO-IF3 Antibody Demonstrated Urinary and Hepatobiliary Excretion

Figure 1A,B shows the urinary and hepatobiliary excretion of [^{89}Zr]Zr-DFO-IF3 after IV administration to the dogs. Most of the excretion took place within 73 h after administration, while after hours physical decay was primarily responsible for the elimination of ^{89}Zr. The dose rate at 30 cm from the dog's body surface fell from 12 μSv/h right after [^{89}Zr]Zr-DFO-IF3 administration to 5 μSv/h at 48 h post administration (Figure 1C), which would allow the dogs to be released to their owners if companion dogs would be used in place of research dogs.

2.2. PET/CT Imaging Revealed Liver, Adrenals, and Bone Marrow as the Highest Uptake Organs

Figures 2–4 display the maximum image projections (MIPs) of the dogs at four time points post [^{89}Zr]Zr-DFO-IF3 administration and the pharmacokinetics information derived from those images. The organs with the highest [^{89}Zr]Zr-DFO-IF3 uptake were, in decreasing order, the liver, adrenals, and marrow in the spine and the shoulders. The antibody was quickly cleared from the heart, and its retention in the testis and whole body was very low.

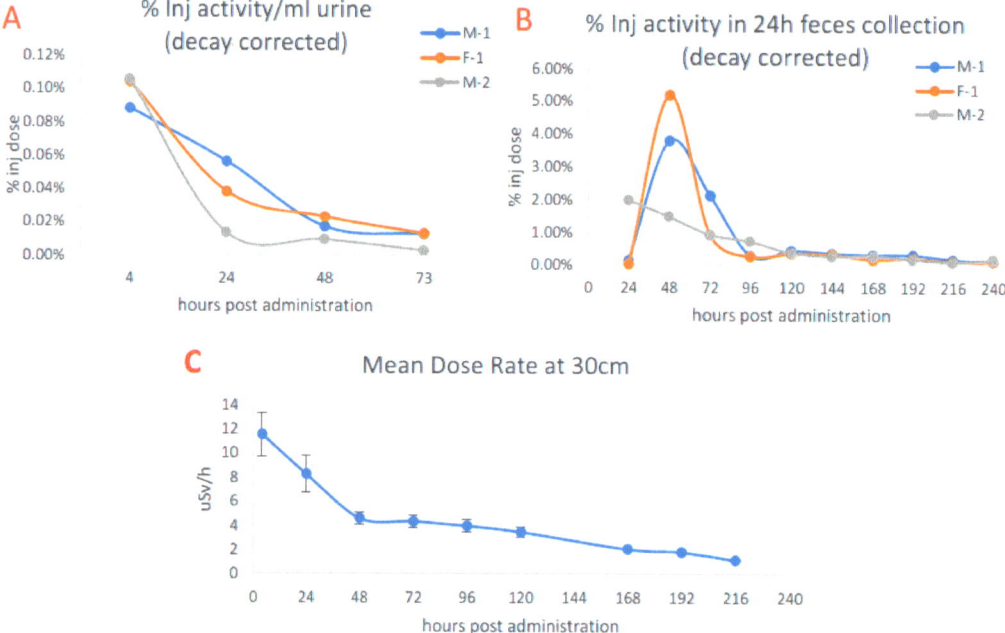

Figure 1. Excretion of [^{89}Zr]Zr-DFO-IF3 after administration to beagle dogs and dose rate at 30 cm from the canine body surface. (**A**) Urine measurement via PET. (**B**) Feces collected over the course of monitoring. (**C**) Average dose measured at 30 cm from the dog over isolation period.

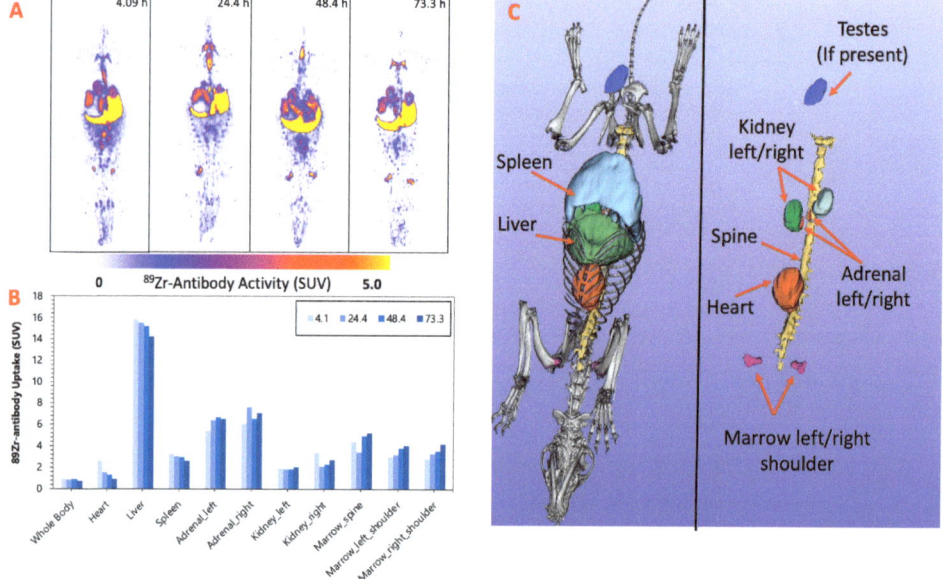

Figure 2. (**A**) F-1—MIPs of PET image volumes. (**B**) Uptake of [^{89}Zr]Zr-DFO-IF3 (SUV) in ROIs as a function of scan times; (**C**) CT-derived position of dog organs.

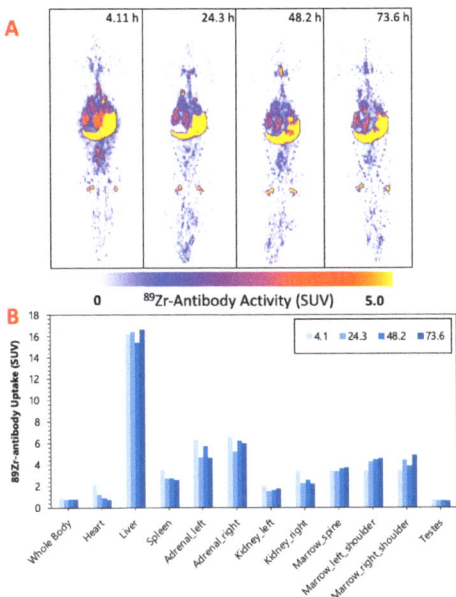

Figure 3. (**A**) M-1—MIPs of PET image volumes. (**B**) Uptake of [^{89}Zr]Zr-DFO-IF3 (SUV) in ROIs as a function of scan times.

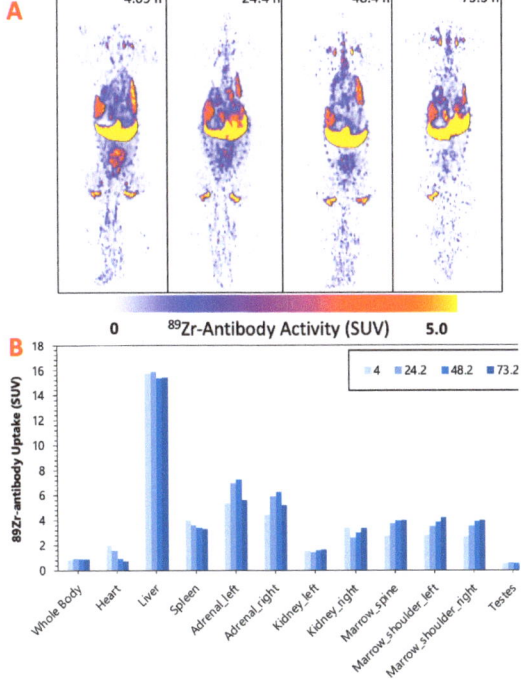

Figure 4. (**A**) M-2—MIPs of PET image volumes. (**B**) Uptake of [^{89}Zr]Zr-DFO-IF3 (SUV) in ROIs as a function of scan times.

2.3. Image-Based Dosimetry Indicated the Bone Marrow as a Dose-Limiting Organ during RIT with [^{177}Lu]Lu-CHXA″-IF3

The results of image-based dosimetry for [^{177}Lu]Lu-CHXA″-IF3 are shown in Table 1. The [^{177}Lu]Lu-CHXA″-IF3 activity for each dog was estimated with the goal of not exceeding a 3 Gy absorbed dose to the bone marrow, which is a dose-limiting organ for this radiopharmaceutical. The therapeutic activities of [^{177}Lu]Lu-CHXA″-IF3 were found to be in the 0.487–0.563 GBq range in beagles.

Table 1. Results of dosimetry calculations for [^{177}Lu]Lu-CHXA″-IF3 for individual dogs.

ROI	F-1		M-1		M-2	
	Rx Dose (Gy/GBq)	0.487 GBq [^{177}Lu]Lu-IF3 (Gy)	Rx Dose (Gy/GBq)	0.555 GBq [^{177}Lu]Lu-IF3 (Gy)	Rx Dose (Gy/GBq)	0.563 GBq [^{177}Lu]Lu-IF3 (Gy)
Heart	2.28	1.11	1.43	0.79	1.66	0.94
Liver	26.89	13.10	23.49	13.04	24.34	13.71
Spleen	5.14	2.51	3.93	2.18	5.31	2.99
Adrenal_left	12.35	6.01	7.42	4.12	9.74	5.48
Adrenal_right	13.52	6.59	9.18	5.10	9.08	5.11
Kidney_left	3.97	1.93	2.75	1.53	2.76	1.56
Kidney_right	5.32	2.59	3.69	2.05	5.41	3.05
Marrow_spine	7.87	3.83	4.44	2.47	5.00	2.82
Marrow_left_shoulder	6.16	3.00	5.40	3.00	5.33	3.00
Marrow_right_shoulder	6.27	3.05	5.67	3.15	5.00	2.82
Testes	-	-	0.90	0.50	0.80	0.45

2.4. Healthy Human Cells Do Not Express IGF2R on Their Surface

Biotinylated B-IF3 antibody produced weak to moderate cytoplasmic/cytoplasmic granule staining of occasional to frequent positive control 143B cells. B-IF3 antibody did not bind in a specific manner to K7M2 cells, which were utilized as the negative control. In its turn, the isotype control antibody, B-hIgG1, did not bind in a specific way to either IGF2R-positive 143B cells or IGF2R-negative K7M2 cells. Taken together, the B-IF3 binding to 143B cells, the absence of its binding to K7M2 cells, and the lack of B-hIgG1 isotype control antibody binding to either proved the specific and sensitive nature of the cell binding assay. Figure 5 displays the representative images of several major organs stained with B-IF3 and control B-hIgG1. Supplemental Table S1 summarizes the intensity and frequency of the staining scores. Binding with B-IF3 was observed in the human tissue panel to the cytoplasm and/or cytoplasmic granules in the following organs:

- epithelial cells in the kidney (tubules), large intestine (colon) (mucosa), liver (hepatocytes), mammary gland (breast) (glands), pancreas (islets, acini, ducts), placenta (trophoblasts), skin (epidermis, sebaceous and sweat glands), small intestine (mucosa), and stomach (mucosa)
- precursor cells in the bone marrow
- mononuclear leukocytes in the esophagus, large intestine (colon) (gut-associated lymphoid tissue [GALT]), ovary, skin, and spleen
- Kupffer cells in the liver
- spindle cells in the placenta (located in chorionic villi and, most likely, Hofbauer cells)
- reticulo-endothelial cells in the spleen
- cells of glomerular tufts in the kidney
- meningeal cells in the brain–cerebrum (falx cerebri)
- arachnoid cap cells in the brain–cerebrum
- neurons in the brain–cerebrum, small intestine (ganglia), and stomach (ganglia)

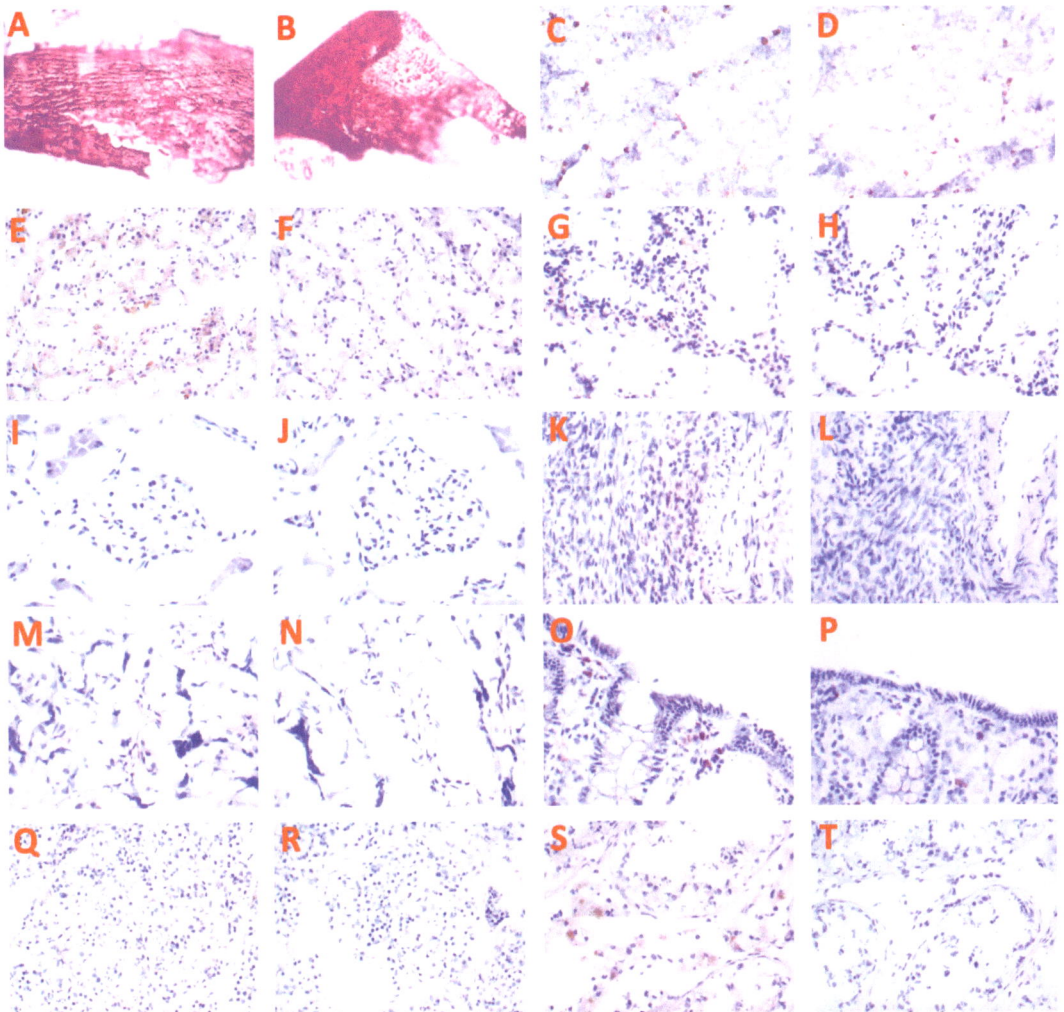

Figure 5. IHC of human tissues (40×) with biotinylated IF3 antibody and human isotype matching control hIgG1. Bone: (**A**) no staining with B-IF3, (**B**) no staining with B-hIgG1. Bone marrow: (**C**) positive staining of precursor cells with B-IF3, (**D**) no staining with B-hIgG1. Liver: (**E**) positive staining of Kupffer cells and hepatocytes with B-IF3, (**F**) no staining with B-hIgG1. Spleen: (**G**) positive staining of reticuloendothelial cells with B-IF3, (**H**) no staining with B-hIgG1. Kidney: (**I**) positive staining of glomerular tuft cells with B-IF3, (**J**) no staining with B-hIgG1. Ovary: (**K**) positive staining of mononuclear leukocytes with B-IF3, (**L**) no staining with B-hIgG1. Placenta: (**M**) positive staining of spindloid cells with B-IF3, (**N**) no staining with B-hIgG1. Large intestine: (**O**) positive staining of epithelial cells with B-IF3, (**P**) no staining with B-hIgG1. Pancreas: (**Q**) positive staining of islet cells with B-IF3, (**R**) no staining with B-hIgG1. Human testis: (**S**) positive staining of germinal epithelial cells and interstitial cells with B-IF3, (**T**) no staining with B- hIgG1.

3. Discussion

As part of the preparation for a clinical trial of OS RIT with [^{177}Lu]Lu-CHXA''-IF3 antibody in companion dogs with OS and subsequently in humans, we performed PET/CT imaging of healthy beagle dogs to enable image-based dosimetry estimations of [^{177}Lu]Lu-

CHXA"-IF3. In addition, the tissue cross-reactivity of IF3 antibody with normal human tissues was evaluated according to the requirements of the FDA Center for Biologics Evaluation and Research (CBER) document "Points to Consider in the Manufacture and Testing of Monoclonal Antibody Products for Human Use".

The imaging performed over the period of 4 days confirmed hepatobiliary clearance of IF3 antibody, which is typical for antibodies as this is where antibodies are catabolized [8]. As the accumulation in the liver is not insignificant, it will need be taken into account for determining future patient dosing regimens to ensure that this organ will continue to remain non-dose limiting. IF3 did not concentrate in the spleen to any degree (Figures 2–4) in contrast to previous murine work, confirming that IGF2R expression is specific for the spleens of Fox Chase SCID mice and, thus, will not be a targeting sink in canine or human patients. There was also no uptake in the normal bone; however, uptake was observed in what is believed to be bone marrow, as the majority of the activity is located within the center of the bone (spine, shoulders). This potentially can be attributed to the osteophilic properties of the ^{89}Zr catabolites or [^{89}Zr]Zr(Ox)$_2$ [8,9]. As an increase in SUV in both the shoulder and spine ROI is observed over time (Figures 2–4), it can support osteophilic catabolite accumulation as a source for this uptake. The RAPID platform used in this work to perform the image-based dosimetry estimations affords the estimation of absorbed doses, which will be delivered to normal organs and tumors [8–11]. Very recently, RAPID was used to calculate the doses of ^{90}Y-small molecule NM600 for treatment of companion dogs with various advanced cancers [12]. For [^{177}Lu]Lu-CHXA"-IF3, RAPID predicted the bone marrow to be a dose-limiting organ, which is often observed for the variety of radiotherapeutic antibodies in humans [13] and, based on this prediction, allowed for the estimation of the projected therapeutic doses of [^{177}Lu]Lu-CHXA"-IF3 in companion dogs with OS.

It is generally accepted that the results from clinical trials in dogs in terms of safety and efficacy can be extrapolated to humans better than any other preclinical models. Companion canines with spontaneous tumors are attractive comparative models to humans for several reasons [14,15], including naturally occurring cancers, many with high recurrence and metastatic potential; strong genetic and molecular target similarities to human cancers; immune competence and native immuno-editing interactions between the tumor and host immune system; relevant tumor histologies with intratumoral and inter-individual heterogeneity; similar environmental carcinogen exposure to human cancers; and a more natural outbred population compared to inbred rodent model laboratory-derived canine populations. The inclusion of companion animals in the development and use of novel RIT agents also has advantages owing to their physical size and spatial distribution of tumors (primary and metastatic) and normal organs/tissues, which more closely mimics that in humans with cancer [16].

The analysis of the binding of biotinylated B-IF3 to normal human tissues revealed that all binding observed with B-IF3 was due to the IGF2R in the cytoplasm with none expressed on the surface of the normal cells. This is in contrast to the high expression of IGF2R on the surface of human and canine OS tumor cells [4–7]. As monoclonal antibodies cannot penetrate through the membranes of live cells, they cannot bind to their respective antigens located in the cytoplasm, and for this reason, such cytoplasmic antigens do not contribute to tissue cross-reactivity [17,18]. The observed staining with B-IF3 in mononuclear leukocytes, Kupffer cells in the liver, bone marrow precursor cells, and neurons was consistent with the reported expression of IGF2R [19–21]. This is an important observation, which means that the radiolabeled IF3 antibody will be binding in vivo only to the cancer cells that express IGF2R on their surface [4–7], while intracellular expression of IGF2R in normal tissue will remain invisible to the antibody, thus avoiding toxicity to normal tissues.

In the past, several bone-seeking radiopharmaceuticals were tried for treatment of OS; however, they cannot be of use for treatment of non-osseous metastases [22]. More recently, two clinical trials have been initiated that will investigate RIT of solid tumors with antibodies to IGF1R and HER-2 antigens labeled with alpha-emitters ^{225}Ac and

^{227}Th, respectively (NCT03746431 and NCT04147819) [23]. Such trials will generate useful information for developing the RIT approach to treatment of OS [23]. While these are also attractive targets in terms of OS, it is beneficial to have a wide variety of potential treatments giving clinicians more opportunity to treat individuals who may have different levels of antigen expression, allowing for a more personalized medical approach.

4. Materials and Methods

4.1. Animal Ethics and Approval

The study design was approved by the University of Saskatchewan's Animal Research Ethics Board and adhered to the Canadian Council on Animal Care guidelines for humane animal use. The study was in compliance with appropriate ARRIVE guidelines.

4.2. Conjugation IF3 Antibody

IF3 human antibody to IGF2R [6] produced at the University of Saskatchewan was conjugated to the bifunctional chelator 1-(4-isothiocyanatophenyl)-3-[6,17-dihydroxy-7,10,18,21-tetraoxo-27-(N-acetylhydroxylamino)-6,11,17,22-tetraazaheptaeicosine] thiourea (p-SCN-Bn-DFO) (Macrocyclics, Plano, TX, USA) via modified literature methods [24]. In short, 800 µg of IF3 was exchanged into carbonate conjugation buffer, pH = 8.5, via spin filtration (30 kDa molecular weight cut off spin filter) and conjugated to the chelator using a 3-fold molar excess of p-SCN-Bn-DFO (2 mg/mL in DMSO) and incubated at 37 °C for 1.5 hrs. The IF3-DFO conjugate was then washed 10 times via spin filtration with 0.5 M HEPES buffer at 4 °C to remove excess p-SCN-Bn-DFO giving the IF3-DFO conjugate.

4.3. Labeling of IF3-DFO Conjugate

A total of 74 MBq of [^{89}Zr]Zr(Ox)$_2$ in 1 M oxalic acid (Sylvia Fedoruk Canadian Centre for Nuclear Innovation, Saskatoon, SK, Canada) was dissolved in 0.5 M HEPES buffer (which was previously passed through a Chelex-100 column to remove any trace metals) and neutralized using 1M Na$_2$CO$_3$. A total of 400 µg of IF3-DFO was then added to achieve a 0.185:1 MBq:µg specific activity. The reaction mixture was heated at 37° for 1 h and then quenched using 3 µL of 0.05 M DTPA solution; the percentage of radiolabeling yield was measured with instant thin layer chromatography (iTLC) (Agilent Technologies, Santa Clara, CA, USA) using 0.5 M EDTA as the eluant. The iTLC was cut in half and measured using a 2470 Wizard2 Gamma counter (Perkin Elmer, Waltham, MA, USA) calibrated for ^{89}Zr emission spectra. Radiolabeling yields were calculated by dividing the counts per minute at the bottom half of the iTLC CPM by the total counts per minute (top + bottom), as the labeled antibody has a Rf = 0 vs. Rf = 1 for [^{89}Zr]Zr-DTPA/EDTA. Radiolabeling yields were greater than 99%. The radiolabeled antibody was then exchanged into sterile phosphate-buffered saline (PBS) prior to injection.

4.4. PET/CT Imaging of Dogs

Animals were sedated with acepromazine 0.02 mg/kg combined with butorphanol 0.2 mg/kg IM with a top-up of a quarter to half of the original dose extra if necessary (if sedation was not adequate). A 20–22 G over-the-needle catheter was aseptically secured into the cephalic vein, and Ketamine 5 mg/kg combined with Midazolam 0.25 mg/kg was injected by IV in increments to achieve a surgical plane of anesthesia. The trachea was intubated with the dog in the sternal position with a cuffed endotracheal tube using a laryngoscope for visualization. The endotracheal tube was secured to the patient with k-ling. The endotracheal tube was attached to the anesthetic machine, which delivered isoflurane at an appropriate concentration to maintain a suitable anesthetic depth using a rebreathing system. Three doses of 11.1 MBq of purified labeled antibody were prepared just prior to injection of three beagle dogs: one female (F-1) weighing 10 kg and two males (M-1 and M-2) weighing 13 kg and 12 kg, respectively. Syringe radioactivity was measured before and after injection giving a total injected activity of 9.88 MBq, 10.0 MBq, and 9.47 MBq for F-1, M-1, and M-2, respectively. PET/CT scans were performed on a

GE Discovery MI DR PET/CT scanner (GE healthcare, Waukesha, WI, USA) at 4, 24, 48, and 73 h post injection of [^{89}Zr]Zr-DFO-IF3 (±0.6 h). The animals were immobilized in sternal recumbency after induction. A 256 × 256 matrix was used, DFOV 40 cm, acquired at 7 min/bed position (49–56 min total), immediately following a full body CT (2.5 mm/slice). The PET/CT images were registered and reconstructed automatically using GE's Q. Clear algorithm, a Bayesian penalized-likelihood iterative image reconstruction, a β value of 550, and incorporating PSF and TOF corrections. A whole-body ROI was drawn around the subject (no excretion was confirmed prior) to confirm that the measured injected activity was consistent with the PET scanner and found to be ±10%.

4.5. Image-Based Dosimetry

Regions of interest (ROI) were drawn manually using the CT data for organ segmentation at each time point using 3D Slicer v5.0.3 (slicer.org) and exported as RTSS DICOM files for dosimetry analysis. The bone marrow dose was measured by drawing ROI on each shoulder and the spine as they showed a high amount of activity concentration. The dose rates were calculated at each of the imaging time points using a Monte Carlo (MC) dosimetry platform called RAPID (Radiopharmaceutical Assessment Platform for Internal Dosimetry) [25]. Following acquisition of the entire imaging series, the PET/CT imaging data were co-registered and resampled to the first time point of the CT image. Next, the activity concentration in each voxel was decay corrected from the imaging radionuclide (^{89}Zr) to represent the therapeutic radionuclide (^{177}Lu). The processed CT and PET imaging dataset was used in the MC simulations to define the geometry and source distributions at each time point, respectively. MC simulations were performed to determine the mean absorbed dose rate at each time point using the MC code Geant4 v9.6. A total of 8000 decays were simulated for each activity-rich voxel so that the uncertainty in average voxel dose rate was 1.07%. The mean absorbed dose rate of the corresponding voxels was integrated using a trapezoidal method to obtain the mean absorbed dose in each voxel. The estimation of activity concentration and standardized uptake values (SUV) were calculated in each ROI at each time point using voxel-level data. SUV was calculated using:

$$SUV = \frac{[A_{voxel}]_{@T_n}/V_{voxel}}{\left[A_{injected}\right]_{@T_0} \cdot e^{-\lambda T_n}/m_{subject}} \quad (1)$$

where $[A_{voxel}]_{@T_n}$ is the tracer radioactivity concentration in ROI voxels at nth time point, V_{voxel} is the volume of the ROI voxels, $\left[A_{injected}\right]_{@T_0}$ is the injection activity, λ is the decay constant of imaging isotope, T_n is the post-injection time, and $m_{subject}$ is the mass weight of the subject.

4.6. Tissue Cross-Reactivity Study with Biotinylated IF3 with Normal Human Tissues

Biotinylated IF3 (B-IF3) and biotinylated isotype control human hIgG1 (B-hIgG1) were generated by adMare BioInnovations (Vancouver, Canada). The human tissue cross-reactivity study was performed by Charles River (Morrisville, NC, USA) (Table 2). Cryosections of human OS 143B cells (ATCC, Manassas, VA, USA) were used as the positive control, while cryosections of murine IGF2R-negative OS K7M2 cells (ATCC, USA) served as the negative control. Positive and negative control cells were stored in a freezer set to maintain −65 °C or below.

A direct immunoperoxidase procedure was performed. Acetone-fixed cryosections were rinsed twice with PBS, pH 7.2. Slides were then incubated with an avidin solution for 15 min, rinsed once with PBS, incubated with a biotin solution for 15 min, and rinsed once with PBS. The slides were then treated for 20 min with a protein block designed to reduce nonspecific binding. The protein block was prepared as follows: PBS + 1% bovine serum albumin (BSA); 0.5% casein; 1.5% human gamma globulins (HGG); and 1 mg/mL heat aggregated human gamma globulins (HAHGG) (prepared by heating a 5 mg/mL solution to 63 °C for 20 min and then cooling to room temperature). Following treatment with the protein block, the biotinylated primary antibodies (B-IF3, B-hIgG1, or none [buffer alone as the assay control]) were applied to the slides at concentrations of 10 µg/mL for 1 h. Next, the slides were rinsed twice with PBS. Endogenous peroxidase was then quenched by incubation of the slides with the Dako peroxidase blocking solution for 5 min. Then, the slides were rinsed twice with PBS, treated with the ABC Elite reagent for 30 min, rinsed twice with PBS, and then treated with DAB for 4 min as a substrate for the peroxidase reaction. All slides were rinsed with tap water, counterstained, dehydrated, and mounted. PBS + 1% BSA served as the diluent for all antibodies and the ABC Elite reagent.

Table 2. Human Tissue (Normal) from One Individual.

Tissues		
Bone	Breast (mammary gland)	Ovary
Bladder (urinary)	Gastrointestinal (GI) Tract [b]	Pancreas
Blood Vessels (endothelium) [a]	Heart	Placenta
Bone Marrow	Kidney (glomerulus, tubule)	Skin
Brain—cerebrum	Liver	Spleen
	Lung	

[a] Evaluated from all tissues where present. [b] Includes esophagus, large intestine/colon, small intestine, and stomach (including underlying smooth muscle).

After staining, the slides were visualized under light microscopy for immunopathology. Each stained cell type or tissue element was identified, the subcellular (or extracellular) location of the staining was recorded, and the intensity (strength) of staining (Table 3) was assigned for each slide. The frequency of cell type staining (Table 4) was also assigned to provide the approximate percentage of cells of that particular cell type or tissue element with staining.

Table 3. Scoring scale for the intensity of IHC staining.

Staining Intensity	
Score	Result
Neg	Negative (no stained cells)
±	Equivocal (very faint stain)
1+	Weak (light stain)
2+	Moderate (light–medium stain)
3+	Strong (medium stain)
4+	Intense (dark stain)

Table 4. Scoring scale for the frequency of IHC staining.

Staining Frequency	
Score	Result
Neg	Negative (no stained cells)
Very rare	<1% stained cells of a particular cell type or tissue element
Rare	1–5% stained cells of a particular cell type or tissue element
Rare to Occasional	>5–25% stained cells of a particular cell type or tissue element
Occasional	>25–50% stained cells of a particular cell type or tissue element
Occasional to Frequent	>50–75% stained cells of a particular cell type or tissue element
Frequent	>75–100% stained cells of a particular cell type or tissue element

5. Conclusions

In this study, we performed image-based dosimetry for ^{89}Zr/^{177}Lu-labeled IF3 human antibody to IGF2R and evaluated IF3 binding to normal human tissues. The results of the study demonstrate that IF3 has a typical human antibody biodistribution profile and does not cross-react with any normal human tissues, thus informing future radioimmunotherapy studies in canine and human patients with OS.

6. Patents

ED and MU are co-inventors on the Provisional US Patent Application "Antibodies to IGF2R and Methods" filed on 30 March 2021.

Supplementary Materials: The following supporting information can be downloaded at: https://www.mdpi.com/article/10.3390/ph16070979/s1, Table S1: Cross-Reactivity of B-IF3 with Normal Human Tissues.

Author Contributions: K.J.H.A., O.K., M.R.H., J.J.G., F.A.C., R.M.V., Y.S.S., L.F. and C.B.P. acquired the data. S.M.C., B.P.B. and E.D. contributed to the conception of the study. K.J.H.A., O.K., E.D., R.D., V.M.-D. and M.U. analyzed the data. K.J.H.A. and E.D. wrote the manuscript. All authors have read and agreed to the published version of the manuscript.

Funding: Funding was provided by the Canadian Institutes for Health Research (CIHR) grant PJT-162433 to E.D. and M.U. and the Centre for Probe Development and Commercialization and adMare BioInnovations Radiopharmaceutical Initiative (CARI). For O.K, J.J.G., and B.P.B., this work was supported by NIH National Cancer Institute (NCI) Grant P01 CA250972.

Institutional Review Board Statement: The study design was approved by the University of Saskatchewan's Animal Research Ethics Board and adhered to the Canadian Council on Animal Care guidelines for humane animal use and followed the appropriate ARRIVE guidelines.

Informed Consent Statement: Not applicable.

Data Availability Statement: Data is contained within the article and supplementary material.

Acknowledgments: The authors acknowledge the support of the personnel at the Fedoruk Center for Nuclear Innovation at the University of Saskatchewan.

Conflicts of Interest: ED has received research support and is a consultant for Actinium Pharmaceuticals. No other potential conflicts of interest relevant to this article exist.

References

1. Ehrhart, N.P.; Christensen, N.I.; Fan, T.M. 25—Tumors of the Skeletal System. In *Withrow and MacEwen's Small Animal Clinical Oncology*, 6th ed.; Vail, D.M., Thamm, D.H., Liptak, J.M., Eds.; W.B. Saunders: St. Louis, MO, USA, 2020; pp. 524–564.
2. Gill, J.; Gorlick, R. Advancing therapy for osteosarcoma. *Nat. Rev. Clin. Oncol.* **2021**, *18*, 609–624. [CrossRef] [PubMed]
3. Poon, A.C.; Matsuyama, A.; Mutsaers, A.J. Recent and current clinical trials in canine appendicular osteosarcoma. *Am. Jew. Hist.* **2020**, *61*, 301–308.
4. Hassan, S.E.; Ba, M.B.; Kim, M.Y.; Lin, J.; Piperdi, S.; Gorlick, R.; Geller, D.S. Cell surface receptor expression patterns in osteosarcoma. *Cancer* **2011**, *118*, 740–749. [CrossRef] [PubMed]
5. Boisclair, C.; Dickinson, R.; Giri, S.; Dadachova, E.; MacDonald-Dickinson, V. Characterization of IGF2R Molecular Expression in Canine Osteosarcoma as Part of a Novel Comparative Oncology Approach. *Int. J. Mol. Sci.* **2023**, *24*, 1867. [CrossRef]
6. Broqueza, J.; Prabaharan, C.B.; Andrahennadi, S.; Allen, K.J.H.; Dickinson, R.; MacDonald-Dickinson, V.; Dadachova, E.; Uppalapati, M. Novel Human Antibodies to Insulin Growth Factor 2 Receptor (IGF2R) for Radioimmunoimaging and Therapy of Canine and Human Osteosarcoma. *Cancers* **2021**, *13*, 2208. [CrossRef]
7. Broqueza, J.; Prabaharan, C.B.; Allen, K.J.H.; Jiao, R.; Fisher, D.R.; Dickinson, R.; MacDonald-Dickinson, V.; Uppalapati, M.; Dadachova, E. Radioimmunotherapy Targeting IGF2R on Canine-Patient-Derived Osteosarcoma Tumors in Mice and Radiation Dosimetry in Canine and Pediatric Models. *Pharmaceuticals* **2021**, *15*, 10. [CrossRef]
8. Berg, E.; Gill, H.; Marik, J.; Ogasawara, A.; Williams, S.P.; van Dongen, G.A.; Vugts, D.J.; Cherry, S.R.; Tarantal, A.F. Total-Body PET and Highly Stable Chelators Together Enable Meaningful ^{89}Zr-Antibody PET Studies up to 30 Days After Injection. *J. Nucl. Med.* **2019**, *61*, 453–460. [CrossRef]
9. Holland, J.P.; Divilov, V.; Bander, N.H.; Smith-Jones, P.M.; Larson, S.M.; Lewis, J.S. ^{89}Zr-DFO-J591 for ImmunoPET of Prostate-Specific Membrane Antigen Expression In Vivo. *J. Nucl. Med.* **2010**, *51*, 1293–1300. [CrossRef]
10. Marsh, I.R.; Grudzinski, J.J.; Baiu, D.C.; E Besemer, A.; Hernandez, R.; Jeffery, J.J.; Weichert, J.P.; Otto, M.; Bednarz, B.P. Preclinical Pharmacokinetics and Dosimetry Studies of ^{124}I/^{131}I-CLR1404 for Treatment of Pediatric Solid Tumors in Murine Xenograft Models. *J. Nucl. Med.* **2019**, *60*, 1414–1420. [CrossRef]
11. Bednarz, B.; Grudzinski, J.; Marsh, I.; Besemer, A.; Baiu, D.; Weichert, J.; Otto, M. Murine-specific Internal Dosimetry for Preclinical Investigations of Imaging and Therapeutic Agents. *Health Phys.* **2018**, *114*, 450–459. [CrossRef]

12. Magee, K.; Marsh, I.R.; Turek, M.M.; Grudzinski, J.; Aluicio-Sarduy, E.; Engle, J.W.; Kurzman, I.D.; Zuleger, C.L.; Oseid, E.A.; Jaskowiak, C.; et al. Safety and feasibility of an in situ vaccination and immunomodulatory targeted radionuclide combination immuno-radiotherapy approach in a comparative (companion dog) setting. *PLoS ONE* **2021**, *16*, e0255798. [CrossRef] [PubMed]
13. der Weg, W.W.-V.; Schoffelen, R.; Hobbs, R.F.; Gotthardt, M.; Goldenberg, D.M.; Sharkey, R.M.; Slump, C.H.; van der Graaf, W.T.; Oyen, W.J.; Boerman, O.C.; et al. Tumor and red bone marrow dosimetry: Comparison of methods for prospective treatment planning in pretargeted radioimmunotherapy. *EJNMMI Phys.* **2015**, *2*, 5. [CrossRef] [PubMed]
14. Khanna, C.; London, C.; Vail, D.; Mazcko, C.; Hirschfeld, S. Guiding the Optimal Translation of New Cancer Treatments from Canine to Human Cancer Patients. *Clin. Cancer Res.* **2009**, *15*, 5671–5677. [CrossRef] [PubMed]
15. National Academies of Sciences, Engineering, and Medicine. *The Role of Clinical Studies for Pets with Naturally Occurring Tumors in Translational Cancer Research: Workshop Summary*; The National Academies Press: Washington, DC, USA, 2015.
16. Vail, D.M.; Leblanc, A.K.; Jeraj, R. Advanced Cancer Imaging Applied in the Comparative Setting. *Front. Oncol.* **2020**, *10*, 84. [CrossRef]
17. Hall, W.C.; Price-Schiavi, S.A.; Wicks, J.; Rojko, J.L. Tissue Cross-Reactivity Studies for Monoclonal Antibodies: Predictive Value and Use for Selection of Relevant Animal Species for Toxicity Testing. In *Pharmaceutical Sciences Encyclopedia: Drug Discovery, Development, and Manufacturing*; Wiley: Hoboken, NJ, USA, 2010; pp. 1–34. [CrossRef]
18. Leach, M.W.; Halpern, W.G.; Johnson, C.W.; Rojko, J.L.; MacLachlan, T.K.; Chan, C.M.; Galbreath, E.J.; Ndifor, A.M.; Blanset, D.L.; Polack, E.; et al. Use of Tissue Cross-reactivity Studies in the Development of Antibody-based Biopharmaceuticals. *Toxicol. Pathol.* **2010**, *38*, 1138–1166. [CrossRef] [PubMed]
19. Barroca, V.; Lewandowski, D.; Jaracz-Ros, A.; Hardouin, S.-N. Paternal Insulin-like Growth Factor 2 (Igf2) Regulates Stem Cell Activity During Adulthood. *Ebiomedicine* **2016**, *15*, 150–162. [CrossRef]
20. Wang, X.; Lin, L.; Lan, B.; Wang, Y.; Du, L.; Chen, X.; Li, Q.; Liu, K.; Hu, M.; Xue, Y.; et al. IGF2R-initiated proton rechanneling dictates an anti-inflammatory property in macrophages. *Sci. Adv.* **2020**, *6*, eabb7389. [CrossRef]
21. Wilczak, N.; De Bleser, P.; Luiten, P.; Geerts, A.; Teelken, A.; De Keyser, J. Insulin-like growth factor II receptors in human brain and their absence in astrogliotic plaques in multiple sclerosis. *Brain Res.* **2000**, *863*, 282–288. [CrossRef]
22. Anderson, P.M. Radiopharmaceuticals for Treatment of Osteosarcoma. *Adv. Exp. Med. Biol.* **2020**, *1257*, 45–53. [CrossRef]
23. Anderson, P.M.; Subbiah, V.; Trucco, M.M. Current and future targeted alpha particle therapies for osteosarcoma: Radium-223, actinium-225, and thorium-227. *Front. Med.* **2022**, *9*, 1030094. [CrossRef]
24. Allen, K.J.H.; Jiao, R.; Li, J.; Beckford-Vera, D.R.; Dadachova, E. In Vitro and In Vivo Characterization of ^{89}Zirconium-Labeled Lintuzumab Molecule. *Molecules* **2022**, *27*, 6589. [CrossRef] [PubMed]
25. Besemer, A.E.; Yang, Y.; Grudzinski, J.J.; Hall, L.T.; Bednarz, B.P. Development and Validation of RAPID: A Patient-Specific Monte Carlo Three-Dimensional Internal Dosimetry Platform. *Cancer Biotherapy Radiopharm.* **2018**, *33*, 155–165. [CrossRef] [PubMed]

Disclaimer/Publisher's Note: The statements, opinions and data contained in all publications are solely those of the individual author(s) and contributor(s) and not of MDPI and/or the editor(s). MDPI and/or the editor(s) disclaim responsibility for any injury to people or property resulting from any ideas, methods, instructions or products referred to in the content.

Article

Radiosynthesis of Stable ^{198}Au-Nanoparticles by Neutron Activation of $\alpha_v\beta_3$-Specific AuNPs for Therapy of Tumor Angiogenesis

Güllü Davarci [1], Carmen Wängler [2,3], Klaus Eberhardt [4], Christopher Geppert [4], Ralf Schirrmacher [5], Robert Freudenberg [6], Marc Pretze [1,6,*,†] and Björn Wängler [1,*,†]

1. Molecular Imaging and Radiochemistry, Clinic of Radiology and Nuclear Medicine, Medical Faculty Mannheim of Heidelberg University, 68167 Mannheim, Germany; guellue.davarci@medma.uni-heidelberg.de
2. Biomedical Chemistry, Clinic of Radiology and Nuclear Medicine, Medical Faculty Mannheim of Heidelberg University, 68167 Mannheim, Germany; carmen.waengler@medma.uni-heidelberg.de
3. Mannheim Institute for Intelligent Systems in Medicine MIISM, Medical Faculty Mannheim of Heidelberg University, 68167 Mannheim, Germany
4. Research Reactor TRIGA Mainz, Institute for Nuclear Chemistry, Johannes-Gutenberg-Universität Mainz, 55128 Mainz, Germany; eberha@uni-mainz.de (K.E.); cgeppert@uni-mainz.de (C.G.)
5. Department of Oncology, Division of Oncological Imaging, University of Alberta, Edmonton, AB T6G 2R3, Canada; schirrma@ualberta.ca
6. Department of Nuclear Medicine, University Hospital Carl Gustav Carus, TU Dresden, 01307 Dresden, Germany; robert.freudenberg@ukdd.de

* Correspondence: marc.pretze@ukdd.de (M.P.); bjoern.waengler@medma.uni-heidelberg.de (B.W.)
† These authors contributed equally to this work.

Abstract: This paper reports on the development of stable tumor-specific gold nanoparticles (AuNPs) activated by neutron irradiation as a therapeutic option for the treatment of cancer with high tumor angiogenesis. The AuNPs were designed with different mono- or dithiol-ligands and decorated with different amounts of Arg-Gly-Asp (RGD) peptides as a tumor-targeting vector for $\alpha_v\beta_3$ integrin, which is overexpressed in tissues with high tumor angiogenesis. The AuNPs were evaluated for avidity in vitro and showed favorable properties with respect to tumor cell accumulation. Furthermore, the therapeutic properties of the [^{198}Au]AuNPs were evaluated in vitro on U87MG cells in terms of cell survival, suggesting that these [^{198}Au]AuNPs are a useful basis for future therapeutic concepts.

Keywords: gold nanoparticles; [^{198}Au]AuNPs; radioactive; tumor therapy; tumor angiogenesis; RGD peptide

1. Introduction

In recent years, gold nanoparticles (AuNPs) have received serious attention since their first use as radioactive ^{198}Au-nanocolloids for nanobrachytherapy in the early 1950s [1,2]. The synthesis of ultra-small AuNPs (<5 nm) [3] with multimerization of target-specific effectors on their surface leads to a new form of targeted AuNPs with higher target avidity compared to the effectors only [4]. The combination of the target-specific accumulation and a phenomenon typically known as the "enhanced permeability and retention" (EPR) effect [5], leads to a higher tumor accumulation [6]. Therefore, AuNPs with a higher renal clearance [7] for theranostic purposes [8–10] were developed in recent years, equipped with small molecules [11], peptides [12], near-infrared dyes [13,14], and radionuclides [15–19]. PEGylation of the AuNPs leads to a higher bioavailability as it prevents the formation of a protein corona around the AuNPs in vivo [20,21]. The high affinity of sulfur for gold surfaces and the formation of stable and covalent Au-S bonds [22] allows a fast and easy functionalization of AuNPs with (di-)thiol-modified (bio)molecules [23]. In addition, the use of dithiols as a surface binding motif leads to a higher stability of the AuNPs [24]. Of particular interest is their therapeutic application [25], especially their ability to be used as radiosensitizers by Auger–Meitner electron emission induced by gamma activation [26–28] or by direct neutron activation of natural ^{197}AuNPs generating [^{198}Au]AuNPs ($t_{1/2}$ = 2.69 d, β^-_{max} 961 keV, 98.99%; γ 412 keV, 95.62%) [12,29–32].

The focus of this work was the development of highly stable targeted gold nanoparticles for neutron activation [33]. Therefore, AuNPs with mono- and di-thiol linkers with low and high loading of target-specific peptides were synthesized to compare their specific avidity in cell binding assays and their stability during and after neutron irradiation. To achieve target-specific accumulation in tissues with high tumor angiogenesis, the AuNPs were functionalized with a c(RGDfK) derivative [32,34]. The Arg-Gly-Asp (RGD) peptide motif is known to bind to the transmembrane $\alpha_v\beta_3$ integrin [35,36], which is overexpressed in tumor angiogenesis in tumors of various origins, for example, on glioma cells (U87MG) [37–39].

2. Results

2.1. Synthesis and Functionalization of Gold Nanoparticles

Integrin $\alpha_v\beta_3$, a transmembrane protein expressed on endothelial cells, binds the RGD triple amino acid peptide motif of extracellular matrix proteins. Growing malignant tumors require continuous angiogenesis, and the integrin $\alpha_v\beta_3$ is overexpressed for this purpose. As a result, $\alpha_v\beta_3$ is preferentially expressed in tumor angiogenesis and is a potential target for AuNPs decorated with RGD peptides [36]. Therefore, ultra-small AuNPs 3 and 6 (3 ± 2 nm) were synthesized by Turcu et al. [40] and Brust and Schiffrin [41], respectively. The AuNPs contained thiol-PEG$_3$-OH or a thioctic acid(TA)-PEG$_3$-OH derivative 2 used as the stabilizing ligands and to achieve enhanced biocompatibility (Figure 1). The AuNPs were further functionalized by ligand exchange with low and high amounts (4–8 mg) of TA-PEG$_4$-c(RGDfK) derivative 5 to obtain mixed AuNP-thio-PEG-dithio-PEG-RGD 7a (high RGD loading), 7b (low RGD loading) and AuNP-dithio-RGD 8a (high RGD loading), and 8b (low RGD loading), respectively. The AuNPs were purified by dialysis and size-exclusion chromatography. The size and stability of AuNPs 7a,b, and 8a,b were confirmed by UV/Vis spectroscopy and high performance liquid chromatography (HPLC).

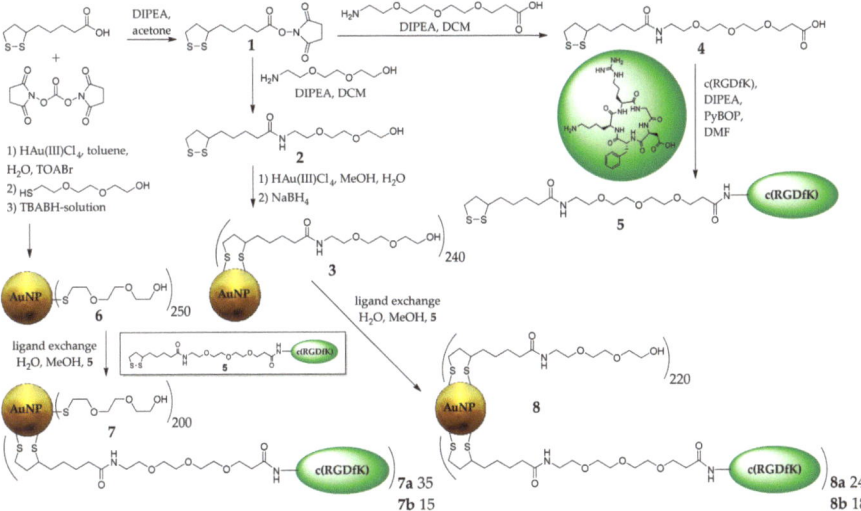

Figure 1. Synthesis of the different RGD-functionalized AuNPs 7a, 7b, 8a and 8b. The synthesis of c(RGDfK) is described in Appendix A.

The organic shell of the AuNPs was characterized by mass loss using thermogravimetric analyses for each functionalization step. After knowing the number of newly attached molecules, a formula by Zhu et al. was used to calculate the total molar mass of the AuNPs [42] (Table 1). A brief description of the synthesis and characterization can be found in Appendix A. All AuNPs were fully characterized by thermogravimetric analysis (TGA) (Table 1), electron microscopy (EM) (Figures A1 and A2), UV/Vis spectroscopy (Figure A9), HPLC (Figure A10), and nuclear magnetic resonance spectroscopy (NMR) (Figures A11–A16). The AuNPs could be stored in lyophilized form at $-20\,°C$ for >12 months without loss of integrity. In contrast, when stored in solution at room temperature, aggregation in the form of precipitation could occur within weeks, especially for peptide-decorated particles [43].

Table 1. Calculated number of ligands and resulting molecular mass of the AuNPs.

Probe	Description	Number of Ligands	Molecular Mass [kDa]
6	AuNP-PEG	250 × thio-PEG	210
7a	AuNP-PEG-RGD$_{high}$	152 × thio-PEG, 35 × 5	239
7b	AuNP-PEG-RGD$_{low}$	196 × thio-PEG, 15 × 5	222
3	AuNP-dithio-PEG	240 × 3	246
8a	AuNP-dithio-PEG-RGD$_{high}$	218 × 3, 24 × 5	262
8b	AuNP-dithio-PEG-RGD$_{low}$	220 × 3, 18 × 5	257

2.2. Neutron Irradiation Experiments

First neutron irradiation experiments with thermal neutrons at the TRIGA Mainz reactor were performed with non-tumor specific AuNP-dithio-PEG **3** (3-1–3-5) and AuNP-thio-PEG **6** (6-1–6-3) in different weights and concentrations. Samples were frozen and removed from the freezer immediately before irradiation. Irradiation was performed at 100 kW for 1–2 h with a neutron flux of 1.6×10^{12} cm^{-2} × s^{-1}. With the reactor running, the background dose rate (DR) at the measurement position was ~2 µSv/h. Gamma measurements were not possible for probes >500 µg on the day of irradiation due to the high activity. The dead time for samples 3-5 (Table 2) was about 30 min at the end of the bombardment and still 7.5 min at 20 cm distance. Therefore, most of the gamma measurements of [^{198}Au]AuNPs had to be performed one day after irradiation. Sample [^{198}Au]3-5 still had ~3% dead time in 20 cm distance (Table 2). Precipitation was observed for [^{198}Au]**6** but not for [^{198}Au]**3** in the solution or on the vessel wall in any case (Figure 2). The activated samples were stored in the freezer for transport and further experiments. In addition, the half-life of [^{198}Au]**3** was determined experimentally (mean 2.80 ± 0.07 d) by measuring the activity of different concentrations with a gamma counter for 28 d (Figure A8). UV-Vis measurements showed a strong broadening of the plasmon bands for [^{198}Au]6-1 and [^{198}Au]6-2, indicating aggregation (Figure 3). For [^{198}Au]3-1 and [^{198}Au]3-2 a typical absorption for AuNPs at 514 nm was observed, indicating stable AuNPs even 5 months after neutron activation ([^{198}Au]3-3, Figure A9). The production of ~100 MBq [^{198}Au]**3** showed stable AuNPs even at high activity concentration for at least 15 d by HPLC measurements (Figure A10).

Table 2. Summary of neutron activation of various AuNPs, mass, and calculated half-life.

Probe	Weight [mg]	DR [1] [µSv/h] in 1 cm/30 cm after				Precipitation Observed	t$_{1/2}$ [d] (Calc.)
		5 min	10 min	30 min	60 min		
[^{198}Au]3-1	0.05	55/4	35/3	25/3	25/3	no	2.6866
[^{198}Au]3-2	0.50	125/5	125/5	115/4	100/4	no	2.8177
[^{198}Au]3-3	0.75	170/5	160/5	155/4	150/4	no	2.8525
[^{198}Au]3-4	1.00	250/6	215/5	210/5	212/5	no	2.7837
[^{198}Au]3-5	2.00	500/8	450/8	420/8	410/8	no	2.8761
[^{198}Au]6-1	0.05	76/3.7	n.d. [2]	n.d. [2]	n.d. [2]	yes	n.d. [2]

Table 2. *Cont.*

Probe	Weight [mg]	DR [1] [μSv/h] in 1 cm/30 cm after				Precipitation Observed	$t_{1/2}$ [d] (Calc.)
		5 min	10 min	30 min	60 min		
[^{198}Au]6-2	0.50	150/n.d.[2]	15/6	n.d.[2]/5.3	n.d.[2]	yes	n.d.[2]
[^{198}Au]6-3	5.06	n.d.[2]	n.d.[2]	1000/n.d.[2]	n.d.[2]	yes	n.d.[2]
[^{198}Au]8a-1	0.05	n.d.[2]	n.d.[2]	15/5	n.d.[2]	no	n.d.[2]

[1] DR: dose rate; [2] n.d.: not determined.

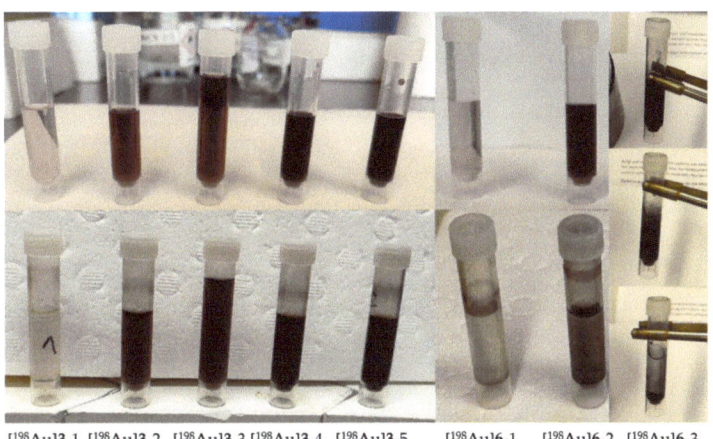

Figure 2. Different amounts of AuNPs before (**top**) and after (**bottom**) neutron activation. [^{198}Au]6-3 (**right**) shows a suspension immediately after irradiation (**top**), followed by precipitation within 0.5 min (**middle**) and 1 min (**bottom**).

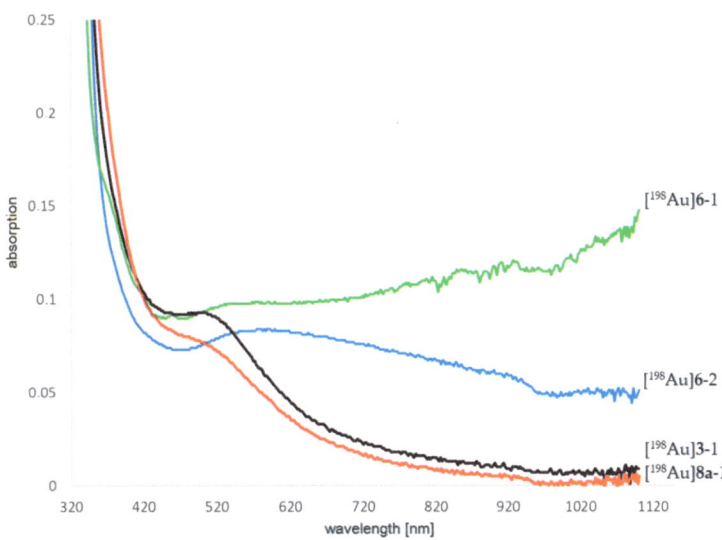

Figure 3. UV-Vis spectra of neutron-activated AuNPs. Intact [^{198}Au]3-1 (black line, 25 μg/mL, irradiation 60 min) and [^{198}Au]8a-1 (red line, 25 μg/mL, irradiation 60 min). Particle aggregation can be seen as broadening of the typical plasmon band at 514 nm for [^{198}Au]6-1 (green line, 25 μg/mL, irradiation 15 min) and [^{198}Au]6-2 (blue line, 25 μg/mL, irradiation 60 min).

2.3. Cell Experiments

2.3.1. Determination of Target Avidities

Several different IC_{50} values for RGD derivatives have been reported in the literature, ranging from 0.1 nM up to 6.7 µM. The main reason for the observed differences is the assay method used to determine the IC_{50} values. IC_{50} values of 0.1–1 nM can be found for RGD peptides having been determined by ELISA assays [38] and IC_{50} values around 20 nM have been reported for solid-phase $\alpha_v\beta_3$ binding assays for monomeric RGD derivatives [37]. Those IC_{50} values were derived by non-living experiments. However, cell experiments are closer to in vivo conditions. Therefore, for the AuNPs **7** and **8**, the $\alpha_v\beta_3$ integrin-avidities were determined by competitive displacement experiments on $\alpha_v\beta_3$-expressing U87MG cells using ^{125}I-echistatin as the $\alpha_v\beta_3$-specific radioligand and competitor. The RGD monomer c(RGDfK) was evaluated as an internal reference. The evaluation of RGD derivatives by displacement experiments yielded IC_{50} values comparable to those reported in the literature [34]. For the c(RGDfK) monomer, a mean IC_{50} value of 0.7 µM was determined (Table 3, Figure A3). The multi-RGD decoration on the surface of AuNPs **7a** and **7b** resulted in a lower mean IC_{50} value of 27.8 and 38.3 nM, respectively (Figures A4 and A5). Mean IC_{50} values of 82.4 and 103.6 nM were found for AuNPs **8a** and **8b**, respectively (Figures A6 and A7). It was observed that the higher the loading with $\alpha_v\beta_3$-specific RGD peptide, the lower the IC_{50} values.

Table 3. Avidity experiments.

Probe	Description	IC_{50} [nM]
c(RGDfK)	$\alpha_v\beta_3$ antagonist	700.4 ± 155.9
7a	AuNP-PEG-RGD$_{high}$	27.8 ± 3.4
7b	AuNP-PEG-RGD$_{low}$	38.3 ± 11.9
8a	AuNP-dithio-PEG-RGD$_{high}$	82.4 ± 9.2
8b	AuNP-dithio-PEG-RGD$_{low}$	103.6 ± 3.5

2.3.2. Determination of Cell Survival

Colony formation assays were performed with [^{198}Au]**3** with U87MG cells. For this proof-of-concept experiment, 5–10 Gy was chosen as the incubation dose. To achieve this dose, 1–2 MBq [^{198}Au]**3** per well in a 24-well plate within a 96 h incubation period was calculated using Formula (1).

$$D(A,t) = S \times \frac{A * T_{1/2}}{\ln(2)} \left[1 - \exp\left(-\ln(2) \times \frac{t}{T_{1/2}}\right)\right] \quad (1)$$

Formula (1)—Calculation of dose to a cell monolayer at the bottom of a multi-well plate or Eppendorf tube for ^{198}Au using Geant4-simulation [44]. D: energy dose, S: S-value, A: activity, $T_{1/2}$: half-life of the radionuclide, t: irradiation time.

This dose corresponds to concentrations of [^{198}Au]AuNPs of 0.515–0.939 µM, which is at least 10 times higher than the IC_{50} of AuNP-dithio-RGD **7** and **8**. It was observed that the survival fraction (sf) of the cells was significantly reduced for [^{198}Au]**3** and that higher doses of 10 Gy (sf = 18.2%) were more effective in damaging the tumor cells than 5 Gy (sf = 33.9%) (Figure 4).

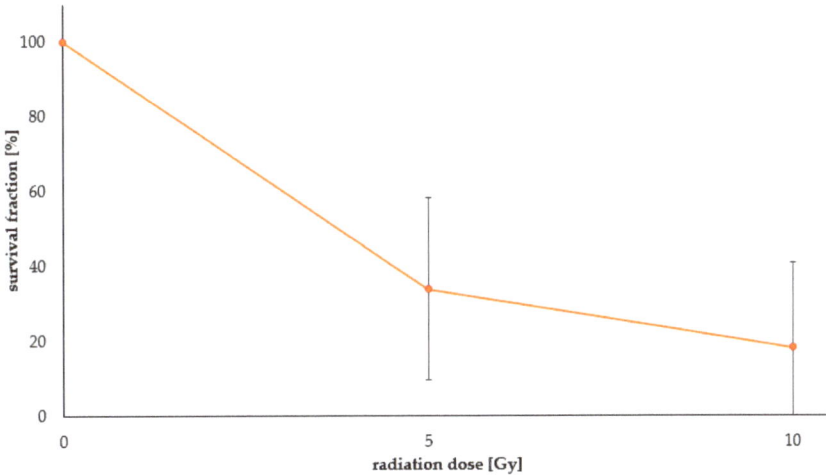

Figure 4. Survival fractions of the colony formation assays of 5 Gy [^{198}Au]**3** and 10 Gy [^{198}Au]**3**.

3. Discussion

c(RGDfK) is a highly potent and selective integrin $\alpha_v\beta_3$ antagonist and therefore could disrupt cell viability by inhibiting angiogenesis [45]. Radiolabeled RGD derivatives can be used as tracers for tumor angiogenesis [46]. Multimerization leads to better tumor accumulation [47,48]. Therefore, AuNPs decorated with a multitude of c(RGDfK) motifs could lead to better tumor accumulation, which is important for therapy.

Methods for the preparation of [^{198}Au]AuNPs are already known in the literature [11,29,32]. However, the synthesis starts with neutron activation of gold foil, which is then dissolved in aqua regia, followed by nanoparticle synthesis and further functionalizations with target-specific ligands. All these steps are performed with radioactive ^{198}Au, resulting in higher dose accumulation for the personnel and more radioactive waste as the consequence. In this work, it was decided to first complete the synthesis of tumor-specific AuNPs with a high target avidity and high stability, and to perform neutron activation as the last step in order to reduce the personnel dose and enable a highly efficient synthesis pathway, which is mandatory for high clinical relevance. The challenge was to synthesize AuNPs that withstand neutron activation without aggregation and loss of the ligand shell.

Stable $\alpha_v\beta_3$-specific AuNPs **7** and **8** were successfully synthesized with a better avidity compared to the monomeric peptide ligand c(RGDfK). During the irradiation experiments, it was observed that AuNPs containing monothiol ligands were unstable against neutron activation. However, all AuNP derivatives containing only dithiol ligands were stable against neutron activation even at the highest concentrations and irradiation times (~7.5 mg/mL within 2 h). It is known that sulfur can also be activated by neutrons via the $^{32}S(n,p)^{32}P$ reaction [49,50]. Presumably, once a sulfur atom is activated to ^{32}P, it loses its covalent bond to the AuNP surface and a monothiol ligand is lost to the environment. In contrast, a dithiol ligand could remain bound to the surface even if a binding interaction is lost by activation of one of the sulfur atoms.

To determine the therapeutic influence of [^{198}Au]AuNPs, cell survival was addressed by a colony formation assay. The activity and incubation time to reach relevant doses between 5 and 10 Gy were calculated for monolayer cell culture in 24-well plates (Formula (1)). To reach these doses of 5–10 Gy concentrations of a factor >10 times higher than the IC$_{50}$ for AuNP-RGD **8a** and **8b** had to be used within 96 h of incubation. Therefore, cell viability should be considered to be very low when using such high concentrations of [^{198}Au]**8** in cell survival experiments, as the antagonist RGD may interfere with angiogenesis and thus cell viability [45]. To circumvent this problem, future experiments should use higher activity concentrations (due to longer activation of AuNPs) or longer cell incubation with lower doses >5 Gy, when evaluating cell survival. However, in the proof-of-concept cell survival experiments, non-specific [^{198}Au]3 showed a significant effect on U87MG cells with a survival fraction as low as 18.2% at 10 Gy. Therefore, the combination of β^--emission from ^{198}Au and the antagonistic effect of RGD could dramatically reduce the therapeutically relevant dose of applied [^{198}Au]AuNP-RGDs.

4. Materials and Methods

General procedures. All reagents and solvents were purchased from commercial suppliers (Sigma, Merck) and were used without further purification. NMR spectra were recorded on a 300 MHz Mercury Plus and a 500 MHz NMR System spectrometer (Varian, Palo Alto, CA, USA). Chemical shifts (δ) are given in ppm and are referenced to the residual solvent resonance signals relative to $(CH_3)_4Si$ (^1H, ^{13}C). Mass spectra were obtained on a microflex MALDI-TOF mass spectrometer (Bruker Daltonics, Bremen, Germany) and HR-ESI-MS spectra on a LTQ FT Ultra Fourier Transform Ion Cyclotron Resonance spectrometer (Thermo Finnigan, Dreieich, Germany). When applicable, purity was determined by HPLC. The purity of all final compounds was 95% or higher. HPLC was performed on a Dionex UltiMate 3000 HPLC system (Thermo Scientific, Dreieich, Germany), equipped with a reverse phase column (Analytical: Merck Chromolith RP-18e; 100 × 4.6 mm plus a guard column 5 × 4.6 mm; semipreparative: Chromolith RP-18e; 100 × 10 mm plus a guard column 10 × 4.6 mm), and a UV-diode array detector (210 nm, 254 nm). The solvent system used was a gradient of acetonitrile:water (containing 0.1% TFA) (0–5 min: 0–100% MeCN) at a flow rate of 4 mL/min, unless otherwise stated. The purity and stability of AuNPs/[^{198}Au]AuNPs were investigated by size exclusion HPLC using a PolySep™-SEC GFC-P 4000, LC column 300 × 7.8 mm, and a 35 mm PolySep guard column (Phenomenex, Aschaffenburg, Germany) with water (0.8 mL/min) as eluent (Figure A10). Purification of AuNPs was performed by dialysis (tubes with molecular weight cut-off of 14,000 g/mol, Visking, Roth, Karlsruhe, Germany) against distilled water and by size-exclusion chromatography using Sephadex G25 PD10 columns (Fisher Scientific, Schwerte, Germany) and distilled water as eluent.

A brief description of the AuNP syntheses can be found in Appendix A.

Determination of the number of ligands on the surface of the AuNPs. The thermogravimetric analyses were performed using a Mettler Toledo TGA 2 STAR^e system. AuNPs (1–2 mg) were weighed into 70-µL-aluminum oxide crucibles (Mettler Toledo, Gießen, Germany) and heated from 25–750 °C (10 K/min) in a stream of N_2 or CO_2 (30 mL/min). The loading of the different AuNPs is shown in Table 1 and was calculated from the different mass losses, which increase as the AuNPs are functionalized. Therefore, the amount of different ligands per particle can be calculated according to the formula of Zhu et al. [42]. Since the nanoparticles have an average diameter of ~3 nm, the calculated amount of gold atoms is ~834 Au atoms per nanoparticle. This gives a molecular weight of an AuNP of 164,298 g/mol. Using TGA, the following ligand numbers were determined:

- The mass loss of the AuNP **6** was ~19.8%. This corresponds to ~250 PEG ligands on the AuNP surface. M~210 kDA.
- The mass loss of AuNP-RGD **7a** was ~24.8% and the RGD accounts for ~5% mass loss (~35 RGD ligands per AuNP). Therefore, the molar mass for AuNP-RGD$_{high}$ **7a** was calculated to be ~239 kDa.
- Furthermore, the AuNP-RGD$_{low}$ **7b** contained ~15 RGD ligands ~222 kDa.
- The mass loss of the AuNP **3** was ~33.27%. results in ~240 PEG ligands on the AuNP surface. M~246 kDa.
- The mass loss of AuNP-PEG-RGD$_{high}$ **8a** was ~37.1% and the RGD accounts for ~4% mass loss (~24 RGD ligands per AuNP). Therefore, the molar mass for AuNP-RGD$_{high}$ **8a** was calculated to be ~262 kDa.
- Furthermore, the AuNP-RGD$_{low}$ **8b** contained ~18 RGD ligands ~257 kDa.

Avidity experiments. The $\alpha_v\beta_3$-binding affinities of the respective RGD peptides and AuNPs were determined using in vitro competitive displacement experiments on U87MG tumor cells (HTB-14, ATCC®, Manassas, VA, USA). U87MG cells were harvested and resuspended in the binding buffer at a cell concentration of 2×10^6/mL to reach 10^5 cells per well.

A special binding buffer in sterile distilled water (Tris·HCl 25 mM, NaCl 150 mM, CaCl$_2$ 1 mM, MgCl$_2$ 0.5 mM, MnCl$_2$ 1 mM, pH 7.4, BSA 0.5%) was used for incubation with 0.25–0.40 kBq/well ^{125}I-Echistatin (81.4 GBq/µmol) as the $\alpha_v\beta_3$ specific radioligand in the presence of increasing concentrations (0–100 µM) of competing c(RGDfK) peptide or c(RGDfK)-modified AuNPs (0–20 µM). IC$_{50}$ values were obtained using GraphPad Prism v6.05 (nonlinear fit) software.

Neutron irradiation experiments. Production of [^{198}Au]AuNPs by neutron activation of 0.05–15.5 mg AuNPs was performed in pneumatic transfer tube one for 1–2 h at 100 kW with a thermal neutron flux of 1.6×10^{12} cm$^{-2} \times$ s^{-1} in the TRIGA research reactor (Mainz, Germany). For calibration of the dose calibrator ISOMED 2010 (NUVIA Instruments, Dresden, Germany) 12.7 mg solid Au was irradiated for 1 h to produce 87 MBq (calculated) [^{198}Au]Au with a measured dose rate of 57 µSv/h. 26 h later, the activity was measured with the dose calibrator, and 60 MBq was obtained (using the ^{137}Cs-channel, 66 MBq calculated). In addition, the solid [^{198}Au]Au (40 MBq) was carefully dissolved in 2 mL aqua regia at 50 °C within 15 min in order to find the correct calibration factors of the dose calibrator for different volumes in vials and syringes.

Irradiation of AuNPs was performed under optimized conditions in 2 mL 10% EtOH/H$_2$O and 25 mg ascorbic acid as a stabilizer against radiolysis [51]. Theoretically, 10 mg of pure ^{197}Au irradiated with a thermal neutron flux of 1.6×10^{12} cm$^{-2} \times$ s^{-1} would produce 48–96 MBq ^{198}Au within 1–2 h of irradiation. In the experiment, neutron activation of 5.0 mg AuNPs **3** and **8** for 2 h produced 48 MBq [^{198}Au]**3** (66.7% Au) and 50 MBq [^{198}Au]**8** (62.9% Au). Neutron activation of 15.56 mg AuNP **3** for 2 h produced ~100 MBq [^{198}Au]**3** (67% Au). The production of ^{198}Au was confirmed by gamma spectroscopy, which found up to three gamma lines at 411 keV (95.6%), 676 keV (0.8%), and 1088 keV (0.2%).

Colony formation assay. Three days before the experiments, 150,000 cells were seeded in 24-well plates. U87MG cells were incubated for 96 h in the presence of the $\alpha_v\beta_3$-specific or non-radioactive AuNPs or 1–2 MBq [^{198}Au]AuNPs to achieve the calculated doses of 5–10 Gy. After incubation, the cell medium was removed, the cells were washed and harvested, and a colony formation assay was performed in triplicate for each irradiation point with 1000 cells per well in a 6-well plate. Colonies were cultured in cell medium for 28 days, then washed with 1 mL PBS, fixed with 2 mL 4% formaldehyde in PBS for 15 min, and incubated with 2 mL 0.5% crystal violet dye solution for 30 min. Afterward, colonies were washed with distilled water, dried, and counted by light microscopy. Colonies of more than 50 cells were considered viable, and the plating efficiency for each sample was estimated based on the initial number of cells seeded. Clonogenic cell survival was calculated as the relative plating efficiency of treated versus untreated samples. Triplicate samples were prepared for each treatment and experimental condition.

5. Conclusions

$\alpha_v\beta_3$-specific RGD-containing AuNPs with a higher target avidity compared to $\alpha_v\beta_3$-specific RGD were successfully synthesized. This proof-of-concept work should demonstrate, that activation of AuNPs with a ligand shell is possible without losing their organic shell and integrity. Irradiation experiments demonstrated the stability and consistency of [^{198}Au]AuNPs with dithiol ligands compared to [^{198}Au]AuNPs with monothiol ligands, which always aggregated at each applied concentration after neutron activation. In vitro experiments determine the therapeutic effect of [^{198}Au]AuNPs by addressing the survival fraction of U87MG cells proved a significant influence on cell death. Therefore, the [^{198}Au]AuNPs could serve as a tool for endoradiotherapy.

Further experiments to determine the therapeutic effects of [^{198}Au]AuNPs in vivo by different modes of application (local vs. systemic) are currently underway.

Author Contributions: Conceptualization, G.D., C.W., M.P. and B.W.; methodology, G.D., K.E., C.G. and M.P.; software (Geant 4 v11.1.2), R.F.; validation, G.D. and M.P.; formal analysis, G.D. and K.E.; investigation, G.D.; resources, M.P. and B.W.; data curation, G.D., R.S. and M.P.; writing—original draft preparation, G.D., C.W. and M.P.; writing—review and editing, G.D., C.W., K.E., C.G., R.S., R.F. and B.W.; visualization, G.D. and M.P.; supervision, M.P. and B.W.; project administration, M.P. and B.W.; funding acquisition, C.W., M.P. and B.W. All authors have read and agreed to the published version of the manuscript.

Funding: This research was funded by Research Campus M^{2}OLIE funded by the German Federal Ministry of Education and Research (BMBF) within the Framework "Forschungscampus: public-private partnership for Innovations", Funding Codes 13GW0091B, 13GW0091E, 13GW0388A and 13GW0389B.

Institutional Review Board Statement: Not applicable.

Informed Consent Statement: Not applicable.

Data Availability Statement: All data can be referred to on request to the corresponding author.

Acknowledgments: The authors are grateful to Karsten Richter from DKFZ Heidelberg for performing the electron microscopy studies of the AuNPs. The NMR measurements performed by Tobias Timmermann at RKU Heidelberg and the HR-ESI measurements performed by Werner Spahl at LMU Munich are gratefully acknowledged. We also want to thank Ulrich Scherer for using the TGA spectrometer and for performing initial neutron irradiation experiments and Thorsten Röder for using the DLS at Mannheim University of Applied Sciences. We thank the mechanical workshop and the staff of the Research Reactor TRIGA Mainz for their excellent support. Moreover, the authors would like to thank Lisa Hübinger for the extensive proofreading of the manuscript.

Conflicts of Interest: The authors declare no conflict of interest.

Appendix A

Appendix A.1. Organic Syntheses

c(RGDfK) [52]

The peptide c(RGDfK) c(Arg-Gly-Asp-D-Phe-Lys) was synthesized according to standard protocols by solid-phase peptide synthesis on solid support using the Fmoc-strategy on H-Asp(tBu)-2-chlortrityl resin (loading 0.73 mmol/g, 137 mg, 0.1 mmol). For amino acid conjugation, HBTU (N,N,N',N'-tetramethyl-O-(1H-benzotriazol-1-yl)uronium hexafluorophosphate) (3.9 eq., 0.39 mmol, 148.7 mg), Fmoc-protected amino acids (4.0 eq., 0.4 mmol) and DIPEA (4.0 eq., 0.4 mmol, 68 µL) were used in DMF as solvent. Each amino acid was coupled for 45 min. After coupling of the last amino acid and Fmoc-removal with 50% of piperidine solution in DMF, the linear protected peptide was cleaved from the resin using 1% TFA in CH_2Cl_2. After removal of the volatile components of the mixture, the crude intermediate was isolated and dissolved in dry DMF (85 mL). After addition of DIPEA (3.5 eq., 0.35 mmol, 59.5 µL) the solution was cooled to 0 °C and DPPA (1.25 eq., 0.125 mmol, 26.9 µL) was added. The reaction was allowed to warm to ambient temperature and stirred for 3 days until the cyclization was complete. The volatile components of the mixture were evaporated under reduced pressure, and the residue was treated with a mixture of TFA/TIS 97.5:2.5 for 3 h to completely deprotect the peptide. The crude product was precipitated in cold diethyl ether and washed twice with diethyl ether and dried under reduced pressure. The product was purified by semi-preparative HPLC and lyophilized to give a colorless solid (yield: 88.79%, 53.6 mg, 0.089 mmol). HR-ESI-MS (m/z) for [M + H]$^+$ (calculated): 604.3 (604.3). MALDI-MS (m/z) for [M]$^+$ (calculated): 603.7 (603.3).

TA-NHS 1 [53]

Thioctic acid (TA) (1 eq., 2.425 mmol, 0.50 g) was dissolved in acetone (12.5 mL) under an argon atmosphere. N,N-Disuccinimidyl carbonate (1.25 eq., 3.031 mmol, 0.78 g) and

DIPEA (1.25 eq., 3.031 mmol, 0.5 mL) were added and the mixture was stirred overnight at room temperature. After removal of acetone under reduced pressure, the residue was dissolved in 10 mL of water and DCM (1:1). The aqueous phase was removed and the organic phase was washed twice with 4 mL water. After drying the organic phase with MgSO$_4$, the solvent, DCM, was removed and TA-NHS was obtained as a yellowish solid. (78.01%, 574 mg, 1.89 mmol). ^{1}H-NMR (300 MHz, DMSO-d$_6$) δ = 3.67–3.58 (m, 1H, H-3), 3.24–3.08 (m, 2H, H-5), 2.81 (s, 4H, H-15, H-16), 2.69 (t, ^3J = 7.2 Hz, 2H, H-9), 2.47–2.37 (m, 1H, H-4), 1.94–1.83 (m, 1H, H-4), 1.77–1.42 ppm (m, 6H, H-6, H-7, H-8).

TA-PEG$_3$-OH 2

TA-NHS dissolved in 3 mL DCM (1.2 eq., 0.96 mmol, 0.29 g) was added to a solution of H$_2$N-PEG$_3$-OH (1 eq., 0.80 mmol, 0.12 g) in DCM (1 mL). After the addition of DIPEA (4 eq., 3.2 mmol, 545 µL) was added and the mixture was stirred overnight at ambient temperature. The solvent was removed under reduced pressure, and the crude product was purified by semi-preparative HPLC. Finally, the product TA-NH-PEG$_3$-OH was isolated as yellowish viscous liquid (yield: 65.04%, 180 mg, 0.533 mol). ^{1}H-NMR (500 MHz, DMSO-d$_6$) δ = 7.89–7.77 (m, 1H, H-11), 3.43–3.37 (m, 12H, H-13, H-14, H-16, H-17, H-19, H-20), 3.22–3.15 (m, 2H, H-5), 2.87–2.71 (m, 2H, H-3, H-21), 2.13–2.03 (m, 2H, H-9), 1.99–1.81 (m, 2H, H-4), 1.60–1.21 ppm (m, 6H, H-6, H-7, H-8). HR-ESI-MS (m/z) for [M + H]$^+$ (calculated): 338.1 (338. 1), [M + Na]$^+$ (calculated): 360.1 (360.1). MALDI-MS (m/z) for [M]$^+$ (calculated): 337.3 (337.1), [M + H]$^+$ (calculated): 338.1 (338. 1).

TA-PEG$_4$-COOH 4

TA-NHS dissolved in 2 mL DCM (1.1 eq., 0.88 mmol, 0.27 g) was added to a suspension of H$_2$N-PEG$_4$-COOH (1 eq., 0.80 mmol, 0.12 g) in DMF (2 mL). DIPEA (4 eq., 3.2 mmol, 545 µL) was added and the mixture was stirred overnight at ambient temperature. The solvent was removed under reduced pressure, and the crude product was purified by semi-preparative HPLC. After lyophilization the product TA-NH-PEG$_4$-COOH was obtained as colorless solid (yield: 48.92%, 160.3 mg, 0.39 mmol). HR-ESI-MS (m/z) for [M + H]$^+$ (calculated): 410.1 (410.1), [M + Na]$^+$ (calculated): 432.1 (432.1). MALDI-MS (m/z) for [M]$^+$ (calculated): 409.4 (409.1), [M + K]$^+$ (calculated): 447.4 (448.1).

TA-PEG$_4$-c(RGDfK) 5

TA-NH-PEG$_4$-COOH dissolved in 0.5 mL of DMF (1.1 eq., 0.055 mmol, 22.4 mg) was added to a solution of PyBOP (1.9 eq., 0.094 mmol, 49.1 g) in 0.5 mL of DMF. DIPEA (3 eq., 0.149 mmol, 26 µL) was added and the mixture was stirred at ambient temperature until the reaction was completed. DMF was then removed under reduced pressure, and the crude product was purified by semi-preparative HPLC. After lyophilization the product TA-NH-PEG$_4$-c(RGDfK) was obtained as colorless solid (yield: 28.91%, 14.3 mg, 0.014 mmol). HR-ESI-MS (m/z) for [M + H]$^+$ (calculated): 995.4 (995.4). MALDI-MS (m/z) for [M]$^+$ (calculated): 994.8 (994.4), [M + K]$^+$ (calculated): 1033.7 (1033.4).

AuNP-dithio-PEG$_3$-OH 3 [40]

Hydrogen tetrachloroaurate (1 eq., 0.525 mmol, 207 mg) was dissolved in 205 mL MeOH to give a bright yellow solution and under stirring a solution of TA-NH-PEG$_3$-OH dissolved in 205 mL of MeOH was added and stirred for 2 h until the reaction color became nearly colorless. A solution of sodium borohydride dissolved in 20.5 mL of water was quickly added to the reaction. The solution immediately turned black. The reaction mixture was stirred overnight, MeOH was removed under reduced pressure, and the residue was redissolved in 9 mL of tracepure water and dialyzed in distilled water for 4 days. After lyophilisation TA-AuNP was obtained as black powder. (39.47%, 180.7 mg).

AuNP-thio-PEG 6 [6]

General procedure for the preparation of PEGylated AuNPs: Briefly, hydrogen tetrachloroaurate(III) trihydrate (1 eq., 0.4 mmol, 157.5 mg, ≥99.9% trace metal basis) was dissolved in 12.5 mL of trace pure water resulting in a bright yellow solution, and then extracted by mixing with 125 mL of a tetraoctylammonium bromide (TOABr, 1.2 eq., 0.48 mmol, 263 mg) toluene solution. The contents were stirred vigorously for 20 min at room temperature to facilitate the phase transfer of the Au(III) into the toluene layer, which resulted in the organic layer turning to a dark orange color and the aqueous layer becoming clear colorless. After the phase transfer was complete, the aqueous layer was removed. The organic layer was dried with $MgSO_4$ and filtered to remove excess of water. The solution was cooled to 0 °C in an ice bath. Freshly-prepared HO-PEG_3-thiol (3 eq., 1.2 mmol, 199 mg) in 6.3 mL of dichloromethane was added and stirred until the orange solution turned to colorless (~1 h). A fresh solution of tetrabutylammonium borohydride (TBABH) (10 eq., 4.0 mmol, 1.03 g) in 6.3 mL dichloromethane was then added to the rapidly stirring toluene solution over 5 s. The solution immediately turned black. The PEG-AuNP began to precipitate from the toluene after 1 h. After stirring the mixture for 16 h from 0 °C to 20 °C, 6.3 mL of trace pure water was added under slow stirring to extract the PEGylated AuNPs for 120 min. The organic layer was decanted and the aqueous layer was washed alternately with 3 × 13 mL toluene/1.3 mL MeCN and 3 × 13 mL toluene/1.3 mL isopropanol. The black aqueous layer was transferred to a Visking cellulose dialysis tube (molecular cut-off 14,000 Da) with 3 × 6.3 mL trace pure water and dialyzed in 3 × 10 L of distilled water for 1 h, 2.5 h and 16 h. The AuNPs were lyophilized to yield 69.5 mg (25.10%) of black powder. ^{1}H-NMR (500 MHz, DMSO-d6) δ = 4.67–4.48 (m, 1H, H-10), 3.93–3.38 (m, 10H, H-3, H-5, H-6, H-8, H-9), 1.36–1.25 ppm (m, 2H, H-2).

AuNP-PEG-RGDs by ligand exchange

General procedure for the preparation of RGD-decorated AuNPs: Briefly, the functionalization of AuNPs **3** and **6** was performed by a place-exchange reaction with TA-PEG_4-c(RGDfK) **5**. TA-PEG_4-c(RGDfK) **5** was dissolved in a mixture trace pure H_2O:MeOH (1:1) and was added to AuNPs **3** or **6** in 2 mL trace pure H_2O and stirred overnight. Purification of AuNPs was performed in two steps: First, the AuNP solution was transferred into a Visking cellulose dialysis tube (molecular cut-off 14,000 Da) with 3 × 1 mL trace pure water and dialyzed in distilled water for 4 days, and second, the AuNP solution was eluted by size-exclusion chromatography using Sephadex G25 PD10 columns and distilled water. The AuNPs were then lyophilized and obtained as a black powder.

AuNP-thio-PEG_3-dithio-PEG_4-RGD_{high} 7a

TA-PEG_4-c(RGDfK) **5** (8 mg, 8.04 µmol) was dissolved in 0.4 mL of trace pure H_2O:MeOH (1:1) and was added to AuNP **6** (20 mg) in 2 mL of trace pure H_2O and stirred overnight. After purification and lyophilization 13.1 mg (57.9%) of **7a** was obtained as black powder. ^{1}H-NMR (500 MHz, DMSO-d_6) δ = 8.43–7.66 (m, 7H, H-11, H -25, H-29, H-34, H-39, H-43, H-47), 7.21–7.18 (m, 5H, H-64, H-65, H-66, H-67, H-68), 6.65 (s, 2H, H-57), 4.58–4.54 (m, 1H, H-j), 4.00–3.42 (m, 16H, H-13, H-14, H-16, H-17, H-19, H-20, H-22, H-23), 3.02–2.92 (m, 1H, H-3), 2.04–1.86 (m, 2H, H-5), 1.78–0.76 ppm (m, 10H, H-4, H-6, H-7, H-8, H-9).

AuNP-thio-PEG_3-dithio-PEG_4-RGD_{low} 7b

TA-PEG_4-c(RGDfK) **5** (4 mg, 4.02 µmol) was dissolved in 0.4 mL of trace pure H_2O:MeOH (1:1) and was added to AuNP **6** (20 mg) in 2 mL of trace pure H_2O and stirred overnight. After purification and lyophilization 14.4 mg (68.4%) of **7b** was obtained as black powder.

AuNP-dithio-PEG-RGD_{high} 8a

TA-PEG_4-c(RGDfK) **5** (8 mg, 8.04 µmol) was dissolved in 0.4 mL of trace pure H_2O:MeOH (1:1) and was added to AuNP **3** (20 mg) in 2 mL of trace pure H_2O and stirred overnight. After purification and lyophilization 20.8 mg (97.5%) of **8a** was obtained as black powder. ^{1}H-NMR (500 MHz, DMSO-d_6) δ = 8.02–7.59 (m, 7H, H-11, H -25, H-29, H-34, H-39, H-43, H-47), 7.22–7.16 (m, 5H, H-64, H-65, H-66, H-67, H-68), 6.65 (s, 2H, H-57), 4.77–4.43 (m, 1H, H-u), 3.61–3.35 (m, 10H, H-13, H-14, H-16, H-17, H-19, H-20), 3.22–3.00 (m, 4H, H-22, H-23), 2.92–2.69 (m, 1H, H-3), 2.13–1.95 (m, 2H, H-5), 1.76–0.73 ppm (m, 10H, H-4, H-6, H-7, H-8, H-9).

AuNP-dithio-PEG-RGD$_{low}$ 8b

TA-PEG$_4$-c(RGDfK) **5** (4 mg, 4.02 µmol) was dissolved in 0.4 mL of trace pure H$_2$O:MeOH (1:1) and was added to AuNP **3** (20 mg) in 2 mL of trace pure H$_2$O and stirred overnight. After purification and lyophilization 19.7 mg (95.1%) of **8b** was obtained as black powder.

Appendix A.2. Electron Microscopy

AuNP samples were diluted at will in deionized water (fade red solution), particles were adsorbed onto glow-discharged carbon-coated EM grids and directly observed by TEM (Zeiss EM912, Carl Zeiss Oberkochen, Germany). Images were digitally captured with a CCD camera (Sharp eye, TRS, Moorenweiss, Germany). Particle number and size were measured using the FIJI software (v1.50e).

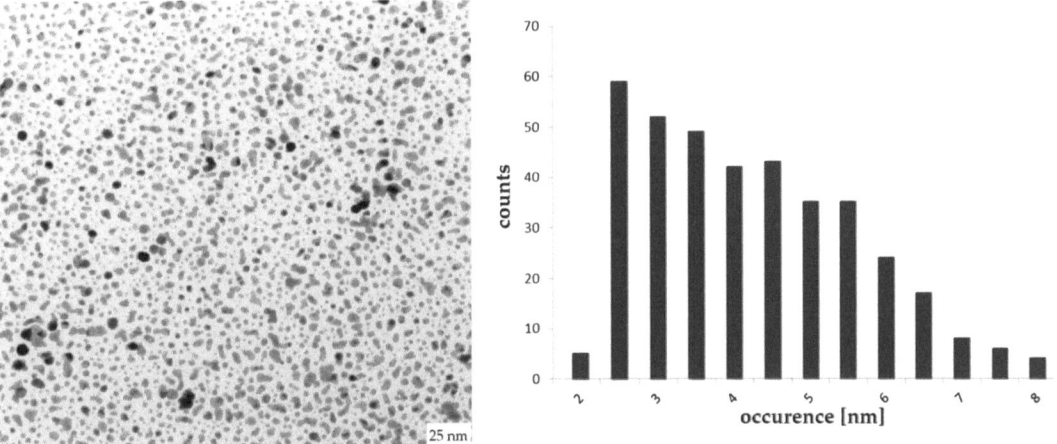

Figure A1. Transmission electron microscope image of AuNP **6** and corresponding histogram of AuNP diameter distribution.

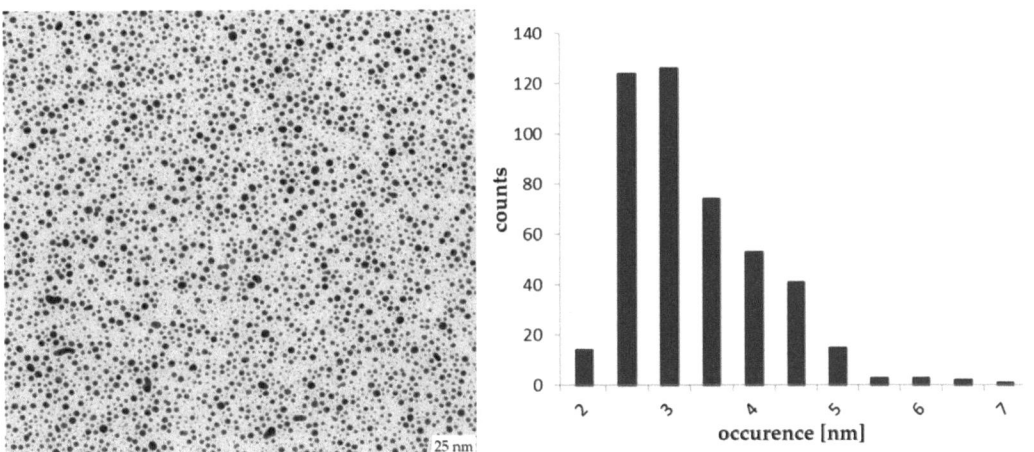

Figure A2. Transmission electron microscope image of AuNP **3** and corresponding histogram of AuNP diameter distribution.

Appendix A.3. Determination of Avidity of Non-Radioactive $\alpha_v\beta_3$-Specific AuNPs

The $\alpha_v\beta_3$-binding affinities of the respective RGD peptides and AuNPs were determined by in vitro competitive displacement experiments with U87MG tumor cells.

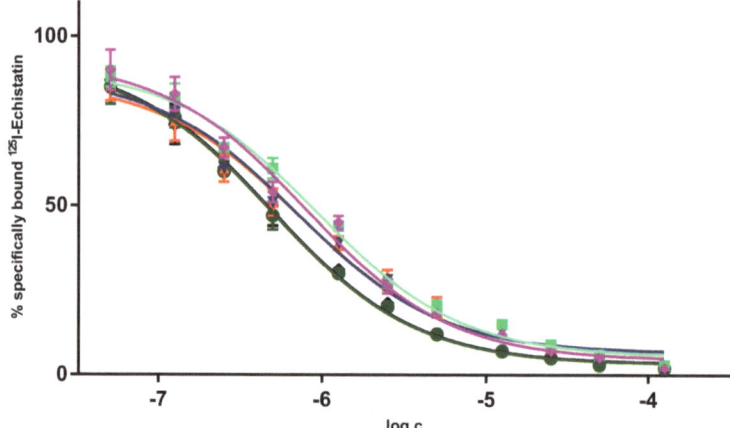

Figure A3. Binding curves of c(RGDfK). Different color means different experiment.

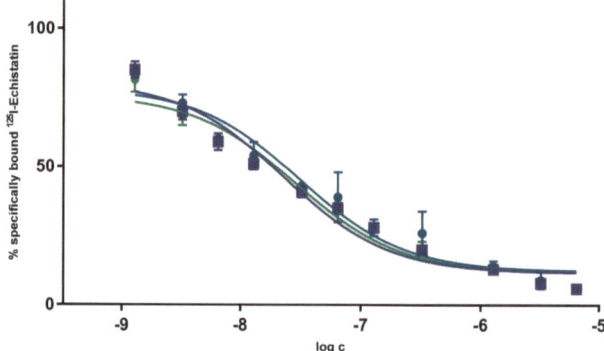

Figure A4. Binding curves of AuNPs **7a**. Different color means different experiment.

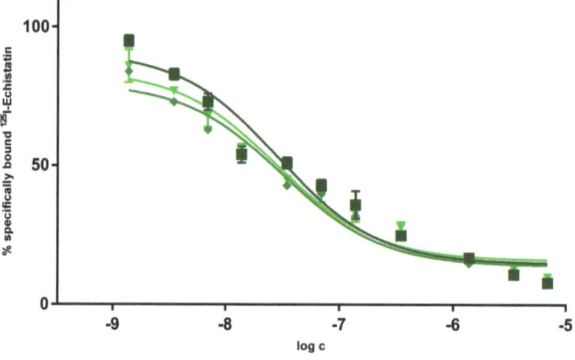

Figure A5. Binding curves of AuNPs **7b**. Different color means different experiment.

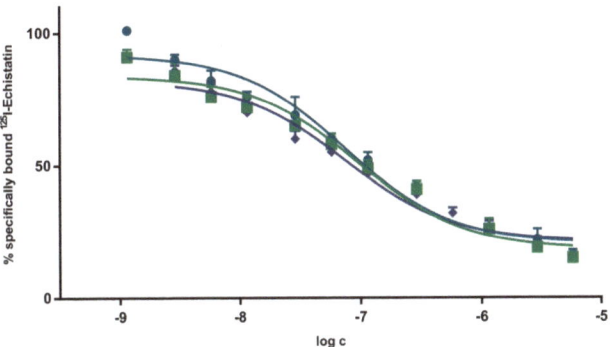

Figure A6. Binding curves of AuNPs **8a**. Different color means different experiment.

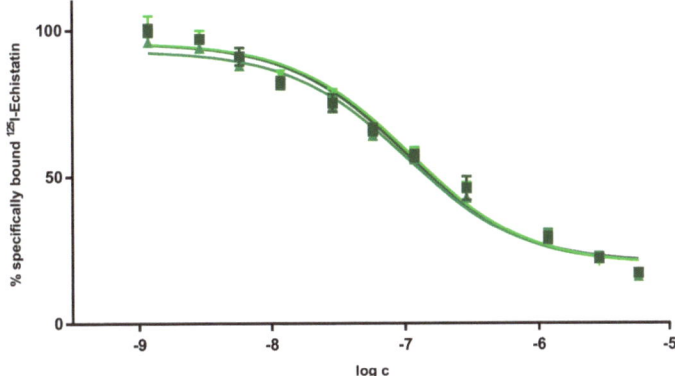

Figure A7. Binding curves of AuNPs **8b**. Different color means different experiment.

Appendix A.4. Determination of Half-Life of [^{198}Au]3

The half-life of [^{198}Au]3 was determined for 0.025–1.0 mg/mL by measuring five different probes for 28 days with a gamma counter (2470 WIZARD^2, Perkin Elmer). A half-life of 2.80 ± 0.07 days was found (real: 2.69 days). Therefore, the half-life found in this experiment deviated by 4% from the real value (Figure A8).

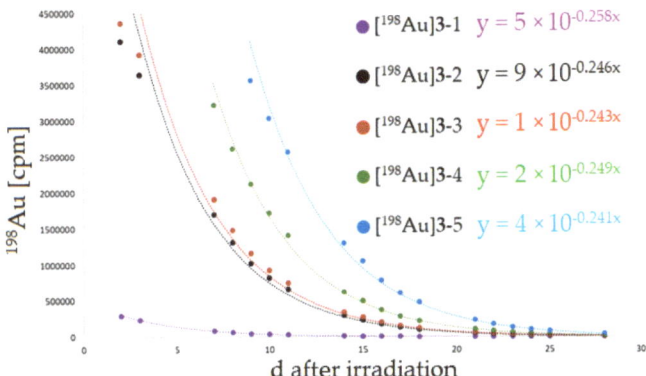

Figure A8. Decay curves of [^{198}Au]3 with different initial activities.

Appendix A.5. Determination of Stability of [[^{198}Au]AuNPs

Appendix A.5.1. UV/Vis Measurements

UV/Vis measurements were performed using an BioSpektrometer Kinetic (Eppendorf, Hamburg, Germany). The absorbance of [^{198}Au]3 at a concentration of 375 µg/mL was measured for up to 5 months (Figure A9) to estimate the particle size and stability. The absorption at surface plasmon resonance (maximum, 514 nm) divided by the absorption at 450 nm (minimum) gives a factor that can be compared with tables from the literature [54].

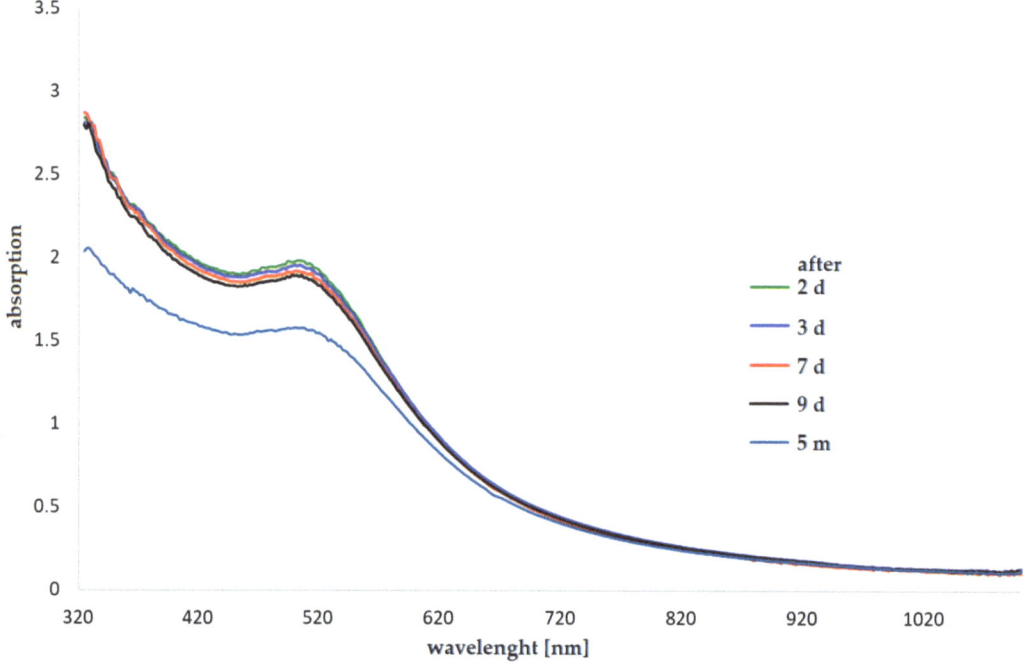

Figure A9. Representative absorption spectrum of [^{198}Au]3 at different time points after neutron activation with a typical absorption maximum for ultrasmall AuNPs at 514 nm indicating no aggregation of the particles.

Appendix A.5.2. HPLC Measurements

10 µL of [^{198}Au]3 (7.75 mg/mL, 50 MBq/mL) was diluted with 50 µL H$_2$O. 10 µL of the diluted solution was injected into an HPLC equipped with a Sephadex column. Measurements were performed up to 77 days after irradiation (Figure A10).

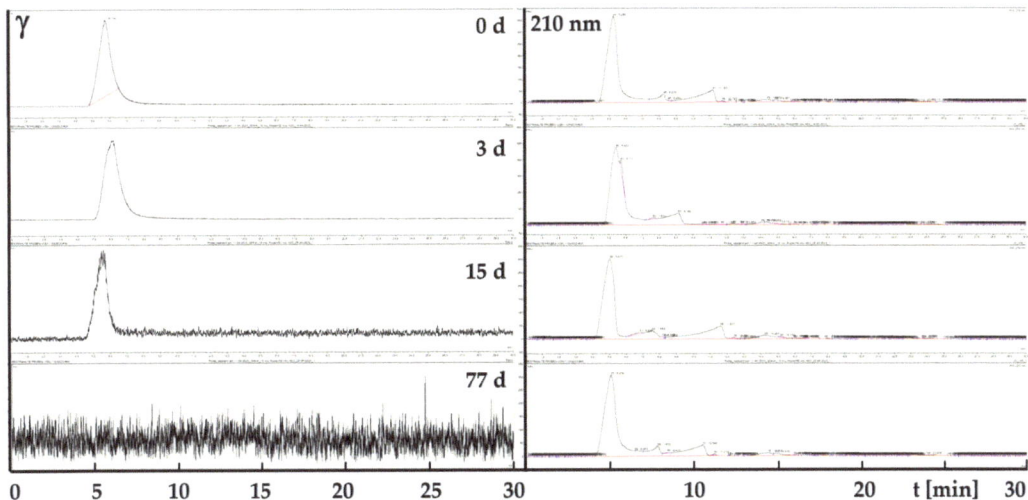

Figure A10. Representative (radio-)chromatogramms of [^{198}Au]3 showing no degradation or aggregation within 77 days. The [^{198}Au]3 t_R = 5.7 min. Ascorbic acid t_R = 11.6 min.

Appendix A.6. NMR Spectra

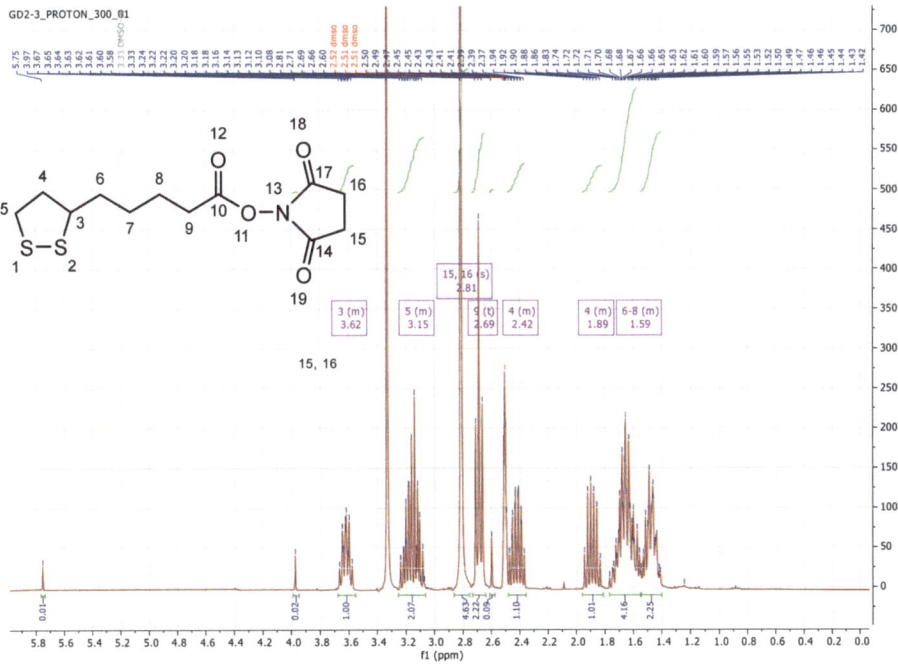

Figure A11. ^{1}H NMR spectrum of TA-NHS **1** in d$_6$-DMSO.

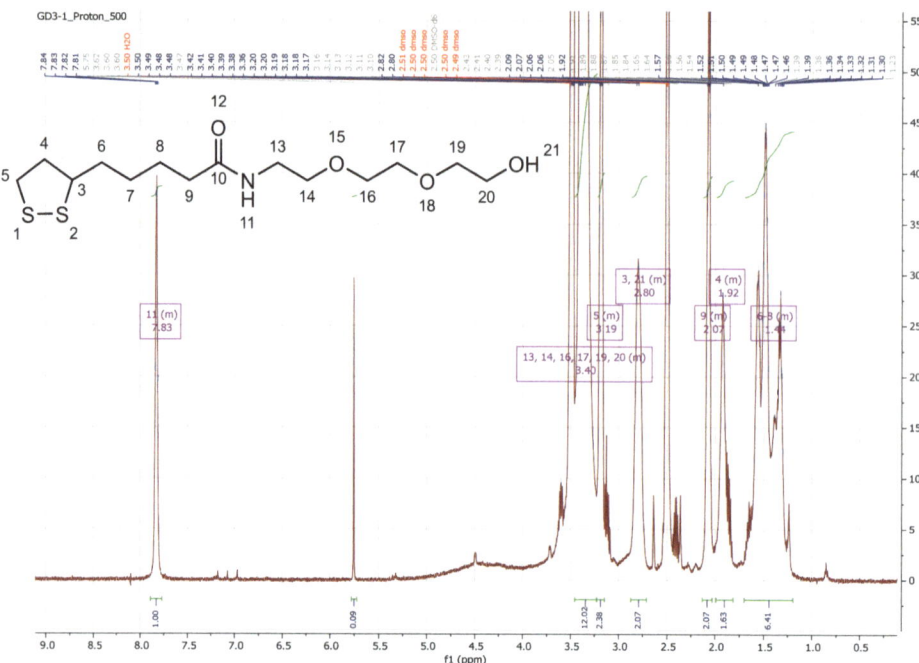

Figure A12. ^{1}H NMR spectrum of TA-PEG$_3$-OH **2** in d$_6$-DMSO.

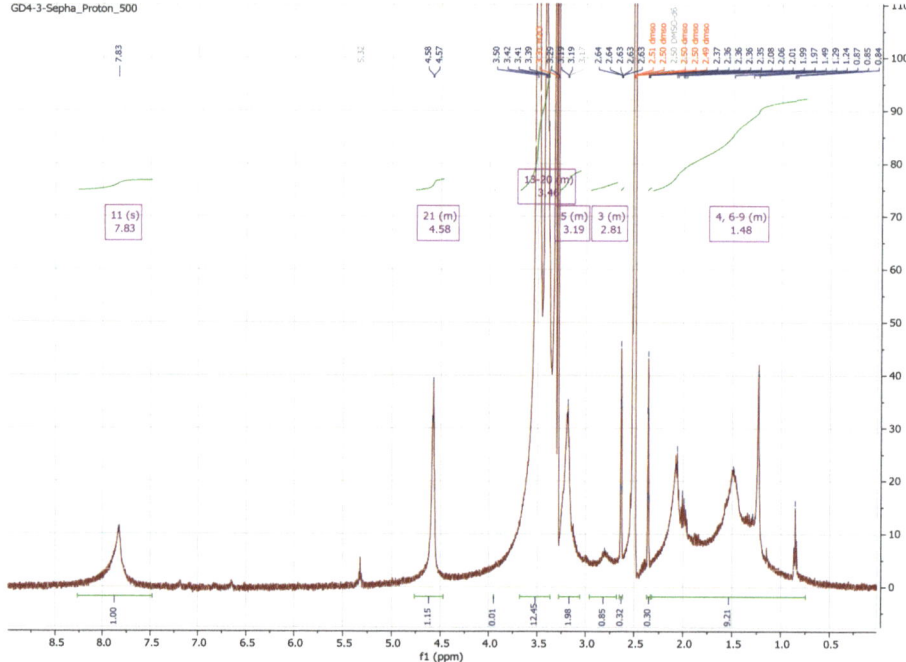

Figure A13. ^{1}H NMR spectrum of AuNP-dithio-PEG **3** in d$_6$-DMSO.

Appendix A.7. AuNP-Dithiol-RGD **8**

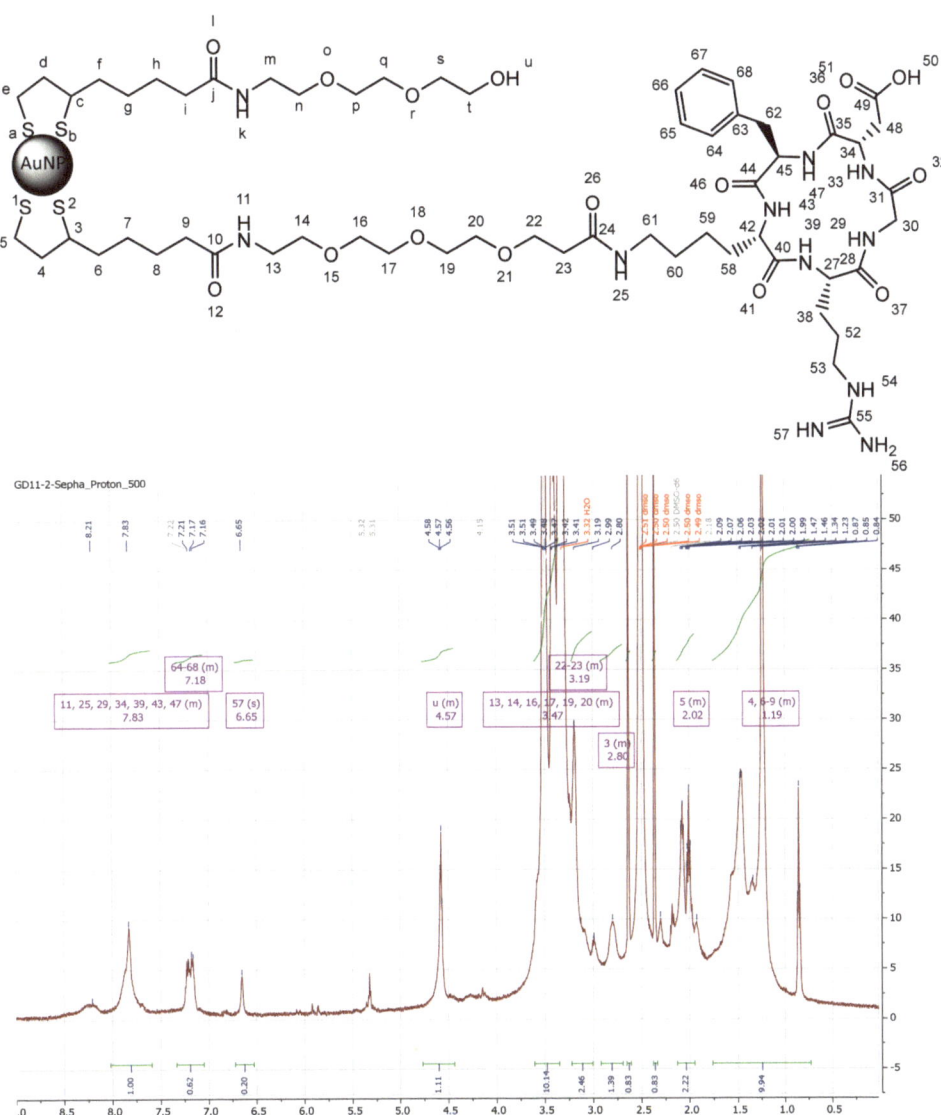

Figure A14. ^{1}H NMR spectrum of AuNP-dithio-RGD$_{high}$ **8a** in d$_6$-DMSO: characteristic signals of peptide-bond-NH (7.83 ppm), Phe-CH$_{arom}$ (7.22–7.16 ppm), Arg-C=NH (6.65 ppm), and Asp-CH (5.32 ppm) can be found.

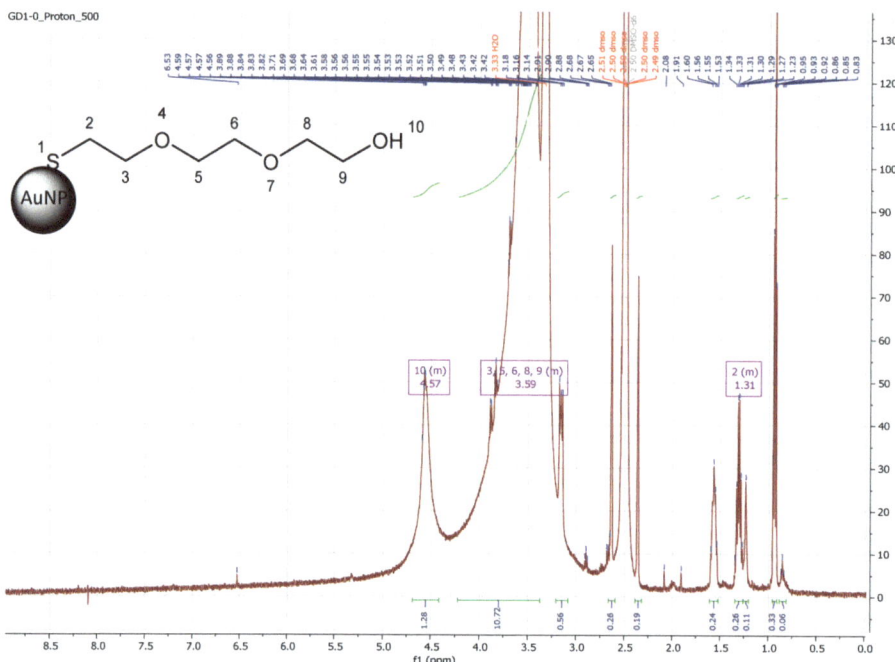

Figure A15. ^{1}H NMR spectrum of AuNP-thio-PEG **6** in d$_6$-DMSO.

*Appendix A.8. AuNP-Thiol-Dithiol-RGD **7***

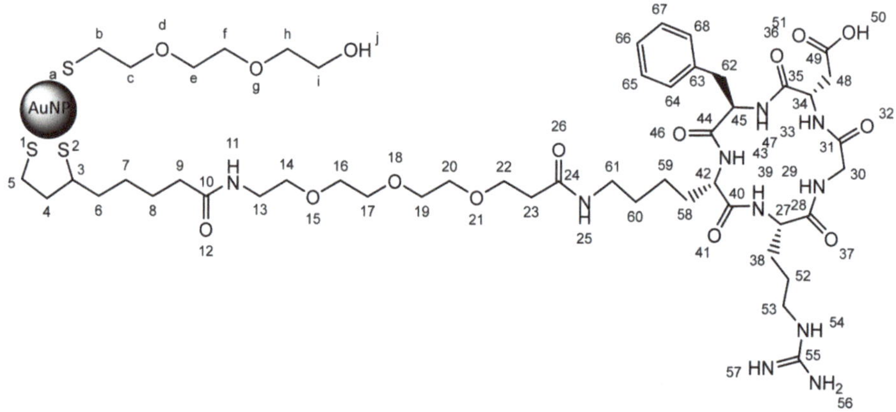

Figure A16. *Cont.*

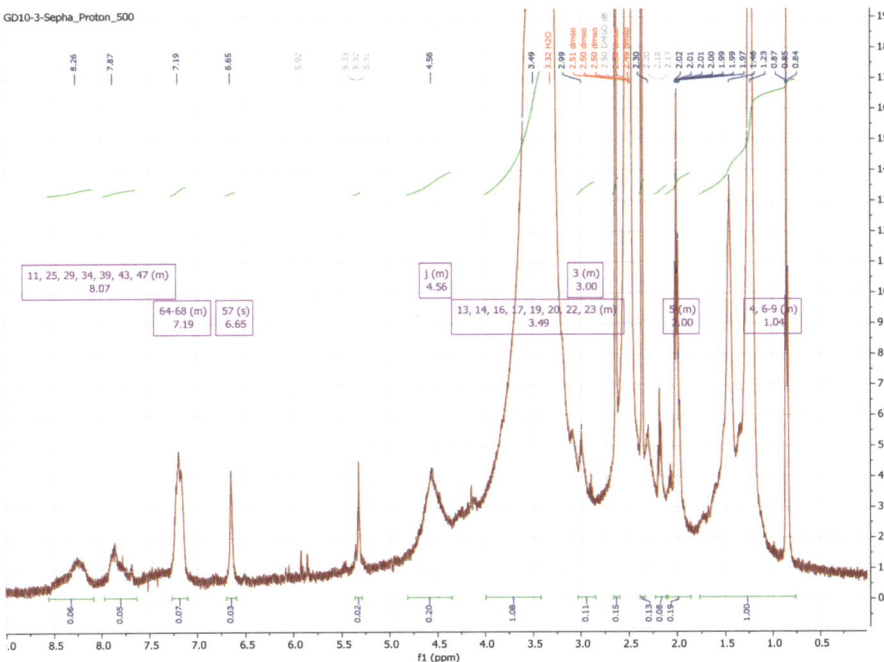

Figure A16. ^{1}H NMR spectrum of AuNP-thio-dithio-RGD$_{high}$ **7a** in d$_6$-DMSO: characteristic signals of peptide-bond-NH (7.87 ppm), Phe-CH$_{arom}$ (7.19 ppm), Arg-C=NH (6.65 ppm), Arg-NH$_2$ (5.92 ppm), and Asp-CH (5.32 ppm) can be found.

References

1. Sheppard, C.W.; Goodell, J.P.B.; Hahn, P.F. Colloidal gold containing the radioactive isotope Au^{198} in the selective internal radiation therapy of diseases of the lymphoid system. *J. Lab. Clin. Med.* **1947**, *12*, 1437–1441.
2. Flocks, R.H.; Kerr, H.D.; Elkins, H.B.; Culp, D. Treatment of carcinoma of the prostate by interstitial radiation with radio-active gold (Au 198): A preliminary report. *J. Urol.* **1952**, *68*, 510–522. [CrossRef] [PubMed]
3. Frens, G. Controlled Nucleation for the Regulation of the Particle Size in Monodisperse Gold Suspensions. *Nat. Phys. Sci.* **1973**, *241*, 20–22. [CrossRef]
4. Pretze, M.; Hien, A.; Radle, M.; Schirrmacher, R.; Wängler, C.; Wängler, B. Gastrin-releasing peptide receptor- and prostate-specific membrane antigen-specific ultrasmall gold nanoparticles for characterization and diagnosis of prostate carcinoma via fluorescence imaging. *Bioconjug. Chem.* **2018**, *29*, 1525–1533. [CrossRef] [PubMed]
5. Maeda, H.; Fang, J.; Inutsuka, T.; Kitamoto, Y. Vascular permeability enhancement in solid tumor: Various factors, mechanisms involved and its implications. *Int. Immunopharmacol.* **2003**, *3*, 319–328. [CrossRef] [PubMed]
6. Pretze, M.; von Kiedrowski, V.; Runge, R.; Freudenberg, R.; Hübner, R.; Davarci, G.; Schirrmacher, R.; Wängler, C.; Wängler, B. $\alpha_v\beta_3$-Specific gold nanoparticles for fluorescence imaging of tumor angiogenesis. *Nanomaterials* **2021**, *11*, 138. [CrossRef]
7. Zarschler, K.; Rocks, L.; Licciardello, N.; Boselli, L.; Polo, E.; Garcia, K.P.; De Cola, L.; Stephan, H.; Dawson, K.A. Ultrasmall inorganic nanoparticles: State-of-the-art and perspectives for biomedical applications. *Nanomed. Nanotechnol. Biol. Med.* **2016**, *12*, 1663–1701. [CrossRef]
8. Kim, M.S.; Lee, E.J.; Kim, J.W.; Chung, U.S.; Koh, W.G.; Keum, K.C.; Koom, W.S. Gold nanoparticles enhance anti-tumor effect of radiotherapy to hypoxic tumor. *Radiat. Oncol. J.* **2016**, *34*, 230–238. [CrossRef]
9. Black, K.C.L.; Wang, Y.; Luehmann, H.P.; Cai, X.; Xing, W.; Pang, B.; Zhao, Y.; Cutler, C.S.; Wang, L.V.; Liu, Y.; et al. Radioactive ^{198}Au-Doped Nanostructures with Different Shapes for In Vivo Analyses of Their Biodistribution, Tumor Uptake, and Intratumoral Distribution. *ACS Nano* **2014**, *8*, 4385–4394. [CrossRef]
10. Cui, S.; Yin, D.; Chen, Y.; Di, Y.; Chen, H.; Ma, Y.; Achilefu, S.; Gu, Y. In vivo targeted deep-tissue photodynamic therapy based on near-infrared light triggered upconversion nanoconstruct. *ACS Nano* **2013**, *7*, 676–688. [CrossRef]
11. Shukla, R.; Chanda, N.; Zambre, A.; Upendran, A.; Katti, K.; Kulkarni, R.R.; Nune, S.K.; Casteel, S.W.; Smith, C.J.; Vimal, J.; et al. Laminin receptor specific therapeutic gold nanoparticles (^{198}AuNP-EGCg) show efficacy in treating prostate cancer. *Proc. Natl. Acad. Sci. USA* **2012**, *109*, 12426–12431. [CrossRef] [PubMed]

12. Chanda, N.; Kattumuri, V.; Shukla, R.; Zambre, A.; Katti, K.; Upendran, A.; Kulkarni, R.R.; Kan, P.; Fent, G.M.; Casteel, S.W.; et al. Bombesin functionalized gold nanoparticles show in vitro and in vivo cancer receptor specificity. *Proc. Natl. Acad. Sci. USA* **2010**, *107*, 8760–8765. [CrossRef] [PubMed]
13. Pretze, M.; Hien, A.; Roscher, M.; Richter, K.; Rädle, M.; Wängler, C.; Wängler, B. Efficient modification of GRPR-specific gold nanoparticles for fluorescence imaging of prostate carcinoma. *J. Label. Compd. Radiopharm.* **2017**, *60*, S601. [CrossRef]
14. Hien, A.; Pretze, M.; Braun, F.; Schäfer, E.; Kümmel, T.; Roscher, M.; Schock-Kusch, D.; Waldeck, J.; Müller, B.; Wängler, C.; et al. Non-contact recognition of fluorescently labeled objects in deep tissue via optimized optical arrangement. *PLoS ONE* **2018**, *13*, e0208236. [CrossRef] [PubMed]
15. Zhu, J.; Chin, J.; Wängler, C.; Wängler, B.; Lennox, R.B.; Schirrmacher, R. Rapid ^{18}F-labeling and loading of PEGylated gold nanoparticles for in vivo applications. *Bioconjug. Chem.* **2014**, *25*, 1143–1150. [CrossRef] [PubMed]
16. Zhao, Y.; Sultan, D.; Detering, L.; Cho, S.; Sun, G.; Pierce, R.; Wooley, K.L.; Liu, Y. Copper-64-alloyed gold nanoparticles for cancer imaging: Improved radiolabel stability and diagnostic accuracy. *Angew. Chem. Int. Ed.* **2014**, *53*, 156–159. [CrossRef] [PubMed]
17. Pretze, M.; van der Meulen, N.P.; Wängler, C.; Schibli, R.; Wängler, B. Targeted ^{64}Cu-labeled gold nanoparticles for dual imaging with positron emission tomography and optical imaging. *J. Label. Comp. Radiopharm.* **2019**, *62*, 471–482. [CrossRef]
18. Jiménez-Mancilla, N.; Ferro-Flores, G.; Santos-Cuevas, C.; Ocampo-García, B.; Luna-Gutiérrez, M.; Azorín-Vega, E.; Isaac-Olivé, K.; Camacho-López, M.; Torres-García, E. Multifunctional targeted therapy system based on ^{99m}Tc/^{177}Lu-labeled gold nanoparticles-Tat(49-57)-Lys^3-bombesin internalized in nuclei of prostate cancer cells. *J. Label. Compd. Radiopharm.* **2013**, *56*, 663–671. [CrossRef]
19. Eskandari, N.; Yavari, K.; Outokesh, M.; Sadjadi, S.; Ahmadi, S.J. Iodine-131 radiolabeling of poly ethylene glycol-coated gold nanorods for in vivo imaging. *J. Label. Compd. Radiopharm.* **2013**, *56*, 12–16. [CrossRef]
20. Cui, M.; Liu, R.; Deng, Z.; Ge, G.; Liu, Y.; Xie, L. Quantitative study of protein coronas on gold nanoparticles with different surface modifications. *Nano Res.* **2014**, *7*, 345–352. [CrossRef]
21. Dai, Q.; Walkey, C.; Chan, W.C. Polyethylene glycol backfilling mitigates the negative impact of the protein corona on nanoparticle cell targeting. *Angew. Chem. Int. Ed.* **2014**, *53*, 5093–5096. [CrossRef] [PubMed]
22. Häkkinen, H. The gold-sulfur interface at the nanoscale. *Nat. Chem.* **2012**, *4*, 443–455. [CrossRef] [PubMed]
23. Li, W.; Chen, X. Gold nanoparticles for photoacoustic imaging. *Nanomed. Nanotechnol. Biol. Med.* **2015**, *10*, 299–320. [CrossRef] [PubMed]
24. Chanda, N.; Shukla, R.; Katti, K.V.; Kannan, R. Gastrin releasing protein receptor specific gold nanorods: Breast and prostate tumor avid nanovectors for molecular imaging. *Nano Lett.* **2009**, *9*, 1798–1805. [CrossRef] [PubMed]
25. Maccora, D.; Dini, V.; Battocchio, C.; Fratoddi, I.; Cartoni, A.; Rotili, D.; Castagnola, M.; Faccini, R.; Bruno, I.; Scotognella, T.; et al. Gold nanoparticles and nanorods in nuclear medicine: A mini review. *Appl. Sci.* **2019**, *9*, 3232. [CrossRef]
26. Mayo, R.L.; Robinson, F.R.S. Auger and secondary X-ray electrons from gold. *R. Soc. Pub.* **1939**, *173*, 192–200.
27. Zhang, X.D.; Wu, D.; Shen, X.; Chen, J.; Sun, Y.M.; Liu, P.X.; Liang, X.J. Size-dependent radiosensitization of PEG-coated gold nanoparticles for cancer radiation therapy. *Biomaterials* **2012**, *33*, 6408–6419. [CrossRef]
28. Hainfeld, J.F.; Slatkin, D.N.; Smilowitz, H.M. The use of gold nanoparticles to enhance radiotherapy in mice. *Phys. Med. Biol.* **2004**, *49*, N309–N315. [CrossRef]
29. Chanda, N.; Kan, P.; Watkinson, L.D.; Shukla, R.; Zambre, A.; Carmack, T.L.; Engelbrecht, H.; Lever, J.R.; Katti, K.; Fent, G.M.; et al. Radioactive gold nanoparticles in cancer therapy: Therapeutic efficacy studies of GA-^{198}AuNP nanoconstruct in prostate tumor-bearing mice. *Nanomed. Nanotechnol. Biol. Med.* **2010**, *6*, 201–209. [CrossRef]
30. Säterborg, N.E. The distribution of ^{198}Au injected intravenously as a colloid and in solution. *Acta Radiol. Ther. Phys. Biol.* **1973**, *12*, 509–528. [CrossRef]
31. Khan, M.K.; Minc, L.D.; Nigavekar, S.S.; Kariapper, M.S.T.; Nair, B.M.; Schipper, M.; Cook, A.C.; Lesniak, W.G.; Balogh, L.P. Fabrication of {^{198}Au^0} radioactive composite nanodevices and their use for nano-brachytherapy. *Nanomed. Nanotechnol. Biol. Med.* **2008**, *4*, 57–69. [CrossRef] [PubMed]
32. Chakravarty, R.; Chakraborty, S.; Guleria, A.; Kumar, C.; Kunwar, A.; Nair, K.V.V.; Sarma, H.D.; Dash, A. Clinical scale synthesis of intrinsically radiolabeled and cyclic RGD peptide functionalized ^{198}Au nanoparticles for targeted cancer therapy. *Nucl. Med. Biol.* **2019**, *72–73*, 1–10. [CrossRef]
33. Aboudzadeh, M.R.; Moassesi, M.E.; Amiri, M.; Shams, H.; Alirezapour, B.; Sadeghi, M.; Sari, M.F.; Keyvani, M. Preparation and characterization of chitosan-capped radioactive gold nanoparticles: Neutron irradiation impact on structural properties. *J. Iran. Chem. Soc.* **2015**, *13*, 339–345. [CrossRef]
34. Lindner, S.; Michler, C.; Leidner, S.; Rensch, C.; Wangler, C.; Schirrmacher, R.; Bartenstein, P.; Wangler, B. Synthesis and in vitro and in vivo evaluation of SiFA-tagged bombesin and RGD peptides as tumor imaging probes for positron emission tomography. *Bioconjug. Chem.* **2014**, *25*, 738–749. [CrossRef] [PubMed]
35. Horton, M.A. The $\alpha v \beta 3$ integrin "Vitronectin receptor". *Int. J. Biochem. Cell Biol.* **1997**, *29*, 721–725. [CrossRef] [PubMed]
36. Liu, Z.; Wang, F.; Chen, X. Integrin $\alpha_v \beta_3$-targeted cancer therapy. *Drug Dev. Res.* **2008**, *69*, 329–339. [CrossRef] [PubMed]
37. Dijkgraaf, I.; Yim, C.B.; Franssen, G.M.; Schuit, R.C.; Luurtsema, G.; Liu, S.; Oyen, W.J.; Boerman, O.C. PET imaging of $\alpha_v \beta_3$ integrin expression in tumours with ^{68}Ga-labelled mono-, di- and tetrameric RGD peptides. *Eur. J. Nucl. Med. Mol. Imaging* **2011**, *38*, 128–137. [CrossRef] [PubMed]

38. Janssen, M.; Oyen, W.J.G.; Massuger, L.F.A.G.; Frielink, C.; Dijkgraaf, I.; Edwards, D.S.; Radjopadhye, M.; Corstens, F.H.M.; Boerman, O.C. Comparison of a monomeric and dimeric radiolabeled RGD-peptide for tumor targeting. *Cancer Biother. Radiopharm.* **2002**, *17*, 641–646. [CrossRef]
39. Zhai, C.; Franssen, G.M.; Petrik, M.; Laverman, P.; Summer, D.; Rangger, C.; Haubner, R.; Haas, H.; Decristoforo, C. Comparison of Ga-68-Labeled Fusarinine C-Based Multivalent RGD Conjugates and [^{68}Ga]NODAGA-RGD–*In Vivo* Imaging Studies in Human Xenograft Tumors. *Mol. Imaging Biol.* **2016**, *18*, 758–767. [CrossRef]
40. Turcu, I.; Zarafu, I.; Popa, M.; Chifiriuc, M.C.; Bleotu, C.; Culita, D.; Ghica, C.; Ionita, P. Lipoic acid gold nanoparticles functionalized with organic compounds as bioactive materials. *Nanomaterials* **2017**, *7*, 43. [CrossRef]
41. Brust, M.; Walker, M.; Bethell, D.; Schiffrin, D.J.; Whyman, R. Synthesis of Thiol-derivatised Gold Nanoparticles in a Two-phase Liquid-Liquid System. *J. Chem. Soc. Chem. Commun.* **1994**, *7*, 801–802. [CrossRef]
42. Zhu, J.; Waengler, C.; Lennox, R.B.; Schirrmacher, R. Preparation of water-soluble maleimide-functionalized 3 nm gold nanoparticles: A new bioconjugation template. *Langmuir ACS J. Surf. Colloids* **2012**, *28*, 5508–5512. [CrossRef] [PubMed]
43. Milne, M.; Gobbo, P.; McVicar, N.; Bartha, R.; Workentin, M.S.; Hudson, R.H.E. Water-soluble gold nanoparticles (AuNP) functionalized with a gadolinium(III) chelate via Michael addition for use as a MRI contrast agent. *J. Mater. Chem. B* **2013**, *1*, 5628–5635. [CrossRef]
44. Freudenberg, R. Monte-Carlo-Simulationen zur Dosimetrie bei der Zellexposition mit offenen Radionukliden in typischen in-vitro Bestrahlungsgeometrien. Ph.D. Thesis, Technical University Dresden, Dresden, Germany, 2012. Available online: https://eltab.ub.uni-kl.de/media/103162/ (accessed on 1 September 2023).
45. Haubner, R.; Gratias, R.; Diefenbach, B.; Goodman, S.L.; Jonczyk, A.; Kessler, H. Structural and functional aspects of RGD-containing cyclic pentapeptides as highly potent and selective integrin $\alpha_v\beta_3$ antagonists. *J. Am. Chem. Soc.* **1996**, *118*, 7461–7472. [CrossRef]
46. Shi, J.; Wang, F.; Liu, S. Radiolabeled cyclic RGD peptides as radiotracers for tumor imaging. *Biophys. Rep.* **2016**, *2*, 1–20. [CrossRef] [PubMed]
47. Wängler, C.; Maschauer, S.; Prante, O.; Schäfer, M.; Schirrmacher, R.; Bartenstein, P.; Eisenhut, M.; Wängler, B. Multimerization of cRGD peptides by click chemistry: Synthetic strategies, chemical limitations, and influence on biological properties. *ChemBioChem Eur. J. Chem. Biol.* **2010**, *11*, 2168–2181. [CrossRef] [PubMed]
48. Quigley, N.G.; Steiger, K.; Hoberück, S.; Czech, N.; Zierke, M.A.; Kossatz, S.; Pretze, M.; Richter, F.; Weichert, W.; Pox, C.; et al. PET/CT imaging of head-and-neck and pancreatic cancer in humans by targeting the "Cancer Integrin" $\alpha v\beta 6$ with Ga-68-Trivehexin. *Eur. J. Nucl. Med. Mol. Imaging* **2021**, *49*, 1136–1147. [CrossRef]
49. McCandless, E.L. Determination of Sulfur in ploysaccharides be neutron activation analysis. *Anal. Biochem.* **1964**, *7*, 357–365. [CrossRef]
50. Vimalnath, K.V.; Shetty, P.; Chakraborty, S.; Das, T.; Chirayil, V.; Sarma, H.D.; Jagadeesan, K.C.; Joshi, P.V. Practicality of production of ^{32}P by direct neutron activation for its utilization in bone pain palliation as Na$_3$[^{32}P]PO$_4$. *Cancer Biother. Radiopharm.* **2013**, *28*, 423–428. [CrossRef]
51. Zamora, P.O.; Marek, M.J. Post Labeling Stabilization of Radiolabeled Proteins and Peptides. U.S. Patent 20010055563A1, 24 June 2001.
52. Dai, X.; Su, Z.; Liu, J.O. An improved synthesis of a selective $\alpha_v\beta_3$-integrin antagonist cyclo(-RGDfK-). *Tetrahedron Lett.* **2000**, *41*, 6295–6298. [CrossRef]
53. Dzwonek, M.; Załubiniak, D.; Piątek, P.; Cichowicz, G.; Męczynska-Wielgosz, S.; Stępkowski, T.; Kruszewski, M.; Więckowska, A.; Bilewicz, R. Towards potent but less toxic nanopharmaceuticals—Lipoic acid bioconjugates of ultrasmall gold nanoparticles with an anticancer drug and addressing unit. *RSC Adv.* **2018**, *8*, 14947–14957. [CrossRef] [PubMed]
54. Haiss, W.; Nguyen, T.K.T.; Aveyard, J.; Fernig, D.G. Determination of Size and Concentration of Gold Nanoparticles from UV-Vis Spectra. *Anal. Chem.* **2007**, *79*, 4215–4221. [CrossRef] [PubMed]

Disclaimer/Publisher's Note: The statements, opinions and data contained in all publications are solely those of the individual author(s) and contributor(s) and not of MDPI and/or the editor(s). MDPI and/or the editor(s) disclaim responsibility for any injury to people or property resulting from any ideas, methods, instructions or products referred to in the content.

MDPI AG
Grosspeteranlage 5
4052 Basel
Switzerland
Tel.: +41 61 683 77 34

Pharmaceuticals Editorial Office
E-mail: pharmaceuticals@mdpi.com
www.mdpi.com/journal/pharmaceuticals

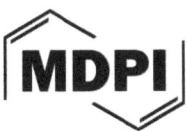

Disclaimer/Publisher's Note: The title and front matter of this reprint are at the discretion of the Guest Editors. The publisher is not responsible for their content or any associated concerns. The statements, opinions and data contained in all individual articles are solely those of the individual Editors and contributors and not of MDPI. MDPI disclaims responsibility for any injury to people or property resulting from any ideas, methods, instructions or products referred to in the content.

www.ingramcontent.com/pod-product-compliance
Lightning Source LLC
LaVergne TN
LVHW072348090526
838202LV00019B/2504